FRONTLINE SURGEON

FRONTLINE SURGEON

NEW ZEALAND MEDICAL PIONEER DOUGLAS JOLLY

MARK DERBY

UNIVERSITY OF NEBRASKA PRESS
Lincoln

The University of Nebraska Press is part of a land-grant institution with campuses and programs on the past, present, and future homelands of the Pawnee, Ponca, Otoe-Missouria, Omaha, Dakota, Lakota, Kaw, Cheyenne, and Arapaho Peoples, as well as those of the relocated Ho-Chunk, Sac and Fox, and Iowa Peoples.

All royalties from the sale of this book will be donated to the Abraham Lincoln Brigade Archives (http://alba-valb.org/), an educational nonprofit organization dedicated to promoting social activism and defense of human rights. ALBA's work is inspired by the American volunteers who served in the Abraham Lincoln Brigade during the Spanish Civil War.

Library of Congress Cataloging-in-Publication Data
Names: Derby, Mark, 1956-author.
Title: Frontline surgeon: New Zealand medical pioneer Douglas Jolly / Mark Derby.
Description: Lincoln: University of Nebraska Press, [2024] | Includes bibliographical references and index.
Identifiers: LCCN 2023053753
ISBN 9781496213389 (hardback)
ISBN 9781496239259 (epub)
ISBN 9781496239266 (pdf)
Subjects: LCSH: Jolly, Douglas W. | Surgeons—New Zealand—Biography. | Surgeons—Great Britain—Biography. | Spain—History—Civil War, 1936-1939—Medical care. | World War, 1939-1945—Medical care. | Surgery, Military—History—20th century. | BISAC: BIOGRAPHY & AUTOBIOGRAPHY / Medical (incl. Patients) | MEDICAL / History
Classification: LCC RD27.35.J643 D47 2024 | DDC 617.092 [B]—dc23/eng/20240123
LC record available at https://lccn.loc.gov/2023053753

Set and designed in Garamond Premier by N. Putens.

CONTENTS

ILLUSTRATIONS

Following page 100

AUTHOR'S NOTE

Proper names are spelled in this book as in the native or local language of the people and places themselves. However, especially during the Spanish Civil War, those names were often written by speakers of other languages and accordingly spelled differently. When quoting directly from archival sources giving such variant spellings, the variants are retained.

FRONTLINE SURGEON

1 The Center of Gravity of the World

Crouched in a shallow foxhole, focusing each of her cameras in turn, Gerda Taro blazed with determination to record the debacle that surrounded her. Across the arid Brunete plain, Republican troops were retreating by the thousands, targeted by artillery and pursued by enemy aircraft. As each wave of heavy Heinkel bombers or smaller pursuit planes approached, Taro ducked below the shrapnel-scarred rim of the trench to take cover and could see her young Canadian companion Ted Allan mouthing terrified pleas to leave the battlefield. She ignored him and continued to juggle her compact Leica and more awkward movie camera, seeking images that might capture the despair of the men fleeing in disarray.

Early that Sunday morning in the searing midsummer of 1937, she had collected Allan, who worked with a Canadian blood transfusion service, from his Madrid hotel. She then persuaded a driver to take them twenty kilometers west of the central city, as close to the disintegrating front as he dared to go. From there they left his car and walked toward the explosions. Taro wore her battlefield outfit of khaki overalls, with a dark beret over her cropped and sun-bleached hair. *La pequeña rubia*, the twenty-six-year-old "little blonde," was already well known and widely adored by Republican troops, and the much younger Allan was just one of her admirers.

The pair reached a dugout, the command post of the shaven-headed former Red Army officer General Walter. It was not his real name, but then neither was Taro's. She had been Gerta Pohorylle in her hometown of Stuttgart. As a fervent anti-Nazi in Paris in the summer of 1935, she had met Endre Friedmann, like herself Jewish, émigré, youthful, undeniably dashing, and ambitious. He was a photographer, a rising star of the Cartier-Bresson school of urgent realism, and she soon became one, too, barely surviving on the occasional magazine commission. To break into the international market, they created a joint brand name devoid of association with national or ethnic origins. For a time both sold their photos under the name "Robert Capa," until Pohorylle's growing ability and vivid personality demanded a distinct identity, one equally succinct and easily pronounced in many languages.[1]

The civil war that fractured Spain in late 1936, after a military coup attempted to overthrow its progressive Republican government, was an irresistible vortex for this passionately leftist couple. In a testamentary series of sparely beautiful black-and-white images, Capa and Taro recorded the exhilaration of newly enlisted Republican troops on the Aragón front, the homeless residents of bombed apartment buildings in Madrid, and an armored column paused in a pine forest in Segovia.[2]

In early July 1937, Capa had returned to Paris to negotiate the couple's next overseas contract, while Taro remained in Madrid, traveling to the front each day in the pitiless heat and earning the admiration even of toughened veterans like General Walter. On this Sunday, however, Taro and Allan found him gray with fatigue and anxiety—harsh, frantic, and in no mood to deal with two youthful idealists strung with cameras. Over the previous two weeks, the Republican forces had pushed their lines five kilometers into enemy territory and captured the small town of Brunete. Gen. Francisco Franco, commanding the Nationalist rebel forces, then ordered reinforcements from the north, including the latest German and Italian fighter and bomber planes. Field Marshal Wolfram von Richthofen's Condor Legion, whose pilots were still reveling in their destruction of the undefended Basque town of Guernica three months earlier, was among the crack squadrons summoned to drive the Republicans back from Brunete. Franco's maneuver succeeded. As General Walter watched the first of his shattered units stumbling back from their lines, he ordered Taro and her companion to turn back immediately. "In five minutes, this will be hell."[3]

Allan was eager to comply, but Taro dragged him to a small trench nearby and began filming in the shadow of enemy aircraft sweeping over them. As fast as she could reload her cameras, she captured the unprecedented spectacle of thousands of infantry and armored troops fleeing before an aerial onslaught. She ignored the bombs and machine-gun bullets landing lethally close to them and gave in to Allan's desperate pleas to withdraw only once she had shot her last roll of film. Choosing a momentary break between bombing runs, the pair scrambled onto a dusty road already strewn with corpses and wrecked vehicles, and joined the mass of dazed and demoralized men trudging toward the small village of Villanueva de la Cañada. At times, to take cover from successive formations of enemy aircraft, they plunged through head-high fields of ripe grain lining the road.[4]

In the village, they found a badly wounded soldier, his legs shattered. A small and battered Russian-made tank rumbled up behind them, and they managed to halt it, load the wounded man on board, and gain a dangerous perch on its fiercely hot hatch cover. The tank stopped at a first aid post where General Walter's long, black Hispano Suiza staff car, now doing duty as an ambulance, was about to carry three other wounded men to a field hospital. In an exchange of shouts, its harried driver agreed to take two extra passengers on the running boards. Taro, exulted with the results of her frenetic day's work, laid her cameras and precious cans of exposed film on the front passenger seat. She and Allan each hooked an arm around a door pillar as the car lurched back onto the cratered road.

"There was some confusion ahead of us," Allan wrote later. "A tank was approaching. It had been strafed by a Nationalist plane and was driving erratically, weaving across the road. Our car swung to the left to avoid it. 'Hold on,' Gerda laughed. The car went out of control; began to roll."[5] The heavy vehicle lumbered off the road and into a ditch, where it overturned, its tires gradually stilling. Allan was flung clear, crushing his leg as he landed, but Taro, lying unconscious on the roadside, was run over by another Republican tank and critically injured.[6]

An ambulance was somehow summoned, and the two crash victims were transferred to it. A British field hospital had been established nearby in a former seminary beside the vast sixteenth-century monastery of El Escorial. At the height of the Brunete battle, three surgeons had worked there simultaneously, but only one now remained on duty to treat casualties of the retreat—a New Zealander in his early thirties named Doug Jolly. It was early evening when Taro's mangled body was carried into the hospital's ground-floor reception room on a stretcher. She was alive, but barely. Irene Goldin, an operating theater nurse from New York, recalled that "her intestines were hanging out."

After she was given a blood transfusion, Taro regained consciousness and pleaded with Jolly to send telegrams to Capa in Paris and to the French magazine

Ce Soir, which commissioned their work. He promised to do this but could see that little more could be done for her, and he instructed nurse Goldin to move the young woman to a room by herself and "maintain her as well as possible without pain." Eviscerated and dying, Taro nevertheless managed to ask Goldin in English, "Are my cameras all right? They're new."[7]

Ted Allan was receiving treatment for his leg on another floor of the hospital when Jolly appeared at his bedside. The two men had already met several times when Allan delivered supplies of preserved blood to the hospital. The young Canadian begged to see his friend, but Jolly told him Taro was in shock and that no visits were possible at that time. Later a nurse brought a message from her, asking whether Allan had managed to save her cameras. He replied that he had not, and a second note was dropped off by Jolly relaying her reaction: "C'est la guerre."[8]

"Doctor Jolly was a very good surgeon," remembered Goldin, "but I don't think he was able to do anything for [Taro] except look at her, put a dressing on her and send her to us. We gave her fluid as much as we could and did all that we could to keep her alive but I doubt very much that anything could have helped her. It was one of those massive wounds that are absolutely lethal, you know. And that night, she died."[9]

*

By the time he lost this courageous patient, Douglas "Doug" Jolly had been serving with Spain's Republican Army for just six months, and he had no prior experience of battlefield surgery. In that brief period, he had already dealt with so much gushing blood and perforated organs that this particular death is unlikely to have struck him as exceptional. In letters to friends in England, he acknowledged that he had become hardened to seeing patients dying on his operating table and to denying them treatment when their chances of recovery had vanished. Yet he was determined, he wrote, not to fall into the habit of regarding the endless flow of mutilated bodies simply as "cases" whose survival or otherwise might be regarded with clinical detachment.

As nurse Goldin noted, even in the few months Jolly had spent operating close to the front lines, his colleagues had come to regard the New Zealander as an outstandingly skilled surgeon and selected him to carry out the most demanding and critical operations. In addition, he had gained a reputation as a humane and dedicated medical officer, known to treat even captured enemy combatants with the same expertise and compassion he gave to injured women, children, old people, and the troops of his own side. After the Republicans' devastating defeat at Brunete, he remained in the physically and emotionally punishing role of frontline surgeon for a further eighteen months, until the Republican Army ordered all its overseas volunteers to withdraw from Spain. During those two years, he developed a breadth of clinical experience, especially in the intricate work of abdominal surgery, that would later be authoritatively assessed as unmatched in the world.[10]

The Spanish Civil War of 1936–39 continues to provoke a lively and seemingly insatiable interest among both academics and the wider public in many countries. Successive generations derive fresh significance from the conflict's distinctive characteristics, such as the geopolitical shock waves generated by the Spanish people's resistance to a military revolt backed by the forces of an expansionist fascism, and the scale of voluntary participation from abroad. After the attempted coup began, would-be fighters and medical workers arrived from more than fifty countries to support the Republic.

The battles fought between Spain's Republican, or pro-government, and Nationalist, or insurgent, forces constitute modern history's earliest instance of a "total war," one in which the entire population was engaged and that incurred many more civilian than combatant casualties.[11] The vast and ever-expanding historiography tracing the course and consequences of the war includes a number of works on the medical services developed to treat both the combatants and the civil population.[12] These works have established that several globally significant advances in health service organization and trauma medicine were initially developed and trialed in Spain under the chaotic conditions of wartime and of the country's own primitive health system, which reflected a society yet to fully evolve from semi-feudalism. Large Republican-held cities such as Madrid and Barcelona endured prolonged and concentrated air raids on some of their most densely populated neighborhoods. The use of high-explosive and incendiary bombs on multistory dwellings produced thousands of casualties, many with injuries that were largely new to medical science. Residents were forced to improvise strategies and structures to withstand these raids, and the underdeveloped civilian medical service was tasked with treating survivors. The local medical staff members in Republican sectors of Spain who addressed these unaccustomed challenges were eventually supported by hundreds of volunteer medical professionals arriving from other countries. Most had no previous experience of the conditions they encountered, but they generally proved dedicated, resolute, and resourceful. Faced with extreme levels of need, they responded by improvising highly innovative techniques and systems that influenced the later course of medical practice.

Of the medical advances originated or greatly developed during the Spanish Civil War, the most significant include the establishment of blood banks and the widespread use of preserved blood for transfusions. In an era shortly before the introduction of penicillin, the Republican medical services also greatly improved on earlier methods for controlling infection in traumatic orthopedic injuries. Jolly made extensive use of these developments in his field hospitals, but he is credited in particular for his contribution to a more general innovation—organizing and linking the various components of army medical services to reduce, as much as possible, the time delay between the infliction of a wound and its treatment. He played a key role in developing a system for strategically positioning each successive stage of treatment, including his own mobile field hospitals, so that injured troops could be admitted and treated within a few hours—a far shorter time span than had been achieved in all previous wars.

This unprecedented method of battlefield health provision, which Jolly named the "three-points-forward" system, evolved in stages as costly lessons were learned from successive battles in the war, including the battle of Brunete in which Gerda Taro died. Jolly energetically advocated for it at medical conferences held during the civil war, publicized it through Republican propaganda channels, and repeatedly refined it. In doing so, he drew both on the surgical training he had received in New Zealand and British public hospitals, and, just as significantly, on his nonsectarian Christian socialist principles. Since his student days at medical school in New Zealand, he had regarded his chosen profession, in accordance with biblical precepts, as a means of relieving social inequity and hardship. Later, in London in the early 1930s, those Christian imperatives were infused with Marxist ideology, and Jolly became a convinced anti-fascist.

That broad-spectrum political standpoint appeared urgently necessary in a period when countries across Europe were succumbing, one by one, to totalitarian rule. When Spain elected its left-leaning coalition government in 1936, it appeared at first a heartening exception to that dismaying tendency. However, six months after the election, the Republican government was confronted by an armed insurrection backed by the most powerful fascist forces in Europe. Both within Spain and around the world, leftists felt compelled to convert their democratic rhetoric into action. "Madrid is the centre of gravity of the world," concluded the Canadian surgeon Norman Bethune, as he made his way there in November 1936.[13] Capa and Taro did the same, and so did Jolly, although to the lasting cost of his later career.

The rampant Axis powers led by Adolf Hitler and Benito Mussolini regarded Spain, coldly and deliberately, as a testing ground for their newest military equipment and strategies. By contrast, the health services hastily assembled to support pro-government forces and their civilian supporters lacked resources of almost every kind apart from determination and inventiveness. Those qualities, however, ultimately proved capable of delivering a standard of medical organization and treatment that exceeded, in some respects, any achieved elsewhere to that date, including in peacetime. Even as Franco's victory appeared imminent and absolute, Jolly could take pride in the advances he and his colleagues had achieved under the worst circumstances imaginable.

When he was withdrawn from the civil war in late 1938, the vastly experienced yet still not fully qualified surgeon faced a watershed in his career. He might have chosen to embark on a prestigious and rewarding civilian practice, but he foresaw that the defeat of democracy in Spain made the prospect of a worldwide conflict against the Axis powers all but inevitable. Jolly therefore took an active part in the campaign to convince British medical authorities of the urgent need to prepare for a new and terrible form of warfare based on massive assaults from the air. He condensed his recent frontline experience into a handbook of military medicine intended to aid those army surgeons who would be treating casualties of battles similar to those Spain, before any other country, had just endured. His book was published as the Luftwaffe was raining bombs on English coastal towns and cities. Jolly then enlisted with Britain's Royal Army Medical Corps and, with customary stoic dedication, served for five years in North Africa and Italy.

After his demobilization as a decorated commissioned officer, Jolly's subsequent peacetime career in Britain was less action-packed than the decade he had spent in uniform, yet it was intriguing in other respects. While he remained highly regarded by former colleagues, and his wartime patients remembered him with profound gratitude, he retreated within the British medical establishment into obscurity to the point of invisibility, and in his country of birth, he was almost entirely forgotten. This book aims to explain and redress that remarkable historical lacuna and reestablish Jolly as a foremost medical pioneer of the twentieth century: an outstanding surgical practitioner, an internationally significant innovator in the field of trauma medicine, and a figure of exemplary courage and compassion.

Although he was a fluent writer who more than once contemplated abandoning medicine for a literary career, Jolly was a modest and unassuming character, and his many press interviews and journal articles contain only fleeting references to his own wartime and later activities. It has been necessary to supplement those sources with official records and with the recollections of his colleagues and patients. Even so, this book could not have been written without the full cooperation of Jolly's relatives in several countries. With great generosity and goodwill, they have made available his extensive personal papers, including letters, photographs, and unpublished writings, and placed no restrictions or other conditions on their use—a rare gift to a biographer.

Through the medium of one outstanding surgeon's experience, this book aims to recount the haphazard, heroic development of medical services under conditions of total war—a conflict between highly mechanized, air-dominated armies deployed across entire countries and continents and affecting all levels of the civilian population. Jolly chose to enter this conflict with no formal military experience but with a family and educational background that prepared him remarkably well for its extreme demands. In particular, his Christian socialist personal ethos, which he retained throughout his life, equipped him to endure emotional pressures that overwhelmed many of those he worked alongside. His nonaligned anti-fascist politics also guided him through the hypocrisies, internecine struggles, and subsequent disillusionments of a low, dishonest decade and enabled him to resolve the swift ethical transition from antiwar activist to noncombatant serving officer. During nine years of near-continuous service in frontline warfare, there is no record of him using, or even bearing, a weapon.

In the course of my researching and writing this book, Douglas Jolly emerged as much more than the one-dimensionally high-minded and admirable figure that he may present at first sight. His personality and career encompassed curious contradictions that both complicated and enriched the project of recording his life. Consequently, further layers of significance were added to the project of retracing the path taken by a storekeeper's son from the remotest corner of a small and remote country to the epicenter of world events, where he made distinguished and enduring contributions to trauma medicine and thereby to the relief of human suffering.

2 The Storekeeper's Son

Otago University's main campus stands in the center of Dunedin, a small city in the far south of New Zealand. Running through its leafy grounds is a clear and meandering stream that occasionally delivers student anglers a sizable trout. These fish are an introduced species, transported from Europe 150 years ago. In fact, almost everything on the campus—the deciduous trees lining the stream banks, the solemn, gray stone lecture halls, the atmosphere of studious tranquillity—suggests that the university was uplifted in its entirety from nineteenth-century Scotland and faithfully re-created in the far South Pacific.

The very name "Dunedin" is a variant of Edinburgh, Scotland's capital city, which provided the model for the planned settlement on the opposite side of the world. In the late 1840s, the first shiploads of settlers, overwhelmingly Scottish and Presbyterian in origin, arrived here to "found a new Edinburgh at the antipodes that shall one day rival the old."[1] The streets of this raw and muddy little township, on a coast swept periodically by freezing antarctic gales, were laid out to mimic its Scottish parent city. The stream running through it was named the Water of Leith after Edinburgh's central river.

For its first decade of life, the new settlement languished, with a small and static population and flimsy wooden buildings lining unpaved tracks that became impassable after rain. Suddenly, in 1861, gold was discovered far inland in the snow-fed rivers of Central Otago, and Dunedin's fortunes were transformed instantly. Its population doubled, then doubled again within a few years. For some decades while the gold rushes lasted, the earnest, upstart little town became New Zealand's most populous and prosperous city, its industrial and commercial center, and its busiest port.[2]

Alluvial gold and Presbyterian rigor were both foundational to Doug Jolly's upbringing, although by the time of his birth in the first years of the twentieth century, the fervor of the gold rushes had largely subsided, and only their economic residue remained. Dunedin's sudden wealth and national prominence proved short-lived, yet they bequeathed the little city a core of handsome stone buildings housing its most significant institutions, including the country's first medical school founded in 1875. This was closely modeled on British lines and proved a vigorous transplant. Its curriculum expanded and teaching standards steadily rose until, by the 1920s, it awarded a medical degree after six years of full-time study, a year more than its British parent schools then considered necessary.

The young Doug Jolly entered Otago University's medical school in 1924 as a resolute nineteen-year-old with no family background in medicine but an upbringing in Otago's stoutly nonconformist values. Every evening after his studies, he would take the tree-lined path that follows the course of the Water of Leith through the town's Botanic Gardens to reach his accommodation, an imposing, red-brick hostel named Knox College after the sixteenth-century founder of the Scottish Presbyterian Church. Jolly and his brothers had also boarded here during their high school years, so for several decades at least one of Knox's sparsely furnished rooms was occupied by a member of the Jolly family.

Knox College provided an austere and socially restrictive environment for its residents, who were predominantly Presbyterian and, until 1983, exclusively male.[3] The head of the college, always known as the Master, was an ordained Presbyterian minister, and other formal terms—"the Beadle," "the Great Hall," "the Buttery"—were deliberately modeled on the traditions of ancient British halls of learning. Hearty outdoor recreation, particularly rugby, was encouraged.[4] The college's physical and spiritual center has always been its chapel, whose bare stone walls are washed with light from a large stained-glass window dedicated to former residents who lost their lives in the Great War. Attending a service here after each evening meal, and a longer one on Sunday mornings, was compulsory for all Knox residents.[5] In the 1950s, a large memorial plaque was installed to honor those "who served King & Country." The long columns of engraved names record twenty-seven college residents who died in the First World War, another twenty-one in the Second World War, and more than two hundred who served in those wars but survived them. In that third category, the name "DW Jolly" appears beside those of two of his brothers.

At the end of every university term, the Jolly brothers returned to their family home in the small Central Otago town of Cromwell. The trip entailed a 150-mile train journey inland across treeless, tussock-covered uplands; Cromwell lies further from the coast than almost any other New Zealand settlement, in the foothills of the country's highest mountain range and at the junction of two swift-flowing, snow-fed rivers. In this exceptionally remote, physically inhospitable, and formerly uninhabited terrain, an instant shantytown arose in 1862 after two American prospectors sieved a quantity of alluvial gold from the icy waters. Within months, several hundred men and a few women made the arduous trek along rough trails to the diggings, flung up crude dwellings with walls of sod and roofs of calico, and pegged out claims along the banks of the Clutha and Kawarau Rivers. One of them was a lanky seaman from the Scottish port of Arbroath named David Jolly. He had arrived in Dunedin at the height of the gold rush as the first mate of a British immigrant ship and promptly abandoned that calling to take the weeklong hike inland, pausing overnight at such ruefully named way stations as Drybread and Drunken Woman Creek.

An early historian of the central Otago goldfields has written feelingly of

> the solemn loneliness of its mountains; the ineffable sadness of its valleys; the utter dreariness of its plains. The weary traveller pursued his lonely way from point to point, always viewing around and before him a continuous and apparently interminable expanse of lofty hills . . . everywhere clothed in a sober livery of pale brown vegetation, relieved only by grim, grey rocks of fantastic form, sharing the desolation to which they contributed—backed by distant mountain peaks, which bounded and encompassed the horizon in every direction, piercing the blue ether, and clad in dazzling snows—an expanse diversified by no pleasant forests; devoid of animal as of human life; where the profound stillness was painful in its prolonged intensity; and the only sound that greeted the ear from dawn to dusk was the melancholy wailing of the wind among the tussocks.[6]

With several partners, the young ex-seaman took up a claim on the banks of the rushing, dangerous Clutha River, some miles downstream from the raw and nascent township.[7] Before they could extract any signs of color from the shingle bed, they were obliged to wait until subzero temperatures froze the headwaters of the river sufficiently to lower its flow. Finally, in the southern winter of June 1863, "each partner took his turn to fish for the precious metal in four feet of water with a long-handled shovel, and the wash dirt was deposited on the beach and cradled [i.e., sieved for gold dust]. The cold being very intense, fifteen minutes was the limit for each man to remain in the water. In this manner we obtained per week about two ounces, enough to keep us in food."[8]

David Jolly eked out a bare living in this way for several years before deciding to reinvent himself once again, this time as a storekeeper, supplying the Cromwell miners with bacon, boots, and the other essentials of their harsh existence. He proved a shrewd and popular merchant, and by 1870 his initial canvas-walled premises had grown to become a spacious, stone-built store on a prominent corner of Cromwell's muddy main street.[9] This building, which still stands, became one of the central institutions of a small town struggling toward respectability. Its stock grew to include wine, furnishings, and fashionable fabrics, and ladies from the neighboring town of Alexandra would make a thirteen-mile journey by horse and gig along the narrow and steep-sided Cromwell Gorge to refresh their wardrobes. The expansive, bearded proprietor was one of Cromwell's leading citizens and served several terms as its mayor. He was known for his tuneful singing voice and played an active part in local theatricals and sporting events, but his greatest enthusiasm was for the town's volunteer militia, the Cromwell Rifles, whose participants paraded resplendent in scarlet tunics and blue serge trousers, and with immense busbies for the officers. They never numbered more than sixty men, but under David Jolly's vigilant command, they developed a ferocious esprit de corps.[10]

Like most South Island towns, Cromwell was far removed from the battles that erupted periodically during the nineteenth century between intransigent Māori and the forces of the Crown, but in 1882 the threat of a new uprising became so acute that the Cromwell Rifles were mustered to face it. Te Whiti, a charismatic chief and pacifist prophet, had attracted thousands of followers from many tribes to his model community of Parihaka in the North Island province of Taranaki. Although his religious teachings and tactics were resolutely nonviolent, tension between the opposing parties grew fierce, and the government declared open warfare was imminent. In far-off Cromwell, the Rifles were summoned to an emergency parade and, one of them later recalled, ordered to hold themselves in readiness to go to the Taranaki front. "Then came the order, 'All those willing to go, take two paces to the front. Quick march!' We all moved forward like one man. Tears of joy ran down the cheeks of fire-eater Captain Jolly."[11]

By the close of the nineteenth century, this bellicose but aging patriot had largely transferred control of his business to his three sons, who jointly operated outpost stores in several small mining settlements around the Central Otago plateau. None of those establishments proved as well patronized and long-lasting as the first in Cromwell, managed by the eldest son, William. He was a steady and reflective character who, in 1901, married Elizabeth Waddell, a teacher at the town's only school. She left that job to raise a family that eventually numbered seven children—a daughter followed by five sons, plus an unofficially adopted niece.[12] The second son, born in 1904, was named Douglas and given both his parents' surnames.

The family home must have been a cramped place in which to raise this sizable family. It was single-storied, built of local stone sealed with mud plaster, and, like its neighbors, had no electricity, town water supply, or flushing toilet. The Jollys were stalwarts of the local Presbyterian church. Doug Jolly's grandfather, father, and mother all gave their time to teach in the church's Sunday school, and the family lived by its sturdy tenets of social service, egalitarianism, and moral rectitude.[13] They abstained from alcohol, and even later in life, when Doug had outgrown his religious upbringing, he drank only occasionally.

The Jolly children were expected to help in the family store almost as soon as they could reach the counter, and they grew up in an aromatic atmosphere compounded of cheese "of prime quality," soaps both utilitarian and scented, tea in foil-lined chests, and three kinds of oil: "salad, castor and kerosene."[14] The store now served a larger and more discerning clientele, prepared to pay for spirits, straw boater hats, and phonograph records. Gold was still extracted from the town's twin rivers but now by giant steam-powered dredges whose crews could work in relative comfort. Many more locals made their living from the orchards spreading over the river flats, where the soil and climate especially favored apricots.[15]

All seven Jolly children received a primary education at the two-roomed, stone-walled school where their mother had taught. Awkwardly sited on a south-facing slope, it was "almost devoid of sunshine and was cool in summer and freezing in winter."[16] When young Doug Jolly began his first lessons there, the building was already more than thirty years old and greatly overcrowded, and its pupils were transferred to a new, larger, and sunnier school nearby in 1915.[17]

Soon afterward the Jollys experienced a devastating dislocation, with unknowable but profound consequences for each of them. Their quiet, good-natured father enlisted for the Great War and embarked in October 1915 with the Otago Infantry Battalion. As a forty-five-year-old pillar of the community with a young family (the youngest son, Ralph, was just four years old), William Jolly would almost certainly have been classified as ineligible for compulsory conscription, and his decision to enlist can best be understood in the light of long service with his father's pride and joy, the Cromwell Rifles. In 1904, the year of his son Douglas's birth, William was appointed the company's commander, and in 1913 he was decorated for "long and distinguished service in the New Zealand Territorial Force," ensuring that when he entered the regular army, he did so with an officer's rank.[18]

In July 1916, Capt. William Jolly headed an infantry company of fellow Otago men who were mostly half his age and inclined to regard him with bemused admiration. They had been posted to the town of Armentières on the western front, considered a "nursery" sector by comparison with the Somme and other charnel houses farther south, and therefore suitable for untested troops such as these. Yet within a month of arrival, they began reinforcing their morale with nighttime raids across the two miles of barbed wire that separated their trenches from the enemy's. Night raids were highly dangerous, but the untried and eager Otago men welcomed the opportunity to take part in them. In preparation for an exceptionally large raid that aimed "to harass and mystify the enemy" and to "do him as much harm as possible," they spent a succession of warm July evenings training in the old town of Armentières under conditions of strict secrecy.[19] The town, however, was buzzing with spies.[20]

At 10:00 p.m. on 13 July, two small scouting companies moved out of their trenches to provide support for the main raiding party. They crouched in shell craters as their artillery sent over a heavy barrage to crush the wire defenses and dishearten the German troops in the trenches beyond them. At precisely midnight, another 150 men and officers led by Captain Jolly, with faces blackened and bayonets sharpened, began their dash across no-man's-land.[21] At the same moment, the night sky exploded with flares from the German side, exposing the Otagos to a storm of fire from machine guns and shrapnel. The raid had been anticipated by the Germans, who had withheld their counterattack until it would prove most devastating. Calling on his long years of military training, Jolly made the snap decision to abort the raid and fired off a green flare, the signal to his men to withdraw. Soon afterward he was wounded by the hail of fire but is said to have left his stretcher to help other injured troops and later suffered a second and fatal shell wound.[22] The barrage continued without pause for two hours, and very few of the main raiding party were able to return to their trenches. Alex Aitken, a sergeant major with one of the flanking parties, spent the entire night crouched in a shell hole with three of his men. When they returned to their base at dawn, he found that 163 of the 180-man company were killed, wounded, or missing, and in a later memoir, he concluded that "the 4th Company might be regarded as extinguished."[23]

Late in his life, Doug Jolly speculated that his father may have opted to leave his family and go to war out of a sense of obligation to all the young men he had trained, first in the Cromwell Rifles and later in the New Zealand (NZ) Territorial Army. "He had 'played soldiers' with all the lads of the country district in a valley of New Zealand's Southern Alps where we lived. . . . Now that war meant killing and maiming and worse, he at the age of 46 could not bear to see them go fatherless, innocent babes to the storming of the bloody beaches of Gallipoli." Doug's mother had consented to her husband's public-spiritedness, and after his death, she felt consumed with guilt that by doing so she had deprived their children of a father.[24] For decades afterward, the family spent each anniversary of Captain Jolly's death in mourning.[25]

The British Army kept a tight lid on reports of this disastrous action, and the patriotic community of Cromwell presumably learned nothing at all of the ill-fated raid except that their punctilious storekeeper had died heroically in action. William's younger brother Lesley assumed control of the family business, and Elizabeth Jolly was left to care for seven dependent children on a war widow's pension of six pounds a week (today approximately $US600) plus a one-eighth interest in the general store that amounted, according to her son, to no more than "pin money." She was nevertheless determined that each of her children would receive a better education than that of their parents, and all seven eventually graduated with a university degree or diploma—an extraordinary record of academic achievement for that time and place.[26]

At the end of 1918, young Doug graduated from Cromwell School as its "dux," or top scholar, and was chosen to ring the school bell loudly and long for the peace celebrations on Armistice Day.[27] At the start of the following year, he left his high-plains hamlet for Dunedin to enroll at Otago Boys' High School, an ornament of the country's public education system. For the previous sixty years, its stone spires, gowned faculty, and solemn traditions had emulated both the English public school and the Scottish academy and produced a large proportion of the young nation's leadership.[28] His elder brother, Leslie, was already a pupil there, and fourteen-year-old Doug, who had inherited his father's level gaze and application to duty, thrived on the school's amalgam of a canonical curriculum, stringent discipline (the cane was readily deployed), and regard for sporting prowess. For the next five years, Doug and at least one of his brothers would board in the school's dormitories, maintain high grades in its classrooms, and distinguish its sports fields. On every holiday, they returned to a devoted mother and resumed familiar duties in the family business or took on casual work in the hayfields and orchards that now surrounded their town.

Several of the Otago Boys' High teaching staff were Great War veterans for whom the surname "Jolly" invoked immediate recognition and hushed respect. One in particular, a young mathematics teacher named Alexander Aitken, had served alongside Captain Jolly at Armentières and commanded one of the flanking units on the night of the fatefully botched raid. Aitken's formidable mathematical gifts and powers of memory made him a legend in the school. It was well known that on the sorrowful day after the July 1916 raid, he learned from his devastated company commander that their casualties could not be fully accounted for since a platoon roll book had been lost. Aitken unhesitatingly recited the names, serial numbers, and next of kin of every member of his platoon.[29] A mind of such capacity could not find its full expression in a school at the far end of the world, and in 1923 Aitken took up a scholarship to Edinburgh University. There he was awarded a PhD in mathematics after a barely believable two years and spent the remainder of a glittering academic career at the university.[30]

Doug gained creditable marks at high school, especially in science subjects, but distinguished himself chiefly as an athlete. He stood a modest five feet six inches (1.7 meters) tall but proved fast, agile, and tireless on the field. For his final three years at the school, he was the fullback of its all-conquering first fifteen rugby team, and he left as its athletics and tennis champion.[31] At least as formative as these achievements was his contribution to the school's military cadet corps. In this postwar period, Otago Boys' High maintained a tradition of martial patriotism upheld by the memory of almost two hundred Old Boys who had died in the conflict overseas and by the staff who had returned from it. The cadets were commanded during Doug's time by a former student and survivor of the Somme, where the cadet had been wounded, attained the rank of major and won the Military Cross.[32] His zealous young troops were drilled in the use of military-style Lee-Enfield rifles, while the artillery section was equipped with a six-pounder field gun. The officers, including platoon commander Doug Jolly, were given further training at regular army base camps.[33]

Doug graduated in 1923, wreathed in formal tributes. In addition to his sporting triumphs, he had passed the university entrance examination with merit, was a prefect for his final two years, and won a trophy for "most efficient Regimental Sergeant-Major."[34] Most significantly of all for his future, he won the Gen. Harry Fulton Bursary, founded to commemorate an Old Boy who had been mortally wounded on the Somme in 1918.[35] Like a Rhodes scholarship in miniature, this bursary recognized both scholastic and sporting ability and was therefore among the most highly prized awards offered by the school.[36]

The bursary provided a sum of money toward study fees, and it must have come as a boon to the financially hard-pressed Jolly household and may have decided Doug on the expensive option of medicine as a course of study. His keen scientific mind and practical bent are also likely to have helped form this decision, but perhaps above all, he was driven by the example of his father's ultimate sacrifice for his country. Brigadier General Fulton's widow wrote from her home in London to congratulate the inaugural scholarship winner. "I am especially interested in the career of a doctor," she told Doug. "It is one of the finest professions with such wonderful possibilities for helping others."[37] A medical qualification offered the prospect of military service of a particularly admirable kind, although other possibilities also presented themselves. Jolly apparently considered carrying out medical mission work for New Zealand's Presbyterian Church, which at that time supported missions in China, India, and the New Hebrides (the South Pacific country later renamed Vanuatu).[38]

As he left his high school, Doug Jolly gave every indication that he had largely overcome the early loss of his father by applying himself with unrelenting determination to both athletic and scholastic goals. The school itself, with its solemn traditions, masculine energy, and elevated expectations of its students, supplied the male parenting he otherwise lacked. It had its own haka, the thunderous Māori war dance performed on occasions such as the interschool rugby matches in which Doug played an adroit game in the backs. This haka ends with the words "Homai te aroha, te pouri kia wete wetea, wete wetea" (Show me love, that sorrow may be released).[39]

3 Attributes Every Battle Surgeon Should Possess

The medical school Jolly entered the following year, 1924, was a prestigious faculty within Otago University and, at that time, its largest. It drew students from around the country, so he was likely to find several of his fellow boarders at Knox College studying alongside him.[1] Unlike the college, however, the medical school had always admitted women, and about one in eight of Jolly's fellow first-year medical students were female, a piquant novelty for a devout young man accustomed to all-male surroundings.[2] He very probably enjoyed their presence, but that attitude was not universally shared. Women students were excluded from many of the medical school's regular events such as the fifth-year dinner, and a Misogynists Society flourished at Knox College throughout this period.[3]

Otago Medical School was, by the 1920s, a pragmatically vocational institution, producing competent, broadly trained physicians for a country comprising mainly rural communities and small towns.[4] The relatively small number of students in each year meant that teaching staff came to know them as individuals. These aspiring doctors spent a first, or intermediate, year taking classes in general physics, chemistry, and biology; then they spent two preclinical years studying anatomy, physiology, biochemistry, and pharmacology. They were followed by two "professional" years of clinical practice, with students moving successively through the hospital departments of medicine, surgery, and obstetrics. This curriculum remained almost unchanged for the next half century.[5]

In parallel with the clinical work were related lectures.[6] Overseas visitors sometimes enlivened the lecture program, and in 1924 they included the American surgeon William Mayo, whose nonprofit clinic and research center in Minnesota was renowned for employing a wide range of specialist physicians.[7]

Classes were initially held in overcrowded and outdated facilities dating from the school's founding years, but a spacious new building named for the medical school's "urbane and resolute" dean, Lindo Ferguson, a graduate of Ireland's Royal College of Surgeons, opened in 1927.[8] Students eager to practice their theoretical knowledge on live patients may have chafed under a hidebound regimen of lectures and demonstrations, but the quality of instruction, especially in anatomy, was high, and Jolly excelled in this field. The school's professor of anatomy, Percy Gowland, had been successively a Lancashire general practitioner (GP), a ship's doctor, and a lecturer at Liverpool Medical School. By the time he began teaching at Otago, he had abandoned the established British system under which a class dissected different parts of a body at the same time, and his students all dissected the same part at once—a novel teaching approach in this period and one that proved far more effective. He also merged the teaching of histology (microscopic anatomy) with conventional anatomy, making Otago one of the first schools in the British Commonwealth to teach in this way.[9] According to one former student, later a professor of neurology at Harvard University, Gowland's highly functional anatomical teaching produced excellent all-purpose surgeons who later proved equally capable of treating severe injuries in peacetime or of repairing facial wounds during the Battle of Britain.[10]

A decade earlier many Otago medical students had volunteered to serve in the First World War at the earliest opportunity, and the war's legacy still hung heavily over the school.[11] Of Jolly's lecturers, a large proportion were veterans whose teaching was greatly influenced by their experiences during the war.[12] Doug Jolly seems to have decided early in his medical studies to become a surgeon, embarking on that masked and gowned branch of medicine that is practiced in a theater and has been described as godlike for its capability to restore patients from otherwise imminent and certain death. The term "surgeon" itself, however, derives from the archaic term "chirurgeon," from the Greek *cheir*, meaning "hand." A surgeon is therefore simply one who works with one's hands, and the storekeeper's son soon displayed a rare gift for doing so.

Otago Medical School's professor of surgery, Gordon Bell, was a New Zealander who had spent four years with Britain's Royal Army Medical Corps (RAMC), much of that time as a surgical specialist at casualty clearing stations near the front line. He received the Military Cross in 1916 for his treatment of the wounded at the Somme and left the British Army with the rank of major.

At times, during the heat of battle, he was obliged to operate for up to twenty-four hours on end and observed:

> As fatigue increases the niceties of judgment and handicraft diminish, but fortunately the relatively crude surgery of war lends itself to automatic surgery. The surgeon scarcely able to stand on his feet can still patch up a lacerated intestine and save a man from inevitable peritonitis: can still excise, and open widely, deep and dark muscular wounds and ward off gas gangrene; and can still find his way to the torn artery temporarily controlled by a tourniquet. . . .
>
> On the credit side, battle surgery provides an immensely valuable exercise in those attributes which every surgeon should possess: prompt decision and prompt action, self-reliance from working with little assistance, and the capacity to get out of difficulties, which stems from imperturbability and resolution.[13]

Those experiences and impressions closely foreshadow the later career of Bell's attentive student from Cromwell.

At Otago Gordon Bell developed his department into several specialist schools, including orthopedics and anesthesia.[14] His assistant lecturer and tutor in surgery, Renfrew White, was yet another World War I veteran who had gained valuable experience in orthopedic surgery as a major with the RAMC in France and later treated injuries to bones, joints, nerves, and muscles at the Royal National Orthopaedic Hospital in London.[15] At Otago White proved a gifted teacher and a memorably colorful personality. In addition to his teaching load, Major White, as he was universally known, built a busy orthopedic practice at Dunedin's main public hospital, where his students were able to develop their experience, especially by treating wounded ex-servicemen.[16]

Another war veteran who had attained the rank of major was Charles Hercus, who enlisted in the New Zealand Medical Corps soon after graduating from Otago in 1914. He was sent to the disastrous invasion at Gallipoli, in the present-day Republic of Türkiye, where thousands of New Zealand, Australian, and British troops toiled in vain to capture a barely accessible stretch of steep coastline from far stronger Turkish positions. He was awarded a Distinguished Service Order (DSO) and the Most Excellent Order of the British Empire (OBE) during his wartime service. Over four years of fighting, Hercus also pursued an enthusiasm for public health. He is said to have gone ashore at Gallipoli carrying a microscope and later succeeded in controlling malaria among New Zealand troops in Palestine.[17] In 1921 he was appointed the professor of public health at Otago and instituted a compulsory fifth-year course of study in preventive medicine and public health. His students undertook a research project of their own choosing, carrying out the main investigation over the summer vacation at the end of their fourth-year studies. They then submitted the results as a dissertation. Hundreds of them are still held by the university, although Jolly's, regrettably, does not appear to have survived.[18]

Hercus was a sterling compound of soldier and scientist, and perhaps no one in the country better understood the specialist training required of armed forces medical officers. In 1927, several years after he joined the medical school's teaching staff, the New Zealand Defence Force appointed him assistant director of medical services for the army's Southern Command. In that role, he began to revitalize a university institution that had long fallen out of favor. In 1909, just a year after the first Officers' Training Corps was set up in Britain, a similar corps, consisting of an infantry company and the Otago University Medical Company (OUMC), was established in Dunedin.[19] The young Charles Hercus served as a corporal in the OUMC, which trained a large majority of the medical and dental officers who served overseas during World War I. The carnage and bungling leadership of that war, however, generated disdain for martial matters among the student body for the next decade until Hercus was called upon to reform this once-hallowed training unit.[20] Subsequently, the OUMC's training took place mainly during a fortnight-long annual camp before the start of the autumn term and was held in an isolated rural area such as Waitati on the Otago coast. Basic military training was combined with instruction in medical and dental military requirements, including lectures on hygiene, sanitation, and field ambulance work.[21] Certificates and trophies were keenly competed for, and Jolly's high school Officers' Training Corps experience and family background must have provided him with a distinct advantage. He is likely to have found the summer military camp an invigorating change from arduous study.[22]

This natural athlete also maintained at least some of the sporting activities at which he had excelled in high school. He played for the university rugby team, turning out for practice on frosty winter mornings, and in his final year was selected for a combined New Zealand Universities team to challenge the Australian Universities team in Auckland. However, another feature of extra-curricular university life proved more important to his future than any other. The Student Christian Movement (SCM) had been active on all the country's university campuses since the late nineteenth century, although Otago was always its stronghold. Nonsectarian but mostly Protestant, the SCM encouraged active engagement with the world beyond the university gates and, in the late 1920s, raised money for causes such as the Austrian (later European) Student Relief Fund, the unemployed, earthquake victims, and crippled children.[23] This boldly progressive organization transformed the social outlook of the unsophisticated medical student from an isolated community and a devout and conservative upbringing, and his early ambition to become a medical missionary quickly evaporated. Jolly's unexamined and inward-looking Presbyterianism gave way to an ecumenical, internationalist, and non-doctrinal practice of Christian socialism that remained the lodestone for his life.

Both at Otago and nationally, the SCM surged in numbers and influence after a new general secretary arrived from Europe in late 1925. Rev. Donald Grant was a dynamic leader of manifest sincerity, with traces of his Highland Scots upbringing in his accent. He and his similarly magnetic wife, Irene (her name was pronounced as three syllables: I-*reen*-ee), and their two children came to Dunedin from Geneva. There Reverend Grant had founded the Austrian Student Relief Fund and spent five years carrying out relief work among "distressed and destitute" students in Europe. Those experiences were reported in stirring terms in Dunedin's daily paper. In famine-struck Russia in 1922, Grant said, "I have seen scores of people in one street after another lying sick with disease and starving and ultimately dying there. . . . I was in one agricultural village where they used to have 117 horses. When I was there, there were seven and the men were pulling the ploughs." He had helped students in Germany to found a self-help organization that ran its own "butchers and dining rooms, loan banks for students, boot and shoe factories and repair shops, laundries. . . . The fact that students are working with their hands alongside ordinary workers and labourers means that they understand in a way never before possible the conditions and the outlook of the ordinary man."[24]

Those words sound more like those of a socialist orator than a preacher, and Grant made no apology for favoring political action over piety. He had spent the final months of World War I in Dartmoor Prison as a conscientious objector, and his religious training was thereafter directed toward international relations in the interests of world peace.[25] "Loyalty to Jesus Christ," he wrote in the SCM's magazine, "has nothing much to do with words, statements, creeds or confessions: but it has everything to do with our character, our spirit, our attitudes, our standards."[26] This unusual and inspiring figure swiftly revived New Zealand's lackluster SCM, traveling the country to visit each of its campuses and breathing "fresh confidence and resolution into jaded spirits . . . the history of the Movement during the next four years is embodied in the person of its general secretary who was to inspire a veritable renaissance among young students."[27] Grant's charismatic leadership soon drew large numbers of students previously uninterested in the SCM into its ranks. He interpreted Christian faith and ethics in the form of practical service to society and placed special emphasis on the importance of an awareness of international issues.

Reverend Grant also served as Otago University's chaplain, encouraging its student body and numbers of academic staff and local political leaders to share an uplifting version of Christian socialism that incorporated Marxist, pacifist, and unorthodox economic ideas.[28] One of those so inspired was Professor Horace Belshaw, perhaps the country's leading economist of that period, who was moved to describe the Christian ethic as "the same as the ideal of communism. . . . Christianity does not, in my opinion, justify itself unless it recognises that the improvement of welfare in general on this earth should be its main objective."[29] These heady opinions were freely offered around the Grants' hospitable dinner table, along with companionship and counsel for any Otago students who happened to call. The young Doug Jolly became a regular visitor and eventually a surrogate member of the family. His close and consequential friendship with the Grants would last for all their lifetimes.

During his fourth and fifth years of study, Jolly and his fellow medical students began to combine the theoretical instruction delivered through lectures and demonstrations with practical skills acquired from dissection and bedside clinical teaching in Dunedin hospitals.[30] Space, staff, and laboratories remained in short supply, and the hospital wards therefore served as clinical workshops.[31] Despite these limitations, the students developed a working familiarity with the principles of surgery and medicine, including an introduction to anesthetics, radiology, and what were then called "mental diseases." The most evident shortfall in their training was in the field of obstetrics and gynecology, where the teaching was described as "chaotic and outdated."[32] Since most women still gave birth at home under the care of midwives in this period, opportunities for practical obstetrics were limited.

The sixth and final year was devoted entirely to clinical work, and a shortage of patients in Dunedin sent many students to work in the central hospitals of other major New Zealand cities.[33] Some found this period the most rewarding of their training. Jolly's contemporary, Russell Chisholm, later a distinguished neuropath, was among six students who spent their final year at Auckland Hospital, where, he said, "we educated ourselves."[34] Jolly appears to have spent part of his final year's training in the small North Island city of Palmerston North. His marks had improved year by year, especially in surgery at which he evidently excelled. He graduated in December 1929, fifth in his class of thirty-seven.

His sense of satisfaction at this achievement may have been muted by the departure from New Zealand earlier that year of the Grant family, now numbering five after the birth of a third child, a boy named after his father. Four years after their arrival in Dunedin, the family returned to Europe so that Reverend Grant could take the post of secretary of the International Fellowship of Reconciliation, an international anti-war body based in Vienna.[35] Jolly likely remained in touch with the family by mail as he gained further clinical experience toward his joint degrees in medicine and surgery.

For three years after graduating, this newly qualified doctor worked in short-term public hospital postings around the country, at first in central Otago, including in his hometown of Cromwell. There his family name remained prominent since two of his uncles had served as mayor, with Ernest Jolly governing during World War I and David Jolly in the 1920s. In this way, and through their continued ownership and operation of the family store, the Jolly family remained leading members of the small and isolated community.

The early 1930s saw intense political pressure for change in the New Zealand health service, as people began seeking inpatient treatment for conditions such as appendicitis that were formerly treated in their homes. Public hospitals faced greater patient numbers and requirements for new medical technologies without a corresponding increase in their funding. The growing demand for a state-funded health-care system soon became a fierce political issue. When the young Dr. Jolly moved in early 1930 to his country's compact, windswept capital of Wellington, he found that its six-hundred-bed, main public hospital was greatly in need of new buildings to accommodate its patients. Plans for additional wards had been drawn up some years earlier, but the sharply deteriorating economic conditions saw those plans shelved; his year at Wellington Hospital was spent in overcrowded and outdated buildings from the previous century.[36] These disadvantages were offset by the hospital's acquisition of the latest X-ray equipment and sophisticated laboratory facilities.[37] It boasted the most advanced surgical department in the country, employing new techniques in the treatment of fractures and nerve regeneration that were increasingly called upon to deal with injuries sustained in motor vehicle accidents.[38]

A large and growing proportion of patients were unemployed men, deserted wives, and other indigent and needy people treated without charge as charity cases.[39] When a deputation from the city's Trades and Labour Council informed the hospital board in early 1930 that a recent rise in patient fees from nine to seventeen shillings a day would entail "considerable hardship for necessitous patients," the board chair replied that the truly destitute would continue to be treated at no charge.[40] Late that year the hospital's Social Welfare Committee drew the government's attention to "the appalling conditions of distress at present existing through prevailing unemployment. Both single and married men now find it impossible to secure work of any kind, with the result that many families are experiencing need."[41]

Jolly worked at this hospital as a house physician and resident surgeon, gaining wide experience in the medical; surgical; eye, ear, nose, and throat; infectious diseases; children's; casualty; and general outpatient departments.[42] Anesthesia did not become a recognized medical speciality until the following decade, and hospital records show him acting as anesthetist for more senior surgeons several times daily during late 1930, administering general anesthetic in the form of ethyl chloride and ether, and nitrous oxide ("laughing gas") and oxygen—all of which he would later administer in wartime.[43]

This period appears to have been a productive and happy one of his early career. His senior colleagues noted his kindness to patients, his conscientious attitude, and his pleasant working manner. Louis Cohen, head of the hospital's eye, ear, nose, and throat department, acknowledged his temporary house surgeon's "sterling qualities as a medical man and a colleague to be associated with." He found Jolly to be "an excellent anaesthetist" and thoroughly reliable.[44] The hospital's pathologist was equally impressed: "I formed the highest opinion of his professional work: he has in addition a personality and qualities of mind which in my opinion are just as important as academic attainments."[45]

After fifteen months of wide-ranging training in this politically charged seat of government, Jolly transferred in 1931 to the much smaller town of Palmerston North, the provincial center for a large rural area. Its two-hundred-bed public hospital had just dealt with an influx of severely injured casualties from a massive earthquake in the port city of Napier, housing them in a marquee and tents, but after this unprecedented emergency was managed, its workload offered few opportunities for clinical experience to match those in Wellington.[46]

While his daily round of cases may have seemed routine, Jolly's social life in Palmerston North was turbulent. At age twenty-seven, he became engaged to marry a "pretty and attractive" woman named Joan King who lived in the rural settlement of Hastings, to the north of his place of work.[47] The only information about this short-lived romance comes from letters he received, including one from Joan herself: "Feeling rather triste because you are not here but are speeding back to Palmerston in a hot, crowded service car." In her fiancé's absence, Joan was evidently delighting in assembling the rudiments of a shared household "against that time when you will have qualified [as a surgeon] and we will have each other for ever, ever and ever."[48]

"Aren't we all lucky young things," wrote another friend named Kitty, who was also evidently either engaged or married. "Do you remember how you and I used to talk about the wonderful love that we knew was just waiting around the corner for both of us—and now we have both found it. . . . It would be perfect if we could all meet in London."[49]

That happy reunion did not take place, since Jolly's engagement was evidently broken off within a few months. Details are lacking, but Joan and Jolly apparently remained on friendly terms. Three years later he received a letter from his former fiancée, written from the ocean liner on which she had recently sailed to Bombay. Joan described the voyage in high-spirited terms and ended by wishing him "happy hunting," presumably a reference to his future marital prospects.[50]

By the time that letter arrived, Jolly had left New Zealand to pursue postgraduate studies in surgery, at that time a necessary prerequisite to gaining a specialist's qualifications. As at Wellington Hospital, his senior colleagues at

Palmerston North bade him farewell with glowing testimonials. David Wylie, the hospital's honorary visiting surgeon and a veteran of both the Boer and Great Wars, could "only speak of his work in the highest terms. He has discharged the usual duties of a house surgeon with conspicuous ability and has been a most agreeable colleague to work with. He has proved himself to be a most careful and excellent assistant at operations, assiduous in his care of patients afterwards and thorough in everything he does. He is much liked by his patients, and I can most cordially recommend him for a resident position at any hospital."[51]

To add to this encomium, Jolly carried a letter by one of his country's leading statesmen, Minister of Finance Downie Stewart, addressed to the New Zealand high commissioner in London. "The bearer of this letter," it said, "is a son of my old friend, the late Captain Jolly, with whom I served in France and who was killed in action." Stewart asked that every possible courtesy be extended to the young colonial doctor, "both for his own sake and for the memory of his father."[52]

In January 1932, Doug Jolly left New Zealand for London on board the liner and former British troopship *Herminius*, paying his passage by working as the ship's doctor. He would never return permanently to his country of birth.

4 Christian Left

The *Herminius* discharged its stocky young doctor, still tanned from the southern summer and the ship's passage through the tropics, into a bleak London winter, and he wrestled his baggage to the first of a succession of temporary lodgings. Jolly was to spend the next five years shuttling between several London hospitals, first as a barely qualified house surgeon and later as a more experienced registrar, to gain the level of clinical proficiency required to pass the legendarily demanding examinations for fellowship of the Royal College of Surgeons (FRCS). To this end, he registered as a medical practitioner in the United Kingdom within weeks of disembarking.[1]

Edinburgh's venerable medical college, the oldest in Britain, was the most obvious choice in this period for an Otago medical graduate seeking qualifications in surgery. Edinburgh had trained most of Jolly's own lecturers, and Scotland was the home of his forefathers. Yet he opted to train instead in London, a decision influenced most likely by the deep and lasting friendship he had developed with the London-based Grant family.

London also proved to be the ideal base for this stage of a novice doctor's career. It was a national hub for medical services of all kinds and a center for innovation. Elsewhere in Britain, the interwar health system retained traces of an earlier pattern of treatment structured largely on social rather than medical grounds. Its hospitals were an uncoordinated mix of Poor Law hospitals for the indigent and municipal and voluntary hospitals funded by patient contributions and donations from wealthy philanthropists. The wealthy classes were generally treated in their own homes or in private nursing homes. London, however, had moved further and faster than anywhere else in the country toward a centrally planned and free-to-all system that, fifteen years later, would become the National Health Service.[2]

By 1932 cooperation was steadily increasing between the city's seventy-four municipal hospitals, which cared for most chronically ill and long-term patients, and its independent voluntary hospitals, funded largely by donations and oriented to treating short-stay patients suffering acute illness. Many hospitals also served as centers of teaching and research with eminent medical schools allied to prestigious general hospitals such as St. Bartholomew's, St. Thomas's, and Guy's.[3] Yet even in go-ahead London, hospitals retained the former distinction between working-class patients, treated for free or at low cost in "the clamour and sociability of the dormitory-style ordinary ward," and the fast-growing middle classes, accommodated in one- or two-bed rooms in wards physically separated from the main hospital and designed to closely reproduce the experience of treatment at home. Those latter patients paid a substantial fee, intended to cover the full cost of their treatment, but could feel reassured that they would not be called on to serve as demonstration patients for teaching purposes.[4]

Despite the harsh economic conditions then prevailing, Jolly was able to find suitable posts with relative ease, thanks in part to a recent development in UK medical schools: Their undergraduate training had been extended from five to six years, producing a temporary shortage of local graduates, and hospital work was readily available to qualified and well-regarded doctors from overseas. One of his former lecturers at Otago believed that New Zealand graduates seeking specialist UK qualifications should aim to work first in a base hospital, "where there is less responsibility and more supervision," and then in a smaller hospital. "There a man is likely to be left more to himself, and with greater opportunity for using his own head and hands."[5] Jolly appears to have broadly followed this advice, and from April 1932, he began working as a house surgeon in the large West London Hospital in Hammersmith. He is likely to have lived on the hospital grounds along with other unmarried junior doctors, who were required to be available at any time of the day or night.

Since its founding in the mid-nineteenth century, the West London had acquired the luster of the main postgraduate teaching hospital in London and was later formally recognized as providing the practice that candidates for membership of the Royal College of Surgeons required.[6] Jolly received instruction and learned by example from its staff while gaining daily practical experience as a house surgeon. His day typically began with a ward round to review each inpatient under his care, whether in pre- or postoperative stage. He then evaluated newly arrived patients, sent either from the hospital's emergency department or from outside consultants' rooms. Surgical operations in the theater generally meant assisting more experienced consultant colleagues, although Jolly increasingly performed solo operations in minor cases. His day's work ended with outpatient clinics to follow up patients after their operations or to see new referrals.

The early 1930s were an ideal period for gaining wide surgical experience since large city hospitals like West London had only two or three consultants in each of its wards. "The consultants and the ward sisters therefore came to know each other's ways, and to trust and be loyal to each other." Newly qualified doctors such as Jolly were taken under the well-starched wing of the ward sister, or senior nurse, who guided them in the practices of the institution and especially those of its "chief," or senior consultant. To ensure continuity of care for patients, junior doctors worked predominantly with just one or two chiefs in each hospital, and this regular contact with their superiors enhanced their education and developed camaraderie under pressure.[7]

Although the wards were divided between the general medical and general surgical, their physicians and surgeons increasingly worked as teams, with patient care crossing the traditional medical-surgical divide. Subspecialties in thoracic, plastic, neurological, and orthopedic surgery had emerged from the carnage of the Great War, but in this interwar period, and especially at the early stage of their training, surgeons such as Jolly were expected to be all-purpose practitioners.[8] By late 1932, he was given the considerable additional responsibility of resident assistant surgeon at West London. His senior surgeon found that the young New Zealander fulfilled this post efficiently and was "a very pleasant man to work with."[9]

Jolly was undoubtedly aware of, and very likely belonged to, the Socialist Medical Association (SMA). This influential body, which remains active today as the Socialist Health Association, had been formed to campaign for a publicly funded national health service that could entirely replace those remnants of the charity-based system that persisted from the Victorian era.[10] Its early members included idealistic and able young doctors such as Reginald "Reg" or "Reggie" Saxton, Alex Tudor-Hart, and Archie Cochrane—all of whom would become Jolly's colleagues and close friends.

In the 1934 local elections, the Labour Party gained a majority on the London County Council, which controlled most of the city's hospitals. The SMA, a party affiliate, was instrumental in shaping its health policy. Following this election, SMA members ran the county council's medical services, acquiring vital administrative experience and the opportunity to develop London's hospitals in the direction of a future national health service.[11] The SMA rejected the established hierarchy of an illustrious surgeon or specialist attended by underlings in favor of the principle that the team, not the individual, was central to providing quality health care. Its membership was open to allied professions such as dentists, nurses, and pharmacists, who were seen as equally vital members of an effective health center. This collective approach may well have influenced Jolly's later work in wartime.

He left his evidently satisfying post at the West London Hospital in January 1933 and for the following four years worked at other London hospitals, especially those—such as St. Peter's Hospital for the Stone, the New End Hospital Goitre Centre, and the Miller General Hospital in Greenwich—that specialized in the treatment of goiter, an unsightly swelling in the neck caused by an under- or overactive thyroid gland. It was a condition sadly common in the United Kingdom at the time, and working-class women were generally the worst affected as they tended to deny themselves an adequate diet to support their families and then typically failed to seek medical assistance until their condition became acute.[12] Jolly's own country had a high incidence of this condition, so he could expect to encounter many cases of it on his return there.[13] In addition, he spent a brief period many miles to the northwest in the ancient county town of Shrewsbury as the locum resident surgical officer at the Royal Salop Infirmary, an elegant Grecian-style building overlooking the River Severn. There, as elsewhere, his superiors reported that Jolly "showed marked ability as a surgeon, both from an operative and diagnostic point of view."[14]

The longest of this series of temporary positions was, like his first, in Hammersmith at the Royal Masonic Hospital, where he spent a year from mid-1934 as a resident assistant surgeon. This private hospital specialized in treating middle-class patients. Its purpose-built, red-brick premises were then brand new, with wards whose southern sides opened onto deep, curving sundecks, exemplifying the most current thinking on the medicinal properties of light and fresh air. The Royal Masonic's two-hundred–plus beds made it the largest independent acute hospital in Europe at that time and an ideal place for a promising young surgeon to advance his career.

Much of Jolly's year in this well-appointed and highly regarded hospital was spent practicing gynecological surgery. As a house surgeon, however, he was required to develop and practice a wide range of surgical skills. Once again, Jolly endeared himself. A specialist obstetrician noted that he had "the knack of securing the confidence of his patients and is agreeable and courteous to patients and colleagues alike."[15] The hospital's senior surgeon found that the young New Zealander "possessed an excellent judgement and in addition he was a most pleasant man to work with. Mr Jolly has already distinguished himself and will, I am quite sure, distinguish himself still further in the future."[16] Another senior colleague found that "he investigates his cases with the utmost thoroughness and is persona grata with patients and nursing staff. I found him a most capable assistant in all my operations and . . . he is well qualified to occupy any surgical post for which he applies."[17]

These glowing endorsements, and others equally admiring, saw Jolly appointed in early 1935 to the post of acting resident assistant surgeon at his former workplace, the nearby West London Hospital. This step was significant in his career since, although only short term, it was a regular staff appointment rather than the latest in a series of temporary training opportunities. Although not yet entitled to call himself a surgeon, since he had still to pass the final FRCS examination, Jolly was now effectively employed in that role, and his colleagues regarded his ascent to the status of fully registered surgeon as imminent and inevitable.

Throughout his years in London, Jolly was focused fixedly on the goal of his final surgical qualifications, and he appears to have devoted little time to romantic, sporting, or other interests. However, after a year in his new country, he was able to renew his treasured friendship with Rev. Donald Grant, his mentor and surrogate father from university days. Although the Grant family had left Otago several years before he did, Jolly is certain to have maintained contact with them. After they returned to London in 1933, their influence on his later life would grow more profound than ever.

The Grant family had left Dunedin in 1929, Jolly's final year at medical school, and traveled to Vienna, where Donald took up the post of director of the International Fellowship of Reconciliation (IFoR). This enduring organization, representing anti-war groups in many countries including Jolly's own, was formed at the outset of World War I and remains active today.[18] The choice of Vienna as its base of operations was both logical and fortuitous. The vibrant Austrian capital spanning the River Danube was, in 1929, undertaking perhaps the most ambitious and exciting experiment in municipal socialism to be found anywhere in the world. Since the Social Democratic Party came to power there eight years earlier, "Red Vienna" had built hundreds of workers' apartment blocks, many with their own kindergartens, maternity clinics, libraries, and other social services. Medical services were free to all, while a special wealth tax was imposed on limousines and servants in private households. Music was everywhere in this urban utopia. Grant's young and multilingual English secretary, Tess Simpson, an accomplished violinist, found that in Vienna "playing chamber music was just taken for granted. It was like cleaning your teeth. Everyone learned to play a musical instrument."[19] These cultural riches were shared by the Viennese working class who, according to one of the city's leading journalists, "achieved a level never reached before by the masses of the people in any industrial society."[20]

These were the words of Karl Polanyi, a Hungarian-born economist and one of the most penetrating voices of Vienna's intelligentsia. As a leading figure at the economics journal *Der Österreichische Volkswirt*, Polanyi established a reputation as a commentator on international affairs and especially on the Soviet Union. He and his wife, Ilona Duczyńska, herself a radical activist and intellectual, had been forced to leave their native Hungary after political repression made it impossible for them to remain there, and they found a congenial haven in the Austrian capital.[21] By the time they encountered the Grants in 1929, the city had become an uplifting experiment in civic socialism. Karl spoke excellent English, and with their six-year-old daughter, Kari, the Polanyis proved ideal guides to introduce the Grant family to their new home.

For much of 1931, the IFoR took an active and outspoken part in preparations for the first-ever World Disarmament Conference, organized by the League of Nations and due to take place in Geneva. With his customary vigor and Highland charm, Donald Grant had convinced young people, both Protestant and Catholic, from all over Europe to take part in a Youth Crusade against the ongoing militarization of mutually hostile nations such as France and Germany. The young marchers came not only from those countries but also from the

United Kingdom, Holland, and Belgium, and proceeded by several routes toward Switzerland, holding public meetings and successively delivering their message of international reconciliation to an estimated fifty thousand European citizens along the way. The Youth Crusade arrived in Geneva by the opening of the conference in February 1932, and twelve representatives from almost as many nations presented a petition to its chairman. The thousands of signatories called for total disarmament as the goal of all states and declared that they refused "to take part in a new war whose victims will be youth."[22] Albert Einstein, a pacifist and internationalist, had predicted that the conference would be "decisive for the fate of the present generation and the one to come."[23] He was among those attending, with Donald Grant acting as his translator.[24]

From this uplifting beginning, the conference degenerated into a cynical stalemate. Although more than thirty countries were represented, including the Union of Soviet Socialist Republics (USSR), the United States, Germany, Britain, France, and Japan, some were only half-heartedly committed to the goal of disarmament, and a few had already embarked on a program of aggressive militarization. "As it went on," Tess Simpson later recalled, "you saw how the conference was being sabotaged. There wasn't any real interest in the disarmament question except by the smallest countries who were quite powerless."[25] Japan, a prominent participant, had recently invaded its neighbor Manchuria and evidently held similar expansionist ambitions toward China and elsewhere. In early 1933, before any real progress had been made toward disarmament initiatives, Hitler was elected chancellor of Germany on a platform of massive rearmament. His country promptly withdrew from the talks, and the conference's high-minded agenda collapsed, fatally damaging the reputation of its parent body, the League of Nations, as a force for world peace.

Within two months of Hitler's election victory, his looming shadow extended across the border to reach the Grants' apartment in Vienna. Two visitors arrived at their door who might have seemed glamorous except that they were both in evident extreme distress. The celebrated actress Helene Weigel and her husband, Bertolt Brecht, had fled their home in Berlin the day after the burning of the Reichstag and left their two-year-old daughter, Barbara, in the care of Brecht's father in Bavaria. They had since learned that the Nazis were searching for the little girl and planned to hold her hostage to compel her vehemently antiauthoritarian parents to return to Germany.

Irene Grant promptly offered to enter the newly Nazi-controlled Germany to find little Barbara and bring her to Vienna. She left by train that night and arrived the following morning in the medieval Bavarian city of Augsburg. "That day I shall never forget. It was the day of the first big Hitler anti-Jewish demonstration in Germany. . . . The city seemed to be flooded by a black and brown wave of terror." Irene found her way to the paper factory managed by Brecht's father, and in a state of great anxiety, he instructed her to take a local train to a small village where, if all went well, she would find an elderly woman with a small child waiting on the station platform.

There indeed, as the train pulled in, was "the poor, weeping nurse and the little two-year-old baby—a curly-haired, bright-eyed, lively little girl." Irene persuaded Barbara to board the train with her, and they sat in a compartment shared with "two homely German women with their full shopping baskets and wearing the local Bavarian dress. . . . They were doing a lot of whispering as the train speeded up, and I know how much denunciations were already the order of the day in Germany." After a journey that seemed interminable, the train neared the Viennese border, and Irene heard the passport inspector approaching their carriage. As he approached, the Bavarian women stood up and pushed past him with their bulky shopping bags. "One of the women patted the child on the head and remarked loudly, 'That's a sweet kid. And such a likeness between mother and child I've never seen in all my life.' Her glance to me explained everything. The subliminal advertising was perfect—clear and effective." The inspector merely glanced at Irene's British passport and pronounced, "Alles in ordnung." Brecht and Weigel were waiting in agonies of anxiety over the border. "The two German women had probably made possible the future, not only for Barbara but for her parents," Irene Grant later concluded, "and they had certainly restored my faith in humankind."[26]

The rise of the National Socialist Party, and its aggressive ambitions, made the closure of the International Fellowship's office in Vienna inevitable, and in advance of that depressing development, the Grant family returned to London deeply dismayed by the war clouds once again hovering over Europe. They had last known Doug Jolly as an earnest, unworldly medical student from New Zealand's hinterland, and four years later, they found him a highly regarded young doctor with broad surgical experience and glowing prospects. He had, however, been living as a somewhat isolated expatriate with a single-minded focus on pursuing his professional studies. Reunion with the Grants in early 1933 effected a transformation in his intellectual and personal life.

Donald and Irene Grant soon assembled around them a circle of friends who shared their lifelong commitment to political engagement. With economic catastrophe continuing to destabilize much of the world, and a bellicose nationalism rising in states barely recovered from the war fourteen years earlier, that commitment veered steadily leftward. Central to this group was the younger and impassioned couple, the Polanyis. Karl's journal, *Der Österreichische Volkswirt*, had resolved soon after the Grants' departure from Vienna that the political situation in Austria had become so tenuous that he could also no longer remain living there. His destination of choice was also decided since the Grant family had clearly indicated when they left Vienna that they hoped to maintain their warm friendship with the Polanyis, possibly by "setting up house together to form an experimental 'social unit' that might . . . perhaps be a model to others for a new society."[27] That adventurous proposal did not eventuate, but when Karl followed the Grants to London in late 1933, he lived at first in the spare room of their home at Pyecombe Corner in north London, becoming one of an endless stream of short-term guests who were sometimes given a bed in the dining room for lack of any other space. Within weeks of his arrival, they arranged for Polanyi to provide firsthand impressions of Austria's increasingly autocratic conditions in a lecture at Chatham House, home of the Royal Institute for International Affairs.[28]

Not long before, in May 1933, the *Times* published a letter signed by an array of renowned academics, among them seven Nobel laureates, announcing the launch of a nonprofit body titled the Academic Assistance Council (AAC). Its objective was "to raise a fund, to be used primarily, though not exclusively, in providing maintenance for displaced teachers and investigators, and finding them work in universities and scientific institutions." One of the signatories was economist John Maynard Keynes. Another was the New Zealand–born physicist and Nobel Prize winner Ernest Rutherford, who became the AAC's first president.

Donald Grant's well-connected secretary at IFoR, Tess Simpson, was ideally placed to understand and aid the quickening torrent of displaced Jewish and leftist intellectuals who were suddenly forced to emigrate to unfamiliar destinations, often lacking adequate means of support. When, in early 1933, she herself was forced to leave her beloved Vienna and return to London, the ACC engaged her at a meager salary as its first assistant secretary and later as secretary.[29] She continued to work for the council and its successor, the Society for the Protection of Science and Learning, for the rest of her career, saving the lives of many hundreds of scientists, philosophers, historians, artists, musicians, and architects who contributed immeasurably to intellectual and cultural life in Britain, the British Commonwealth, and the United States.[30]

Operating from the attic of a large house in Piccadilly, central London, the AAC acted as a conduit between the expatriate academics endangered by Nazi policies and the foreign universities that might employ them. They included eventual luminaries of postwar Britain such as the architectural historian Nikolaus Pevsner, art historian Ernst Gombrich, and some two hundred German and Austrian doctors. By late 1933, Dr. Somerville Hastings, the first president of the Socialist Medical Association, met almost daily with these medical refugees and sought financial help for them.[31] From 1935 the influx of emigré scholars overwhelmed the positions available for them in UK universities, and the council looked abroad, particularly to the United States but also to other countries. A young Austrian-born philosopher, Karl Popper, was dispatched to a teaching post in far-off New Zealand.[32]

By 1934, when Karl Polanyi's wife, Ilona, joined him in London, the impact of Nazi hostility toward the visionary socialism of Red Vienna had reached a devastating crisis. In February that year, the magnificent new workers' apartment block named in honour of Karl Marx, the pride of the city's municipal housing complexes, became a symbolic stronghold when anti-fascist resisters barricaded themselves inside it. The Karl-Marx-Hof was shelled by artillery fire and badly damaged, and in the aftermath of this uprising, the Social Democratic Party's leaders were executed or driven into exile and the party itself declared illegal.

In this cheerless political climate, the Grants engineered a productive meeting of minds between the ascetic, unorthodox Marxist economist Polanyi and another of their close friends, an iconoclastic Scottish philosopher named John Macmurray, whose slender stature, Vandyke beard, and searching gaze reminded some of "a healthier DH Lawrence."[33] Macmurray had known Irene Grant since their student days, when both belonged to the Student Christian Movement. He then served in World War I as a nursing orderly and later as a junior officer in a Highland regiment. Two years after Jolly's father was killed at Armentières,

Second Lieutenant Macmurray was severely wounded near the same battlefield and awarded the Military Cross for gallantry. He later became a professor of philosophy at London's University College, grappling with issues of freedom in the modern world, the title of his first book. His practice of basing his classes on his students' own lived experience made him a dissident philosopher in relation to his colleagues. His early publications were intended primarily for students and the wider public rather than for his fellow academics, and in their emphasis on the primacy of action over theory, they echoed the precept of early Marx: It was necessary to change the world, not merely to explain it.

By 1933 Professor Macmurray was also a prominent public intellectual with a nationwide profile after giving a series of talks on BBC radio that addressed key philosophical concepts in straightforward lay terms. The talks were hugely popular, but the revelation that Macmurray's own intellectual direction inclined toward a merging of Christianity with Marxism proved so controversial that the BBC canceled the series.[34] He was nevertheless able to provide vital assistance to the work of Tess Simpson by supplying assessments of the work of emigré colleagues such as the philosopher and avant-garde composer Theodor Adorno, who arrived in London as a political refugee from Frankfurt in 1934.[35] In that year, Macmurray and his wife, Betty, accompanied by the fluent-German-speaking Irene Grant, even made the dangerous journey from London to Nazi-occupied Vienna "to help get socialists out."[36]

The unlikely collaboration of the instinctively rational journalist Polanyi and the priestly soldier-philosopher Macmurray proved exceptionally fruitful. The unprecedented crisis of their times—the failure of both socialism and liberalism to prevent a worldwide economic breakdown and the rise of fascism, with capitalism as its economic engine—had brought them by quite different intellectual trajectories to a historic junction. Both men now believed that social change required a spiritual basis as well as a theoretical framework. Through Donald Grant's socialist reading of the New Testament, they found a new way of understanding history and contemporary problems and the potential for a new social and economic order. Grant's vision of a humanist Christian socialism provided inspiration and grounds for optimism in the face of despair. Over the course of endless discussions between 1933 and 1935, Polanyi and Macmurray developed these mutual philosophical insights into a remarkable synthesis.[37] They came to believe that if the intellectual positions of Marxism and Christianity, popularly assumed to be mutually antagonistic, could be reconciled, then the combined efforts of their adherents might achieve the vital political goal of effective popular resistance to fascism and eventually the establishment of a democratic socialist economic order.[38]

Even before Polanyi arrived in London, Macmurray had envisaged producing a multiauthored collection of essays that would confront the crisis of fascism by exploring the relationship between Christianity and communism. He now enlisted Polanyi as one of the book's three editors. The emigré Hungarian also contributed an essay on the essence of fascism, which he described as a counter-religion to Christianity and an affront to Christian values.[39] A victorious fascism, his essay insisted, would mean "the end of Christianity in all but its most debased forms."[40]

Christianity and the Social Revolution appeared in 1935. Publisher Victor Gollancz ran a headline on the cover calling on readers to give "special attention for this very important book." The eminence of some of its contributors may have had even greater publicity benefit. They included the American theologian Reinhold Niebuhr, the Cambridge biochemist and historian of science Joseph Needham, and the poet W. H. Auden. Other contributors ranged in political affiliation from a serving Anglican minister to the Cambridge philosopher and "avowed communist" John Lewis. The preface acknowledged that the book's contributors held an array of philosophical and theological positions but agreed on the central issue of the necessity for greater understanding and dialogue on what they had in common. "Christianity cannot be ignored by Socialists. It is . . . too deeply penetrated with social idealism to be scorned either as a foe or an ally." Similarly, readers were invited to decide for themselves "whether or not communism is the true heir of the Christian tradition."[41]

John Macmurray supplied a chapter on recent developments in Marxist thought and in a concluding essay proposed a synthesis of Christian and communist ideas to address the emerging crisis in world affairs. "There is one very strong reason for suggesting that Christianity cannot stand in such essential opposition to Communism as most Christians and nearly all Communists suppose. It is the fact that Christianity stands in precisely such an essential opposition to Fascism."[42] The book sold a respectable twelve thousand copies, aided by an admiring review from the historian and social critic R. H. Tawney, who singled out Polanyi's contribution as particularly timely and insightful.

There can be no doubt that the teetering diplomatic and political edifice of mid-1930s Europe produced this unprecedented rapprochement of ideas. Facing the prospect of the annihilation of their entire political project, democratic socialists were urgently seeking the support of any anti-fascist constituency they could find, and those in the religious Left were especially sought-after allies. From the other direction, since at least the 1920s, progressive Christians had participated in a widespread questioning of the existing social order. Many were ready to accept profound structural changes in society and found socialist analysis highly relevant to their prospect of the future.

The Grants and their tiny radical coterie were now determined to establish an institutional presence that could further advance an alliance between the traditional Left and anti-fascists within the church. An existing organization was identified as the most likely vehicle from which to build a nationwide movement—the Auxiliary (known as the "Aux") of the Student Christian Movement, comprised of alumni who wished, in their post-student lives, for the same Christian challenges and community they had known at university. The SCM had expanded to include these former members because, as Irene Grant put it, "so many people couldn't bear to lose touch" with the parent organization.[43] Both she and her husband were active and influential figures in the London Aux. So also was the widely revered economic historian R. H. Tawney, who had already declared his admiration for Karl Polanyi's work in particular. Jolly, along with Polanyi, Macmurray, the Grants, and others, took part in an influential Aux summer school in mid-1934 that was held in the Cheshire village of Parkgate. Another enthusiastic participant found the speakers and leading figures of the summer school "a stimulating and attractive group of folk . . . many of whom became lifelong friends."[44]

In late 1935, Tawney was asked if he would support a project to win over the entire national membership of the Aux to the political program that Christianity should be an active force in the transformation of society toward socialism.[45] Although he remained personally equivocal, Polanyi, Macmurray, and Irene Grant were sufficiently encouraged to form a group that began meeting early in the following year and was eventually named the Christian Left. "In our day the socialist movement has everywhere asserted that . . . universal brotherhood is the only solution of the actual political and economic problems of the world," its first newsletter declared. "We believe as Christians that they are right. Russian Communism is carrying out this task in practical politics. We believe that it has discovered the *true* political task; we also believe that it cannot complete and maintain this work if it rejects Christianity."[46] The new group's activities included studying Marx's early writings, which were not then available in English. According to Irene Grant, it was Karl Polanyi's "heretical view that Marx's fundamental philosophical position was expressed in his early writings from about 1846 and later works, such as *Das Kapital*, were simply more developed expressions of it."[47] Polanyi translated these early writings for the group by reading them in German and reciting them aloud in English as he went.[48]

Most early members of the Christian Left were socialist intellectuals and activists in the Labour and Communist Parties. Its bulletins addressed subjects such as Trotskyism, Russia and the world, and the Chartists, Levellers, and Diggers. The group held training weekends on "getting ready to be a Christian Leftie" and more wide-ranging "Q Camps" that dealt with social relations—that is, "questions of sex and freedom of lifestyles." Irene Grant noted with some surprise that "although we took everyone," no Roman Catholics joined the organization.[49] She states explicitly, "Doug was at the heart of the Christian Left," and he associated closely and warmly with its leading figures, including the "court philosophers" Polanyi and Macmurray.[50] Jolly would also have followed with similar interest and satisfaction the recent election in his homeland of its first Labour government. A Christian socialist strand of thought had prevailed in New Zealand's Labour Party from its formation, and its first parliamentary cabinet included freethinkers such as Walter Nash (an Anglican influenced by Tawney's ethical approach), former Salvation Army preacher Harry Holland, Presbyterian minister Arnold Nordmeyer, and others whose political consciousness was shaped equally by intensive, self-guided reading of both the New Testament and the first volume of *Kapital*.

5 Bread, Peace, and Liberty

By the early months of 1936, Jolly had reached the final stages of his surgical training and, after a demanding daily routine of ward rounds, spent his free time preparing for the fearsome oral final examination for membership of the Royal College of Surgeons. He had passed the preliminary entrance exam without difficulty in 1933 and showed every prospect of doing the same at the final exam, but he was taking no chances. If, in addition to these onerous professional duties, the studious young doctor gave up his evenings to engage in earnest debate at meetings of the embryonic Christian Left, he did so willingly and enthusiastically. From the time of his reunion with the Grants four years earlier, Doug Jolly had been reincorporated into their family and admitted to their circle of left-wing idealists. In that select company, he appeared as something of an anomaly, with his unfamiliar foreign upbringing and inclination toward practical actions rather than the battle of ideas. Yet he was able to hold his own in conversation with the likes of Macmurray, was respected for his dedication and abilities as a doctor, and was admired for his athletic appearance and easygoing Antipodean manner.

During 1934–35, he also revealed a surprising and immoderate enthusiasm for writing fiction. Over the course of many late nights in his bachelor rooms in the arty environs of Earls Court, he produced *Sand*, a full-length historical novel set on the Otago goldfields during his grandfather's time. Its plot was based on a real-life tragedy in October 1878 when the unruly, snow-fed Clutha River rose forty feet and carried away bridges, buildings, and entire settlements in Cromwell and other areas many miles downstream. Growing up in the town thirty years later, Jolly would have heard accounts of the early gold-mining days, the devastating flood, and other old-timers' stories firsthand, and he drew on these anecdotes to produce a vivid and historically accurate account of his hometown's origins. There are traces of the author's homesickness in his evocation of a landscape with "clear, sharp, broiling days" that was "a tropical suntrap in summer and an arctic waste in winter. Two hundred miles from the sea in any direction and surrounded by mountains towering up to eight thousand feet, the goldfields existed through the three months December, January and February with the thermometer much of the time in the region of a hundred [thirty-eight degrees Celsius]."[1] The novel's catalog of the town's four churches, each catering to an ethnically and socially distinct congregation, plus "a Buddhist or Confucian temple in Chinatown," echoes the contemporary deliberations of Jolly's friends in the Christian Left. His ship-jumping grandfather is a central character, along with a clog-wearing, phlegmatic Yorkshireman and a stalwart Chinese miner and market gardener named Ah Wee Gow. Although overly heavy on factual detail, the *Sand* manuscript reads today as an intriguing and engaging first novel, and in another era, it may well have found a willing publisher.

Jolly appears to have been so inspired by his creation that he seriously considered abandoning his ten years of medical studies in favor of a career as an author. Fortunately, he first sought advice on this caprice from a long-standing mentor, his former high school teacher and his father's onetime comrade in arms, Alexander Aitken, by then a professor of mathematics at Edinburgh University. Professor Aitken received Jolly's typed and heavily annotated manuscript in the mail, read it with evident care, and composed a reply that filled twelve pages of notepaper and revealed a depth of understanding acquired from both a lifetime of teaching and his innate qualities of insight and humanity.

Aitken referred to his wartime acquaintance with Jolly's father ("we all knew, liked and respected him") and gently and sympathetically deflated the novice author's expectations for his book's critical reception while finding aspects of it to praise. "Certainly the story of the ups-and-downs of your family is to me of compelling interest," he assured Jolly, before adding:

> You are far from being the first who at some turning in his life has been seized by a powerful impulse to break away in a new direction. . . . I don't know how strongly you feel called to your profession of doctor; but of this I am quite certain, that with the floods of books now issuing from the presses of the world, it is increasingly difficult for young and unknown writers, especially if not born in this country and without influence behind them,

to make the barest living by writing. It would therefore, in my opinion, be rash to throw up your profession in order to try another, literary, one; especially as the art of writing is really extraordinarily difficult. On the other hand, there is nothing to stop you keeping on in your profession and doing writing which might turn up trumps later on. Other doctors have done this; Brett Young, Somerset Maugham and so on.

Aitken then astutely noted:

Many people have a nervous upheaval, culminating sometimes in a breakdown, during which they are actually exalted above their usual level, and may create something worthwhile; the vast majority, on returning to the normal trend, lose this hyperaesthesia. I don't intend this to be unduly damping; once again I merely urge caution. Write away (and the best thing is to write plenty and leave the polishing, which inhibits momentum, till later), but (i) don't overdo it by burning the midnight oil, and (ii) don't overwork either in your ordinary routine, for a nervous breakdown is a serious matter. . . . Don't do anything rash then, Doug; don't let "Sand" become quicksand.[2]

Jolly followed this kindly and insightful advice, and *Sand* remains unpublished to this day. He continued to write in various genres throughout his life, but thereafter, with one very notable exception, he generally regarded that activity as recreational rather than vocational.

The would-be novelist's decision to consult Aitken rather than Donald Grant, his first and most influential mentor, on the worth of his writing seems initially surprising. However, by 1935 Grant was less often present in Jolly's life. He was developing a new career as a freelance commentator on international affairs, a role requiring frequent travel, especially to the United States. Irene was left in London for long periods with their children and, as a result, found a new degree of freedom for exploring her own interests, political and otherwise.[3] She not only devoted much time and energy to her work with the Aux and its activist offshoot, the Christian Left, but also embarked on more personal areas of exploration.

Although rather more Christian and rather less wealthy than the intellectual aristocracy of the Bloomsbury Group, the Grants and their friends had certain characteristics in common with that set of progressive thinkers who, it was said, "lived in squares and loved in triangles."[4] In accordance with their comprehensive rejection of codes of behavior and morality that they saw as outdated and repressive, some members of the Aux were willing to venture into social territory that to others seemed peculiar, transgressive, and sometimes shocking. During one of Donald Grant's return visits to London, John Macmurray's wife, Betty, revealed to her husband that she had formed a sexual relationship with their mutual friend. Both of their spouses came to accept this situation, albeit with some difficulty.[5] Macmurray and Irene Grant may themselves have formed a connection that "ventured beyond the normal bounds of friendship."[6] Later, Irene informed Macmurray that her relationship with yet another mutual friend, the vigorous New Zealand doctor almost a decade younger than herself, had reached a new and more intimate level. "You will mean a great deal to him, I know, and he to you, I hope," Macmurrray replied, adding "I like him a lot."[7]

This couple's sexual relationship, which was certainly known to and presumably accepted by Donald Grant, was alluded to several decades later in a controversial pamphlet titled *Towards a Quaker View of Sex*. Published in 1964 by the British Society of Friends and written by a "group of Friends," it presented a startlingly advanced case for multifarious forms of sexual expression, including sex outside marriage. One of the authors, Kenneth Barnes, had been a member of the Christian Left before the war and is likely to have known of the relationship between fellow members Irene and Donald Grant and Doug Jolly.[8] "Sometimes the very happiness and security of a marriage may attract a young man or young woman from outside. . . . [All] these situations can, but need not, destroy the marriage. For, more often than is recognized, the three people concerned behave responsibly, are deeply conscious of difficulties and are equally anxious to avoid injury to others. . . . At all times the belief of the husband and wife that they are fully committed to responsibility for each other's good, and to a joint creative family enterprise, will bring them through their difficulties and enrich their marriage."[9]

These diversions took place in the shadow of an ever more dire international situation, as fascist leaders in Germany and Italy employed greatly enlarged and technically advanced armies to intimidate, control, and invade less powerful nations in which they claimed an interest. The Italian dictator Mussolini saw himself as a modern-day Caesar, destined to restore a vast empire. In early 1935, he began building up troops in Italian colonies on the borders of the ancient desert kingdom of Abyssinia, as Ethiopia was then known. Although both countries were members of the League of Nations, that body signally failed to prevent the military buildup, and its most powerful members, including the United States, did not enforce even the feeble sanctions the league imposed. In October 1935, Mussolini's troops invaded Abyssinian territory, employing armored vehicles, aerial bombing, and mustard gas against a people armed, if at all, with pre–World War I weapons.

For Doug Jolly, reading of this grotesquely asymmetrical conflict in the London papers, its most meaningful feature is likely to have been the intervention of a remarkable British surgeon named John Melly. A devout Christian, Melly had served with an artillery unit in World War I when aged just seventeen, and by 1935, he was working, like Jolly, as a house surgeon in London general hospitals. News reports of the suffering of Abyssinia's people compelled Melly to intervene, and he swiftly organized the British Ambulance Service in Ethiopia. Initially funded largely from his own pocket, the service was later integrated with the British Red Cross, becoming that organization's first international humanitarian operation since 1918.

With Melly as commandant and four other doctors, the service traveled to this disordered, almost roadless country with two specially designed tents to use as portable operating theaters. It soon found that its field hospitals were repeatedly bombed by Italian aircraft, whose raids killed and injured civilians of all ages. One of the hospitals was moved into a cave high on a mountaintop. "There was a good deal of gas about that day. There were crocodiles of the blind. They stumbled forward, the hand of one on the shoulder of the one in front."[10] Melly struggled to describe the enormity of the humanitarian disaster: "This isn't a war—it isn't even a slaughter—it's the torture of thousands of defenceless men, women and children, with bombs and poison gas." Six months after his arrival in Abyssinia, he was treating a wounded man in the capital, Addis Ababa, when he was shot and killed by drunken looters.[11] His ambulance service was highly praised for its professionalism and dedication, and later it was cited as a role model for similar initiatives in Spain.[12]

Italy's brutal intervention in Abyssinia conclusively demonstrated the impotence of the League of Nations. Its half-hearted sanctions against this fascist regime were widely ignored, and other member states flouted its authority by negotiating with Italy and other aggressor nations. France proved so desperate to enlist Italy's support against the looming threat from Germany that it declined to condemn Italian war crimes in Abyssinia, while Britain refused to close the Suez Canal to Italian troopships.[13] Those concessions proved worthless. After seizing control of most of this impoverished country, Mussolini was emboldened to develop much closer military relations with Hitler's Germany, which was then exercising its own bellicose territorial ambitions. In the same month that Melly was killed, Hitler's troops breached the Treaty of Versailles by occupying the demilitarized Rhineland.

One of the most insistent and authoritative British voices warning against the threat from these developments was a left-wing agitator and journalist named Tom Wintringham. Slim, bald, and bespectacled, he retained a military briskness that revealed his World War I service with the Royal Flying Corps, the forerunner of the Royal Air Force (RAF). During the early 1930s, Wintringham drew on that experience to write several books warning of a forthcoming world war that would be dominated by aircraft and result in civilian casualties of unprecedented scale and severity. In *The Coming World War*, he warned of the "bombing of localities which in many cases will be densely populated. . . . It is this ruthless bombing that will distinguish, and set apart from all other battles in world history, the first phases at least of the second World War."[14] By 1935 these efforts had succeeded in establishing Britain's Air Raid Precautions Department, but Wintringham continued to inveigh in print against the threat of total war and the government's unpreparedness to adequately defend its most vulnerable citizens.

The seemingly inexorable march to war in Europe was periodically countered by encouraging developments on the left. In February 1936, the general election in Spain's fragile new republic produced a narrow victory for a Popular Front government of fifteen liberal and left-wing parties promising "Bread, Peace and Liberty."[15] Three months later, France also elected a Popular Front government. Throughout Europe, apprehensive democrats found reason to hope that the political tide had finally turned in their favor. This cautious optimism was soon shattered when, four months after the Spanish Popular Front's election victory, a conspiratorial group of army generals launched a military revolt against the new government. The attempted coup d'état was resisted, sporadically but fiercely, by supporters of the Republic, including elements of the Spanish Navy and its other armed forces.

At first this chaotic and often hand-to-hand fighting appeared to have crushed the military coup. Then the European press reported that in early August 1936, in a crucial and historically unprecedented airlift, convoys of German and Italian military aircraft had ferried elite units of the Spanish Army from Morocco across the Mediterranean to reinforce the insurgent generals. The rebel army, eventually under the command of General Franco, advanced swiftly northward toward Madrid. The men encountered little effective opposition from the local militias and other disparate elements ranged in support of the Republican government that now found themselves confronting not only Spanish rebels but also thousands of well-equipped and highly trained troops from the armies of Italy, Germany, and, to a lesser extent, Portugal. The governments of those countries, anticipating only a short, sharp engagement, had agreed to supply military aid to the Nationalists. The term "Axis powers" in reference to the alliance of fascist Italy and Nazi Germany was first coined in this period.

Overnight, a faltering coup had been transformed into a nationwide civil war in which only one side enjoyed the backing of professional troops and advanced military hardware from foreign allies. Hoping to prevent further escalation of the war, the governments of Britain and France drew up a Non-Intervention Pact, whose signatories agreed not to supply arms and troops directly to Spain or to allow their passage en route through their own countries. This pact, eventually signed by almost thirty nations, treated both warring parties in Spain as equally legitimate, although the Republicans led a duly elected government that their opponents had illegally attempted to overthrow. Germany and Italy added their signatures to the pact even as they continued to deliver fighter planes, bombers, naval vessels, heavy artillery, and other military equipment, along with battalions of their finest combat troops, to reinforce Franco's forces. For some months afterward, they persistently denied providing such aid. In November 1936, from his bachelor rooms in London, Doug Jolly read guarded and conflicting British news reports of the "alleged intervention of Germany and Italy in the Spanish war."[16] The Non-Intervention Pact proved a charade of willful diplomatic apathy and hypocrisy that, more than any other factor, decided the ultimate outcome of the civil war.

The Republican government, seemingly abandoned to its fate by the remaining democratic countries of Europe, appealed desperately for international support elsewhere. On the grounds that the Non-Intervention Pact was already being flouted by the Axis powers, Soviet Russia and Mexico responded by sending arms to Spain on a relatively small scale. They were the only nations to do so. However, thousands of individual anti-fascists from throughout the world also chose to defy the pact by volunteering to support the Republican forces. Few were professional soldiers, and many had no military experience at all. Their numbers soon overwhelmed the chaotic and under-resourced Republican military facilities, and from October 1936, they were provided with their own base in the town of Albacete in southeastern Spain and organized into the first of several *brigadas internacionales* (international brigades). They were a colorfully amorphous legion, speaking at least a dozen languages and avowing all shades of left-wing political coloration and none at all. While many were hardened activists who had already spent years fighting totalitarian domination in their own countries, a small number were "holiday boozers," attracted by the prospect of adventure and a tiny daily wage to a war they wrongly assumed would be brief and exhilarating and from which they could leave whenever they chose.

For the Grants and their idealistic London circle, the news from Spain meant the chilling realization that an international war had again erupted in Europe. Like all those who upheld democratic values and sought nonviolent solutions to political disputes, they had continued to hope the tide of fascism might yet be turned. The ugly spectacle of war between supporters of an elected government and those seeking to overthrow it showed that democracy itself was now under direct threat in Europe. Nonviolent strategies, they quickly concluded, must now be abandoned in favor of a "just war." The Christian Left's *News Sheet* urged in October 1936 that "the British Government ought to conform to international law and allow the export of arms of all kinds to the Spanish Government, while prohibiting their export to the insurgents. . . . If we fail now, the last chance of upholding Democracy against a conspiracy of international law-breakers may have disappeared."[17]

Military aid, however, was not the only desperate requirement of the beleaguered Spanish government. One of the first British organizations to respond in a practical manner to the turmoil in Spain was the Socialist Medical Association. Just days after the coup began, its secretary, a London GP named Charles Brook, learned that the Spanish Republicans were pleading for medical aid. He immediately called together all the influential figures he could contact, and a

Spanish Medical Aid Committee (SMAC) was rapidly formed. Its membership exemplified the Popular Front's approach to anti-fascist action, as it included union leaders, eminent Quakers, Labour and Liberal ministers of parliament (MPs), and "a charming Italian-born peeress" named Lady Hastings.[18] Most SMAC members, however, were doctors and members of the SMA. One was a twenty-three-year-old medical student named Kenneth Sinclair-Loutit, then finishing his second year of clinical studies at St Bartholomew's Hospital in London. An unaffiliated leftist, he was active in the Inter-Hospitals Socialist Society, the student wing of the SMA.

Sinclair-Loutit contributed to the committee by drawing up a list of essential equipment and, with the funds that had begun pouring in, to buy "drugs, dressings, sterilising equipment, hospital ward equipment, kitchen stores and field cookers" from around the country and at great speed. He found that he received "a lot of miraculous help. The peerage would telephone the top when things got stuck while the warehousemen, hearing it was for Spain, would service no other orders until ours were satisfied."[19]

Popular opinion in the United Kingdom regarded the sudden outbreak of factional warfare in Spain as an odd aberration by excitable Latins and assumed that it would be over within weeks. Nevertheless, public support for the SMAC initiative proved so enthusiastic that the committee soon expanded its initial modest intentions and prepared a more ambitious plan to send a fully equipped and professionally staffed medical unit to the battlefront. An advertisement called for "offers from doctors, students and nurses who are prepared to undertake service in Spain." Of the many replies received, it chose four doctors; four medical students, including Sinclair-Loutit; and four nurses.[20] Several others joined the unit in support roles, including two young Australian women then living in London. One of them, Margot Miller, had grown up in Australia and New Zealand and was working in London as an advertising copywriter when the civil war began. She had no medical training but proved a dedicated and valuable team member.

Doug Jolly, deeply engaged in preparations for his final FRCS exam, was not among those who volunteered for this hastily planned and untried project. He is certain, however, to have watched its emergence with interest and admiration.

Just three weeks after the SMAC was formed in mid-July, the first British Medical Volunteer Unit was ready to leave the country. This remarkable logistic feat was, says Sinclair-Loutit, made possible by three combined forces: The first was "the sheer energy of young people working together for something they really want to do; the second has been given the uninspiring name 'working-class solidarity' but it's real enough; and the third is disparagingly referred to as the 'old boy network.'"[21]

The young medical student had been placed in charge of a twenty-member unit tasked with setting up an advanced field hospital to provide emergency surgery close to the front—a daunting responsibility even for a veteran military doctor. However, "none of the eminent, well-placed and experienced doctors who helped set up the unit felt able to go themselves and there was I, untouched by their constraints, who was foolhardy enough to get the job."[22] It was also a plan riddled with uncertainties. Loutit-Sinclair found that "the only reference model available in 1936, apart from the Great War which was still very much in people's minds, was Dr Melly's Ambulance in Abyssinia at the time of the Italian invasion. Since very little was known about the latter we had been happy to recruit two ex-orderlies from Dr Melly's Ambulance. They were good men but had nothing new to tell us."[23]

Despite his youth and inexperience, Sinclair-Loutit had a keen appreciation of the political complexities of his team's mission and the murky loyalties of some members of his team. Amid the rush to leave for Spain, he found time to meet the shrewd general secretary of the British Communist Party, Harry Pollitt, and found him "an immensely likeable man who made personal contact very easy." Sinclair-Loutit explained to Pollitt the concern he felt both for the members of his unit and for the many shades of British political opinion that had backed it, and he accepted a personal letter of support typed on white silk "requesting that I should be given every help."[24]

With this informal visa carefully concealed on his person, Sinclair-Loutit assembled at Victoria Station "a friendly group of relative strangers all dressed in khaki drill from Millet's Army Surplus stores."[25] The drivers took the trucks and ambulances ahead by road and ferry, while the unit members—"farewelled" at every stage by large and vociferous crowds—traveled by rail to Paris and then across the Spanish border. Few members of this would-be battlefield surgical team had any significant experience of working under fire. A somewhat mysterious military veteran joined their train at Paris and engaged Sinclair-Loutit in conversation. Tom Wintringham was also bound for Barcelona in the capacity of war correspondent for the Communist Party's *Daily Worker* newspaper. He gave the young and anxious medical student practical advice on how to survive ground and aerial attacks. Sinclair-Loutit found that "you do not forget someone who shows you how to stay alive."[26]

The British Medical Volunteer Unit arrived by train in the key Republican city of Barcelona, where it was received tumultuously. "The arrival of our unit had for the Spanish Republic immense political significance because we were the first really visible sign of international support since the start of Franco's revolt. Here were a group of photographable men and women in neat uniform proving that Spain was not alone."[27]

The city had been transformed by the militias of the anarchist and communist trade union confederations that had converted the Ritz Hotel into a public canteen. The nearest fighting was taking place some 250 kilometers inland, on the plains of Aragón, where the Nationalists held the western half of the province and the Republicans the eastern. In the country overall, the Nationalists controlled a small area around Gibraltar in Spain's southwest and a swath of the country's north and center. The larger area that included the main industrial and port cities remained loyal to the Republican government.[28]

The local Republican military leaders favored attaching the British unit to a hospital in Barcelona, but its members were determined to base themselves closer to the front line. "The more [the Republican attaché] said it was crazy to go to the ill-defined front, the more we were all determined to do so." By poring over the map, they selected the small village of Grañén, a strategic location on an isolated and barren plateau about eighteen kilometers behind the Aragón front, as the most suitable base. On arrival the medical team found the village lacked any modern comforts, but "a large, rambling house of feudal design" was available for its use. The house was "indescribably dirty and only half of it fit for habitation," but those rooms were rigorously cleaned and fitted out as a field hospital. The drivers and orderlies installed electric lighting and heating stoves.[29] As a visible declaration of the team's noncombatant status, Sinclair-Loutit took a large Red Cross flag into the garden outside the new hospital and began pegging it to the ground where the Nationalist planes could clearly see it. "We were violently interrupted by some of our Spanish helpers. Some were really frightened, all were emphatic that it was insane to mark the place as a hospital. The minute it was spotted from the air Grañen would be machine-gunned."[30]

Those anxieties proved well founded. Although the hospital never received a direct hit from the German bombers sent to reinforce Franco's ground troops, their bombs fell close enough that the hospital staff felt the ground shake under their feet. Villages around Grañén were bombed without regard for their military significance, and surviving residents, including one blinded woman in her eighties, were brought to the hospital for treatment.

In September the twenty-four-year-old Margot Miller ran to the aid of a wounded militiaman and was hit by bullets in both legs. She lay under machine-gun fire for twenty minutes until she could be carried to safety. As soon as she was well enough, she was invalided back to England and spoke fervently at a large public meeting about the need for greater international support for the Republican forces. This intrepid Antipodean returned to Spain several months later, where she married an English volunteer.[31]

At first, according to Sinclair-Loutit, the Grañén hospital's methods were "pure 1914," but it soon began to function under an improvised system that Doug Jolly would later adopt and develop. A first aid post staffed by a doctor, stretcher-bearers, and one of the nurses was based at the front. From there the ambulances took the wounded to the field hospital along roads "little more than cow-tracks" and, if possible, by night to avoid aerial attacks. All those patients fit to be moved simply had their wounds cleaned and dressed, were fed if hungry, given a tetanus injection, and sent by train to base hospitals in Barcelona or other towns.[32] Most were German anti-fascists who had fled Hitler's regime and, in the first days of the war, formed themselves into the Centuria Thälmann, named for a German left-wing leader then held in prison by the Nazis. However, the hospital staff treated anyone, regardless of their condition or political affiliation, including enemy combatants. On one occasion, a young soldier who had been lying wounded in the sierra for days was brought in with a gangrenous leg. He proved to be one of the eighty thousand Moorish troops from the Spanish protectorate of Morocco who made up Franco's most feared and ruthless forces. When the Grañén villagers learned of his presence, "they wanted to lynch him, but although he was past saving, the hospital performed the amputation and gave him the best treatment until he died."[33]

The hospital had two operating theaters and eventually also surgical, medical, and venereal disease wards. Initially it provided thirty beds, but as many as seventy patients were accommodated at times of peak activity, with the staff giving up their own beds and sleeping on stretchers or mattresses on the stone floors.[34] Patients arrived sporadically as action on the Aragón front surged and subsided. At the most desperate times, as many as two hundred might be admitted over three days, and the staff worked almost without rest. In between were long lulls.[35]

One of the doctors, the Scotsman Archie Cochrane, came from a wealthy family, and throughout his time in Spain, he received prized luxuries such as English tobacco, which he invariably distributed among his colleagues.[36] To the astonishment of the Grañén locals, he also bathed in the nearby river every morning regardless of workload or weather, even when he had to break the ice to do so. Some of his fellow doctors were less disciplined and returned to London, willingly or otherwise. Sinclair-Loutit learned that an organization staffed by volunteers must anticipate a very uneven standard of ability and commitment from them. "We were strong nurse-wise but lamentably weak medically."[37] Urgent calls to London for reinforcements produced six more nurses and two doctors, including Reginald Saxton, a blood transfusion specialist whom a colleague described as "slim, tall, blond and soft-spoken."[38] His first impressions were of "dirt and filth and rats and a stinking courtyard."[39] The staffing difficulties were finally resolved when the team acquired its first Spanish member, a brilliant young Catalan surgeon named Moisès Broggi, who had recently headed the emergency department of a large Barcelona public hospital.[40]

Inexperienced and unsuitable volunteers were found in the firing lines as well as behind them, as Sinclair-Loutit found when he went up to reconnoiter the Huesca battlefront together with a visiting Tom Wintringham.[41] The volunteer fighters and their peasant supporters did not lack courage, but the routine business of soldiering—digging trenches, fortifying positions, standing watch—was carried out "in a lacklustre fashion, if at all."[42]

Wintringham came away convinced that this haphazard, amateurish form of warfare would condemn the Republic to defeat at the hands of Franco's troops and their well-trained and well-equipped fascist allies. In September 1936, he sent a report to Britain arguing for a more rigorous, military-style organization of the volunteers preparing to come to Spain and for the systematic recruitment of ex-servicemen.[43] The situation, he declared, was critically urgent. The Spanish Republic was defending democracy against tyranny and retained the support of the bulk of the population, but it was confronted by an efficiently led and well-supplied army that was rapidly sweeping toward Madrid, brushing aside the undisciplined and poorly armed militias that stood in its way.

Kenneth Sinclair-Loutit must have felt the sting of his older friend's harsh assessment. Like the militias, his own medical team had been formed and then functioned in a dedicated but ad hoc manner without regard for Spanish command structures. He nevertheless felt proud of their achievements, as the Grañén hospital had proved remarkably efficient at providing a frontline surgical and medical service, and eventually even a GP service for the local villagers.[44] As the first overseas medical unit to come to the aid of Republican Spain, it had also demonstrated a practical example of foreign support for the Spanish Republicans. "Our mere presence on the Aragon Front and our persistence in an exposed and hazardous position helped to keep Spaniards in good heart and to bring people at home to understand what the Civil War was about."[45]

As evidence of that heightened awareness in Britain, the Spanish Medical Aid Committee was fielding a steady flow of applications from volunteers to work in new frontline hospitals of the type that Grañén's had pioneered. The successful applicants were told that although they would remain noncombatants, they were now required to enlist in the Spanish Republican Army. Their medical units, even though largely funded from abroad, would officially form part of that army's medical services. Symbolically at least, this would require British medical volunteers to abandon entirely the traditions of peace and reconciliation that Donald Grant and others had been working for since World War I. After that war, the British Left had been overwhelmingly anti-militarist and pacifist in outlook and intent, but by late 1936, it had become apparent that the world faced an enemy that could only be resisted by force. For the high-minded idealists of the Christian Left, the time had come to put intellectual propositions into action.

To the Socialist Medical Association, one of the first UK bodies to unequivocally back the Republican military effort, medical volunteers in Spain were practicing the fundamental principles of their profession. The SMA's magazine, *Medicine Today and Tomorrow*, declared that medicine was "international in the highest sense of the word." Fascism, by contrast, represented a refutation of "the universal spirit that has developed in the medical profession during the past centuries." Doctors and nurses repaired the human carnage caused by warfare; therefore, they understood its real cost better than politicians.[46]

Doug Jolly was living at this time in the north London suburb of Hampstead and preparing to take the final examination that would complete the long course of study that had brought him to Britain. He had passed the preliminary exam three years earlier and could confidently contemplate his admission to the Royal College of Surgeons within months. He decided on a different course of action. "As soon as I was convinced that right was predominantly on the 'Government' side, and that the action of the insurgent generals was probably a prelude to a Fascist v. anti-Fascist war in Europe, I began to think that, unmarried and uncommitted as I was, I might be of some help to the Republican cause by volunteering to go to Spain as a surgeon, even if it meant postponing my final FRCS."[47]

The young doctor may have felt an additional and personal impulse to volunteer for service in a country he had never seen. In 1916 his father, driven both by his Presbyterian conscience and by the heightened patriotism of a distant colony, left his business and family to go to war. Now his son, twenty years later and compelled by anti-fascist sympathies, broke off his surgical studies to do the same. In a prescient message to fellow members of the Christian Left, later published in their *News Sheet*, Jolly wrote,

> I believe deeply that the conflict between Fascism and Democracy in Spain may decide the fate of Europe and the world for many years to come. It is no longer a Spanish "domestic" war; in this conflict are ranged the forces contending for the shaping of the future of mankind. It is a war of religions, between two conceptions of the nature of man. And so, because I am a Christian, and because I believe that true Christianity must be on the side of those who struggle to extend the brotherhood of man, I must do something about it, when and where the need is.[48]

With the blessing of the Grant family and others in the Christian Left, Jolly deferred his surgical career and joined the British Medical Volunteer Unit of the International Brigade.

6 Nine Months of Winter

> This La Mancha town, nestled in the dusty path of the errant knight [Quixote], yesterday monotonous, peaceful and gray, today has the polychrome, polyglot and nomadic charm of an Asian port.
>
> —JUAN RAMÍREZ DE LUCAS

The transformation of the drowsy provincial town of Albacete exemplified the turmoil, shifting fortunes, and frantic improvisations of wartime. Until the summer of 1936, when the insurgent Spanish generals issued their call to overthrow the Republican government, Albacete was simply the undistinguished capital of a quiet agricultural province of the same name in the La Mancha region of south-central Spain, where great numbers of landless farmworkers toiled on the plains of its giant estates. A major crop was the labor-intensive, pink-flowered saffron, harvested for the spice that is a vital ingredient of paella.

Within days of the military leaders' call to arms, Nationalist troops took control of the entire province. The surrounding region, however, remained loyal to the Republic, leaving Albacete an isolated and vulnerable island of insurgency. Loyalist militias backed by small companies of regular troops advanced from the coast and seized the main town after a few hours of street fighting. Albacete, both the province and the town, then remained under Republican control for almost the entire duration of the civil war.

Although it was distinctly lacking in civic facilities, the town was conveniently sited on the main railway line between Valencia and Madrid and safely distant from the multiple battlefronts. It therefore became the training base for the thousands of foreign volunteers pouring into Spain to strengthen local resistance to the military takeover. They came at first mostly from France, Germany, and eastern Europe, but eventually more arrived from at least fifty other nations including Turkey (Türkiye), the Philippines, Ethiopia, Vietnam, and China.[1] The overcrowded town became a polyglot mayhem, somehow sustained by a shared camaraderie and political fervor. The bullring, of a flamboyantly Moorish design, was used as a makeshift parade ground where new arrivals formed into disheveled ranks based on their nationalities and language groups. The unmartial enthusiasm of this period is captured by a photograph of a young bugler signaling to troops while holding a small dog under his other arm.[2] The new arrivals were then trucked to surrounding villages where they received a cursory training using mismatched and outdated weaponry before being thrown into battle against the armored columns converging on Madrid from several directions. Each instructor tended to issue orders according to his own country's practice, and linguistic, cultural, and political misunderstandings abounded.

The pressure to turn these disparate and largely untrained volunteers, in a matter of weeks, into an efficient fighting force was heightened daily by disturbing news from the several battlefronts west of Albacete. As Franco's well-armed columns headed for Madrid, they crushed the defiant but poorly equipped resistance they encountered along the way with relative ease, massacring civilians together with Republican troops. In late October, word reached Albacete of the aerial bombing of Getafe, a town just south of Madrid and the site of a Republican airfield. An English volunteer, nineteen-year-old James Albrighton, witnessed a heavy bombardment by German Junker bombers that destroyed several buildings including the local elementary school and killed sixty of its pupils. "I find it very distressing to even try and describe the picture that I saw. . . . The remnants of limbs, the particles of flesh and blood splattered against whitewashed walls, fragments of all that remained of what only a few minutes before had been innocent, carefree, joyful toddlers playing in the morning's sun."[3]

By the time of this air raid, some two thousand foreign volunteers had been recruited at Albacete and organized into two brigades—the Eleventh, named after the anti-Nazi leader Ernst Thälmann, and the Twelfth, the Garibaldi. Although made up predominantly of German and Italian speakers, respectively, both included a number of English-speaking volunteers, mainly from Britain but also a few Canadians, Australians, and New Zealanders. One of these Englishmen, a Byronic young Cambridge University student and rising poet named John Cornford, had previously written on "what Communism stands for" in *Christianity and the Social Revolution*.

By late October 1936, Franco, the Nationalist military commander who now held the dual titles of generalissimo and chief of state, ordered what he assumed would be a final offensive to take Madrid. Four columns of troops—each with their own artillery, anti-aircraft guns, and medical and transport units, and backed by German and Italian aircraft and tanks—advanced on the city from different directions. His compatriot, Gen. Emilio Mola, famously claimed that a *quinta columna* (fifth column of sympathizers) was already at work inside Madrid, secretly providing information to the rebels to prepare for their arrival. This boast—the first use of the term "fifth column" to refer to clandestine internal opposition—aimed to demoralize and provoke discord among the defenders of Madrid, but it undoubtedly had a basis in fact. In Albacete the French quartermaster of the International Brigades, responsible for issuing all supplies, was a covert fascist, and he and his cohorts ensured that trucks and machine guns left the base with highly abrasive emery powder added to their lubricating oil.[4]

In preparation for the four-pronged attack, Madrid was bombed repeatedly in the same series of air raids that destroyed the outlying town of Getafe, just eight miles from the capital's center. The city's population, swollen by refugees arriving from towns already overrun by Franco's troops, fled to underground train stations or specially built *refugios* (air raid shelters) as motorcyclists with wailing sirens raced along streets obstructed with barricades, and a few anti-aircraft guns on the tallest buildings fired futile volleys of light shells.[5] Only the wealthiest residential areas, where fifth columnists were most likely to be found, escaped the systematic bombing aimed at breaking the morale of the population.[6] In its targeting of civilians, the Nationalist siege of Madrid was a historically unprecedented exercise in total war. Never before had a major city been subjected to intense air as well as artillery bombardment.

As the number of shattered apartment blocks, mutilations, and deaths rose, "everyone who can flee the city is fleeing," noted one Russian war correspondent. "By means fair or foul, all the rich people, all top officials escape. . . . The streets are completely dark in the evenings. Everywhere patrols are checking people's passes, and it's become dangerous to drive around unarmed."[7]

A week after the first air raids, the Republican government also abandoned its official premises and reestablished an administration in the town of Valencia on the Mediterranean coast, far distant from the front lines. Franco's victory appeared so certain and imminent that several of the foreign journalists who remained in Madrid reported the city's capture in advance of the fact to scoop their rivals.[8]

Yet Madrid's citizens held firm, extended their trenches, and swore to defend their city to the last. Their hopes were raised when modern and powerful Russian tanks arrived to defend the outskirts. As the Soviet Union had belatedly and reluctantly added its name to the list of nations upholding the risible Non-Intervention Pact, it tried to keep evidence of its involvement in the war from reaching the foreign press. The tank drivers described themselves as Mexicans but proved unable to speak Spanish.[9]

The Nationalist infantry had now reached the outer suburbs of the city itself and threatened to overrun the large military hospital at Carabanchel on its southern fringe. In early November, the Republican military command ordered the evacuation of this hospital, and a fleet of trucks and ambulances transferred more than two thousand patients to the enormous Palace Hotel in the city center. Its main dining room, hung with great crystal chandeliers and lined with gilt-framed mirrors, was converted into an operating room with eight tables, each with two surgeons, an anesthetist, and a nurse. This site became the city's new Surgical Hospital No. 1, and its staff worked day and night to the sound of nearby explosions.[10] Chickens were raised on the roof to supplement the food supply.[11] All the city's public hospitals were requisitioned to treat military as well as civilian patients, and their operating theaters were moved to the cellars as a protection against the daily fusillade of bombs.

Suddenly, on 7 November, an additional and highly visible form of international support for the Republicans appeared: Some two thousand members of the newly formed Eleventh International Brigade marched through Madrid's main street, the Gran Vía, with their officers issuing shouted orders in French, German, and Polish. The handful of English speakers among them included John Cornford and a young mathematician from New Zealand named Griffith McLaurin. The brigade had been rushed from Albacete to reinforce Spanish troops fighting desperately to block the Nationalist advance on the northwestern outskirts of the city. Franco's troops were battering Republican defenses in the Casa de Campo, a large park that had once been the royal hunting grounds and adjoined the newly built Ciudad Universitaria (University City).

From high ground within the Casa de Campo, Nationalist artillery batteries could hurl shells right into the city center, some hitting the sleek, new fourteen-story Telefónica tower, the heart of the city's communications systems. As the tallest building in Europe at that time, it was an excellent target. Many shells were incendiaries and sparked massive fires that roared through the old section of the city and its financial district.[12] Throughout November 1936, an unrelenting series of attacks, counterattacks, and close-quarter battles took place along a trenched front line that ran through the streets to the south and west of the central city. The Nationalists established fixed positions along this front but were unable to break through the line, and the city's defenders held out until the very end of the war, almost three years later.[13]

By early December, the defense of Madrid had settled into a frigid, resolute siege. Intermittent air raids, artillery bombardments, and skirmishes continued, but the Nationalists' almost unbroken series of victories en route to Madrid was finally halted. Six months after the coup d'état was launched in the height of summer, it had mutated into an intractable civil war, now with foreign intervention on both sides. The rebel generals were forced to acknowledge that the Republican defenses were well established and strongly held and that their direct frontal attack on the capital had failed. They required a new strategy.

At this significant turning point in the war, Tom Wintringham was training novice machine gunners at Albacete. In December 1936, the little town seemed to him "a menagerie" of Slavic strangers in sheepskin capes, loping through the unlit cobbled streets and barking commands in a babel of tongues.[14] One evening he noticed a new arrival seated at one of the town's café tables, "a man whose bearing and appearance seemed English without any possibility of doubt. . . . He was a surgeon and a New Zealander. He was also thoroughly lost, having come out on his own from London with a minimum of papers and less knowledge of foreign languages than even an Englishman of his sort can usually muster. I was able to set him on his road to the right bureau."[15]

Among the characteristics that so distinctively marked Jolly as "English" (a term then loosely extended to all white subjects of the British Commonwealth) was his toothbrush mustache. While it may have been de rigeur among

Londoners of his class at that time, in the vehement political atmosphere of revolutionary Madrid, it was a signifier of bourgeois sympathies.[16] He quickly removed it.

Jolly had offered his services to the Republican government through its embassy in Paris, where they were "gladly accepted." He arrived in Spain more swiftly and comfortably than other foreign volunteers, flying to the port city of Alicante on the southwest coast and then traveling inland to Albacete with a convoy of British ambulances "to be in time for the siege of the capital."[17] He carried a letter from the Spanish ambassador in London that, in the stiff and archaic phrases of international diplomacy, asked "officials of all levels, and the military of the Popular Front, to facilitate the entrance and transit through national territory of Comrade Doug Jolly, supplied with passport number #55963 of New Zealand, as he is travelling to Spain to join the medical section of the International Brigade."[18]

This earnest young doctor's political affiliations, a matter of utmost importance in the torrid political environment of besieged Madrid, were uncertain since he had never belonged to any political party. However, like Sinclair-Loutit, he had taken the precaution of securing a letter from Harry Pollitt, the general secretary of Great Britain's Communist Party, that introduced Jolly as "a fully qualified surgeon who we have appointed to take charge of the Field Ambulance that we have sent to Albacete for the use of the International Legion. This comrade is not a member of the Communist Party, but is a very warm sympathiser with the cause of the Spanish Government, and has been highly recommended to us."[19]

Although this documentation appeared minimal to Wintringham, it indicates that the bearer was well connected and well spoken for. Pollitt's description of Jolly as a fully qualified surgeon was not entirely accurate, but paper credentials counted for much less than life-saving knowledge in the daily turmoil of the winter war. Jolly was, in fact, at that time one of a tiny number of foreign surgeons—including a Parisian surgical team that arrived in Albacete on the same day—available to the Republican forces.[20] Most of the Spanish Army's medical staff had joined the Nationalist forces at the outbreak of the coup or defected to them soon afterward. Providing an adequate medical service for its troops was among the most urgent requirements of the motley, under-equipped, and critically menaced Republican Army.

By late 1936, it had also become apparent that the growing numbers of international volunteer soldiers required a health service distinct from that of the regular army. At first, sick and wounded internationals had been treated in the same hospitals and by the same medical staff as their Spanish counterparts. Even when these bed-bound casualties of the war were placed in their own wards, their exclusion by a nearly impenetrable language barrier from other patients and staff led to a sense of loneliness and incomprehension that proved a major obstacle to their recovery.

Of the small but significant numbers of international medical volunteers such as Jolly who arrived daily at Albacete alongside the foreign fighters in this period, almost none had any prior experience of military medicine, and they were in desperate need of skilled organization and leadership. Their first chief medical officer, Rudolf Neumann, recalled by Archie Cochrane as "a charming, intelligent Viennese doctor,"[21] vividly described some of the challenges he and his colleagues faced:

> We had to quickly create a Medical Service that would be responsible for the life and health of a growing army of volunteers that would soon consist of 30,000 men. With military hospitals in the rearguard, and on the front line, its own system of transport, the prevention of epidemics, the question of food and clothes for the troops—all these were problems that had to be solved very rapidly. We shared out among us the few books on military medicine that we had brought. Each of us was responsible for a chapter. And we sat on boxes, suitcases still not unpacked, and we gave talks to each other, we studied![22]

Under the pressure exerted by Franco's remorseless advance on the capital, these inadequately prepared young medics drew up the framework for a nationwide International Brigade health service to be based at Albacete. One of its founders, a French doctor named Pierre Rouqués, left for Paris to create an overseas office, the Centrale Sanitaire Internationale, that could coordinate the supply of further staff and medical equipment from abroad.[23] The Albacete base of the Servicio Sanitario (Sanitary Service) was headed briefly by Rudolf Neumann and then by Oscar Telge, a nom de guerre adopted by the Bulgarian-born Tsvetan Kristanov, who was one of the most enigmatic and impressive of all the medical volunteers who traveled to Republican Spain.[24]

Within days of Jolly's arrival in Albacete, he was enlisted in this newly formed servicio with the rank of *teniente* (lieutenant). In early December 1936, he advised the Grants,

> There is already here a French ambulance corps with which we will combine—two French Surgeons and myself will form a surgical team. In four or five days we will go to set up a casualty clearing station—in the meantime we are overhauling equipment and making all preparations for the work ahead. There is much to be done before we can begin the real work. I have been speaking so much mongrel French that I now find it very difficult to write decent English. . . . Am missing you all and would that I might come this night to Pyecombe Corner.[25]

His first orders, which changed very little over the following two years, were to form a surgical team to set up and staff a fifty-bed mobile field hospital based just behind the front line and capable of moving at short notice as the tide of battle shifted. The hospital would "deal with those wounded men who could not safely be transported over a long distance. These cases were mainly in the abdomen and chest, and bleeding wounds."[26] This mobile unit was required to "move frequently with troops, and send our wounded men to Madrid which lay some ten miles in our rear and to the south."[27] Jolly was issued with a high-level military *permiso de viaje* (travel pass), essential in the distrustful milieu of the besieged city, that permitted him to "travel freely through Madrid and the battlefront front and receive information, strictly in accordance with the instructions of the military command. It is obligatory to submit . . . proof of the information that has been obtained."[28]

Jolly's first field hospital had a staff of twelve, representing seven nationalities and almost as many languages. Several of its members remained his lifelong friends. They included his assistant surgeon, a young French doctor named André Dervaux, whose pointed black beard made him look "like a young pirate."[29] One ambulance driver (probably Robert Francis Allen) was a playwright from Boston; another was a Czech mechanic named Joe Edenhoffer. Three of the nurses—whom Jolly recalled only as Demetria, Martinez, and Mercedes—were Spanish, while the fourth was a prematurely silver-haired Hungarian named Anna-Mária Basch. Her husband, Endre, and their sixteen-year-old son, János, were both fighting with the International Brigades. All three had previously been active in Belgium's anti-fascist Popular Front and were among the first volunteers to leave Belgium in October 1936 to defend the Spanish Republic.[30] The anesthetist was a dapper young South African–born aristocrat named Peter de Sarigny who, just weeks earlier, had been training as a chef at London's Savoy Hotel.[31] A national daily paper then reported that the "handsome young count" had suddenly disappeared from his Bayswater flat.[32] He initially planned to report on the war as a foreign correspondent, but Jolly asked him to become the field hospital's anesthetist and gave him an extremely brief training in administering the highly flammable chloroform and ether gases. The two men worked closely and amicably together for the following year.[33]

This polyglot ensemble had no common language and communicated in a frantic pidgin for several months until "we all picked up a smattering of Spanish."[34] They were attached to the newly formed but already battle-hardened Eleventh and Twelfth International Brigades, composed mostly of French, German, and Polish anti-fascists, that had suffered appalling losses the previous month in defending Madrid's western fringe.[35]

In mid-December, just two weeks after his arrival in Spain, Jolly's field hospital went into action. The Nationalist strategy had shifted from a frontal assault on Madrid to an attempt to cut Republican supply lines and reinforcements in the sierra northeast of the city.[36] The rebel offensive on the northern outskirts of Madrid tightened, and Franco's forces took the outlying townships of Majadahonda and Las Rozas. The field hospital was therefore posted to the nearby town of Fuencarral, where a new Hospital de Primera Urgencia (Hospital of Primary Emergency) was established. It was based in the Casa Nazaret, a former orphanage and school for the children of this very poor working-class borough.[37] "At 10.30 a.m.," reported a French member of the unit, "we set to work, and by 5 p.m. everything had been moved in. We had knocked down a wall to get the truck in, repaired the heating system and running water, washed the entire building, set up the operating theatre and two patient rooms, a storeroom, a waste disposal chute, an office for the operating theatre and a meeting room for our own use."[38]

This hastily installed field hospital was equipped and staffed to treat only the most critical and life-threatening injuries, and all others were redirected to more permanent hospitals, especially the Palace Hotel in the city center that had become Madrid's main base hospital. The Casa Nazaret's upper floor was used to house very seriously ill patients and to accommodate the staff. Their workload fluctuated daily depending on the intensity of combat, but in the first week, they performed more than twenty major operations, mainly treating crushed limbs but including two trepannings, or skull operations, on men with severe head injuries. One of them, a "Moor" (i.e., Moroccan) Nationalist soldier, did not survive the procedure. Six laparotomies, or abdominal operations—Jolly's speciality—were also carried out that week. "The morale of our team is good—the quality of our work is not yet perfect, but we are improving every day," their first report read. "We have been provided with everything we wanted, in particular a second ultramodern operating table, and all the equipment, linen, dressings, bedding, etc. so that as soon as possible [our unit] can be put on standby for the eventuality of having to leave. We believe we would be ready to move out in 3 to 4 hours if need be."[39]

W. F. Hawkins, a London schoolteacher and councillor, described the work of this hospital for Britain's *Daily Worker* newspaper:

> The wounded were pouring in, some of them carried on the most primitive of ambulances. Stretchers had been tied to the sidecars of motor-cycles and the wounded were carried on these, shrieking in agony as they were bumped and bruised over the rough tracks and uneven roads.
>
> Dr Jolly and his staff were kept hard at work for hours on end in their improvised hospital. They were fortunate enough to have running water at this spot, a blessing which has sometimes been lacking in other places. I watched breathlessly while Dr Jolly attended to the wounds of a young Spaniard shot through the stomach. . . . Fifteen minutes after the conclusion of that operation the young Spaniard was again conscious, struggling in his agony, and crying for the water they dare not give him.[40]

The midwinter weather proved as debilitating as the German dive-bombers. Freezing winds swept down from the mountains, and the troops fought from trenches knee-deep in icy slush. "One needs all available clothing," Jolly reported. "We are wearing by day warm corduroy velvet pants and jacket, caught with elastic at waist, wrist and ankle (like Skiing suits). They are very roomy and enable one to have many layers underneath."[41] These harsh conditions were far from most foreigners' expectations of the Spanish climate, but to Jolly, they may have seemed oddly familiar. "The central plateau on which Madrid is situated has a climate not unlike that of Central Otago; intense, dry heat in summer and months of snow and frost in winter." He learned the old and mordant saying that Madrid has "nueve meses de invierno, tres meses de infierno" (nine months of winter, three months of hell), adding, "I can subscribe to this opinion."[42]

"There is a spirit of optimism and directed purpose here—no mistaking it," Jolly wrote to the Grants as his team departed for the front. "Persons do things when and where required, just because they are required. There is scarcely any questioning of a request to do some particularly unpleasant or dangerous job. I tell you again that something big and enduring is being given expression to in the setting up and working of this International Brigade."[43] More medical equipment and personnel were urgently needed from Britain, he told his friends, but it would no longer be possible, as with the first Grañén hospital, for the donors to circumscribe those resources and direct their use for a specific purpose. "Any English doctors or nurses and any equipment will go to the Medecin Chef de Brigada Internacional at Albacete [at that time Dr. Rudolf Neumann] and will be drafted by him to the various unit organisations on the different fronts."[44]

7 A River of Blood

Among the inundation of injured men carried in day and night by the stretcher-bearers during the battle of Las Rozas in the first week of 1937 were many with machine-gun and shrapnel wounds to the abdomen. They required immediate and very painstaking treatment. Prior to World War I, British military surgeons were frequently instructed not to bother treating abdominal wounds under wartime conditions due to both the woeful success rate of such expensively time-consuming operations and an official reluctance to operate close to the firing line. In World War I itself, they applied this principle to such wounds: "If they could be treated within six hours, the chances were in favour of the patient. If not, they were always against him."[1]

Lengths of intestine had to be lifted out of the abdominal cavity and minutely inspected for fragments of shrapnel as well as any small perforations. "Such an operation," wrote a colleague and friend of Jolly's, "leads to considerable shock, and both for shock and loss of blood the best treatment is transfusion of blood, and plenty of it."[2] These were the words of Canadian surgeon Norman Bethune, eventually perhaps the best known of all the foreign doctors to serve in the Spanish Civil War. Although he was fourteen years older and vastly more egotistical than his New Zealand colleague, the two men appeared to recognize each other's qualities and became closely acquainted during the brutal battles around the city's perimeter. Bethune had arrived in Madrid in November 1936 and quickly grasped that the unprecedented nature of the warfare, in particular the heavy aerial bombing and shelling of civilian as well as military targets, called for bold and innovative medical strategies.

A forceful and ebullient figure, Bethune was determined that, rather than be assigned to a multinational medical unit such as Jolly's, he would direct a stand-alone Canadian unit. After investigating Madrid's military hospitals and the outlying field hospitals, he concluded that their most urgent need was improved facilities for blood transfusion.[3] Bethune himself was a thoracic surgeon with little, if any, knowledge of transfusing blood, but he discovered that the Republican stronghold of Barcelona had already created a world-leading blood transfusion facility on which he could model his own.

Shocked and exsanguinated men had been revived on the battlefield with transfused blood, including stored blood and plasma, since World War I, and blood grouping became standard in the following decade. Yet the technique remained experimental and highly risky at the outbreak of the Spanish Civil War; knowledge of the appropriate volume and timing of transfusions was scant.[4] In mid-1936, as gun battles between loyalist and rebel sections of the army raged in Barcelona's streets, a young hematologist and ardent socialist named Frederic Duran i Jordà, together with his surgeon colleague Moisès Broggi, remained on duty day and night at the Hospital Clínico in the city center. Many of the wounded and dying brought to them for surgery could not be saved due to massive blood loss, and just weeks after the war began, Duran i Jordà was appointed to set up a network of blood banks to provide a frontline transfusion service.[5]

He was allocated space above the basement morgue of a former civilian hospital on the outskirts of the city; there he and his team rapidly built up the first military blood transfusion service in the world. By September 1936, their first stored blood was delivered to the Aragón front, three hundred kilometers to the west, in a refrigerated van formerly used by a fish vendor.[6] Duran i Jordà and his assistants developed a simple and reliable technique, and invented their own equipment, to enable even barely trained medical staff working under the spartan conditions of the field hospitals to administer the stored blood safely to their wounded patients. Since blood typing was rarely possible at the front line, only the universal type O blood was initially supplied, and it was stored as briefly as possible before its use.[7]

Bethune obtained permission from the military authorities to travel to Barcelona, where he visited this pioneering transfusion center and its blood bank stocked with donations from thousands of Barcelona's citizens. Through his supporters in Canada, he arranged to buy a refrigerator, an autoclave, and other essential equipment in France, including a Ford station wagon to provide a mobile transfusion service. His vigor and air of authority sufficiently impressed the Madrid medical authorities that he was given the rank of colonel and the use of the luxurious premises that had formerly housed the German Embassy in Madrid's diplomatic quarter. Bethune was a heavy drinker with a flair for publicity, and he informed the foreign press corps that they were welcome to enjoy his hospitality there. Frequent guests included a South African photographer and filmmaker named Vera Elkan and a red-haired and flamboyant Swedish journalist, Kajsa Rothman. Both eventually became his lovers.[8]

By 19 December, the Madrid center was ready to receive donated blood, and that evening Bethune broadcast an appeal for donors on the local radio station. The following morning one of his staff saw from his office window "a long, long line of people right around the corner of the block. . . . It was something which appealed to the Spanish very deeply emotionally, the replenishing of blood at the Front."[9] For the duration of the war, the malnourished citizens of Madrid risked aerial and artillery bombardment to donate their blood to the troops and received vouchers for food in exchange. Their blood was typed and collected in glass bottles sealed with a rubber bung, and Bethune and his team delivered these day and night wherever they were most needed, initially to the military hospitals in and around Madrid.[10]

Jolly later described the system that enabled him to provide life-giving transfusions to his severely wounded patients:

> In 1936 research in Barcelona and Madrid established the fact that blood taken from a donor and kept at zero temperature could be used without ill effect for a recipient up to 18 days afterwards. . . . Centres for the collection of blood were set up in those cities, the blood being grouped and put up in glass ampoules containing half a pint. To these ampoules was attached a rubber tube with a sterile needle wrapped and sealed in cellophane. The blood was delivered daily to the field hospitals in special vans equipped with frigidaires [i.e., refrigerators] run by small petrol motors (rather like a milk delivery service). We received and stored the blood in our own frigidaires, run off our lighting dynamos or during the day, by alcohol burners.[11]

With an eye on his postwar medical practice, he noted that a large-scale transfusion service of this kind would likely prove valuable not only in wartime but also for civilian medicine, "especially in a country like New Zealand with its scattered population."[12]

One of the Madrid blood bank's very first frontline transfusions was given at Jolly's hospital at Fuencarral in the early hours of 3 January 1937.[13] In this and in typical later cases, the recipient was lying on a stretcher "as white as paper . . . shocked, with an imperceptible pulse."[14] After quickly checking for the correct blood type, Bethune or an assistant would expose a vein in the forearm, insert a cannula (a thin glass tube), and deliver the blood by gravity. "You would get that vein in the arm and start pumping blood into him and the change was miraculous. You'd see the man come around and it was the greatest reward you could ever ask for. . . . They became alive right in front of your eyes within the space of several minutes."[15]

Bethune was also a passionate propagandist for Republican Spain, and at 2:00 a.m. on Christmas Eve 1936, he, Jolly, and others made their way through the darkened and frozen city to the cellar of a building on the main thoroughfare, the Gran Vía, whose windows were soundproofed with mattresses.[16] From a radio station run by the country's largest trade union body, the Unión General de Trabajadores, they delivered an impassioned international shortwave broadcast in numerous languages. The Swedish journalist Kajsa Rothman, "a handsome giantess with flowing red-gold hair," was among those who "on the waves of the air . . . sent a call to the whole civilized world."[17] In addition to Jolly and Bethune, doctors from Poland, France, Germany, Romania, and Spain addressed their compatriots in their native tongues. Jolly's Hungarian nurse Anna-Mária Basch was joined by nurses from Italy, Bulgaria, China, and New Zealand.[18] According to Jolly's own account, he "spoke of the conditions here and of the needs of the Spanish people in their war against Fascism. Spoke of what I had seen in this city and in our Advanced Field Hospital—of the medical needs of the International Brigade. Said that we needed *fully* trained nurses and doctors, ambulances, stretchers, surgical equipment of all kinds, including Hospital beds and surgical linen."[19]

Later that day ("I believe this is Christmas Eve though I'm not quite certain. The day and the date here are mostly unknown quantities"), he sent a long and poignant letter to the Grants in Britain, making the same plea for medical supplies. "Any hospital or Ambulance equipment that can be sent . . . (how I know not) would be like manna in the desert. Stretchers, metal hospital beds, surgical instruments, surgical linen and medicaments—*fully* trained nurses and of course qualified medical men."[20]

At that time, a month after arriving in Madrid, he had received no letters from his friends or family, and he sounded rather homesick. Due to both the risks inherent in a wartime international mail service and the unceasing demands of his work, he wrote all his outward letters only to the Grants, with instructions to forward them to other friends and to his family in New Zealand. "I've been sending letters off into the blue and hope that at least one with the above address has reached you; that you may be assured as to my well-being and that you have somewhere to send letters [in reply]. The receipt of them here is very uncertain for many reasons. It's a long way from Albacete even if they arrive there safely. . . . We are not directly in touch with a post office so that most of my letters have been given into the pockets of men going city-wards—many may fall by the wayside."[21]

The Grants faithfully followed his instructions regarding his outward letters. Each of them, handwritten in a legible boyish script, was typed out once it reached London—probably by Irene Grant's younger sister Gladys, a shorthand typist by profession—and several copies made and distributed. One set of the typed copies was eventually deposited with the Imperial War Museum in London.[22]

The constraints of wartime censorship ("I am always careful not to infringe the allowed content—it apparently takes little to have letters held up as unsuitable") gave Jolly's correspondence a somewhat forced and breezy tone.[23] Nevertheless, he clearly felt hugely enthusiastic about his unfamiliar and very challenging circumstances:

> The days here are just grand. Hot sunshine with never a cloud in the bluest of skies—the nights cold, the stars ever so large and shining bright. In lulls of work it is so peaceful that one can hardly imagine that there is a war going on only a few kilometers away. It's impossible however to forget the reality as the boom, boom, crack, crackle, boom is ever present. . . .
>
> We are doing good work and are now smoothly organised to deal with the casualties as they arrive. . . . It is good to be thus effective—to know quite certainly by results that we are able to do a little in this bloody business to make it less of a Hell.
>
> My French medical colleagues are good chaps and we get over the difficulty of communication increasingly easily as my stock of French words grows. There are many languages spoken and anyone who has two or three

languages is a boon—providing of course that they have other contributions to make to the working of the unit.

Don't worry about me. I will take good care of myself and accept only the necessary risks that are in the situation.[24]

On Christmas Day 1936, a party was given in a large cinema for the predominantly Italian, French, and German battalions of the International Brigades. "If you listened carefully," wrote Kajsa Rothman, "in spite of the music and all the laughing and talking you could hear bursts of gunfire, and now and again the dull thud of a cannon. The enemy was not even a kilometre away. But no-one was listening. . . . For the space of a few hours, we had tried, and perhaps managed, to forget all the atrocities of war—the daily bombing attacks that without any military target in mind were devastating entire neighbourhoods just for the sake of something to destroy."[25]

For Jolly and his medical team (he was learning to refer to it by the local term *equipo*), their first Christmas in Spain passed with little to mark the day.

> We each received a box of sweets, cigarettes, matches (very precious) and a bottle of Cognac—from the Spanish S.R.I [Socorro Rojo Internacional (International Red Aid)—a Spanish trade union relief group that, for the first six months of the civil war, organized the medical services of the Republican Army]. The guns boomed and the rifles and machine guns cracked as usual, and the wounded were none the less wounded or fewer in number. We now have a wireless set and listen in at some hour each day to the English news. It is very amusing and informative to hear from the English announcers news about the progress of the fighting on this sector of the front. . . .
>
> In spite of the great difference in race and the language difficulties, we are a very united group. It's good to be with so many from different countries who are politically conscious. So different from the condition that one imagines in an ordinary war. Here we are all united not only against a common enemy, but by a deep conviction—there is scarcely any discipline or the need for it.[26]

The reference to tobacco in this letter strikes an odd note in the present day when its physically harmful properties are taken for granted. On the front lines in Spain, however, the importance of cigarettes could not be overestimated. Photographs of Jolly show him smoking whenever not actually at work at the operating table. Everyone, men and women, smoked "not only to relieve tension and allay boredom or hunger pangs but also as a way of helping to overcome one of the most pervasive accompaniments of war—smell."[27]

Franco's artillery rang in the new year by firing twelve shells into the heart of Madrid on the stroke of midnight, ten of them hitting the Telefónica building.[28] Its largely female staff continued to direct phone calls with a sangfroid that Jolly found astonishing and impressive. "The courageous contempt shown for the fascist bombs and bombardment is epic. Far from creating panic in the city (as must be the intention, for there is no other sane reason) these air raids and artillery bombardments seem only to strengthen the purpose of the people. There is no possible doubt that they are a brave and worthy people. Great things are in store for Spain when this war is over. My increasing regret is that I have not yet enough Spanish to discuss with the milicianos [militia fighters] the meaning for them of this war."[29]

Later, reflecting on the Madrileños' death-defying contempt for the daily artillery and aerial bombardment, Jolly concluded, "One has to go to Spain's national sport in the bull ring to find the analogy of this seeming indifference to death. . . . This attitude of scorn for enemy bombs and disdain for the shelter of the deep bomb-proof chambers provided by the government and municipal councils in all the larger cities and towns, or of the open trenches dug on all clear land around the villages, was responsible for much loss of civilian life in the first year of the war."[30]

After the relentless street fighting and near-constant air raids of November and December, "something like a truce prevailed on the Madrid front" by mid-January.[31] The shattered city managed to present a superficial air of normality with its regular tram services still running even up to the front lines of the conflict. Its citizens thronged the streets each day as they made their way to work, dodging the periodic shelling and cratered sidewalks. There were long queues for food, and trenches and sandbags surrounded strategic points, but the cinemas and theaters remained open.

Jolly's equipo celebrated New Year's Eve with "an hilarious and vinous party in the mess," then spent much of January enjoying a rare respite from their duties while the Nationalists regrouped for a further attempt on the city.

"I've spent the last two days laying in the warmth of the Spanish winter sun," he reported. "Warm enough to sit in it for hours without being cold—but as soon as the sun goes down it begins to freeze."[32] More vinous social occasions took place with Bethune, his colleagues, and other notable visitors such as the renowned biologist J. B. S. Haldane, whose son was serving with the International Brigades; journalist Claud Cockburn; and photographer Vera Elkan. The still and moving images she recorded of the International Brigades included several of Jolly's team at work.[33]

The troops defending Madrid were largely "en repos" (on a break) in this period, he told the Grants, "and so are we more or less. A number of Spanish wounded continue to arrive. The time hangs heavily when there is no work to be done. For obvious reasons I cannot go far from this place as I never know when I may suddenly be wanted."[34]

Throughout January 1937, Jolly wrote several times a week, sometimes at considerable length, to Irene Grant. His letters confirm both the deep affection between the two and his unflagging interest in her reports of the activities of the Aux and the CL (Christian Left), to which he clearly expected to contribute as soon as he was no longer needed in Spain. He was at pains to reassure her that "I am very well and contented. I wonder how long this will last—I'd like very much to see you all—seems so much more than a month since I left England."[35]

Setbacks such as a defeat for the International Brigades at Córdoba in southern Spain appear to have only strengthened Jolly's commitment to the Republic, although his hopes that Britain and its European allies would enter the conflict in its support were starting to fade.

> I wonder more and more whether Britain will wake up to the reality of her position in the European political conflict—whether she will see before the last moment that her destiny *must* be linked with France and Russia. . . . The issues in this conflict and Britain's interest in the outcome are so simple from the left viewpoint, that all one reads in such papers as the Times and the Telegraph is the most utter bilge. . . . In England I was never really touched by the right wing press—it was just a matter for superficial sneering. Here in Spain it is a matter for tears.[36]

More satisfying English-language reading matter was evidently hard to come by, and Jolly was delighted when, in mid-January, three volumes of Shakespeare and Ernest Hemingway's novels *The Sun also Rises* and *Death in the Afternoon* appeared. He considered that Hemingway, a high-profile visitor to Madrid in this period, "has a grand vivid style and his settings are those in which *we* now live."[37] Later he was able to buy D. H. Lawrence's *The Plumed Serpent* and James Joyce's *Ulysses* and *Dubliners*. Like many others before and since, he found *Ulysses* a challenging read. "The flights of ideas of all his people are like moving in a world of schizophrenics. Perhaps our minds all work that way, but it's strange to read the expression of this working in black and white. Some passages of Joyce are reminiscent of Picasso's portraits."[38]

By the end of January, the weather reverted to bitter cold and driving rain, and Jolly's team, "cooped up together, all beginning to get on one's nerves a bit," studied Spanish systematically to pass the time. "A Spanish school teacher comes out from the city on alternate days, and from five to seven o'clock half a dozen of us struggle with the subjunctive and suchlike. It's a pleasant language to hear spoken well and not terribly difficult to learn—the French make much more rapid progress than I and the other English."[39]

Although Jolly's limited Spanish frustrated his efforts to communicate with the local people, his admiration for them and his affection for the children are evident. "Spanish children are the sweetest things—very friendly, wide open, dark eyes. I wish I could speak with them—'mucho bueno' and things like that only take one a short distance on the way. If one uses any Spanish at all they conclude that they will be understood and rattle away—it's much better just to be dumb and use sign language."[40]

News from the battlefront arrived only sporadically and was often unreliable. In late January 1937, Jolly learned that both "W. H. A." (the poet W. H. Auden, a contributor to *Christianity and the Social Revolution*) and "S. S." (the writer Stephen Spender) had arrived in Spain.[41] Other war news was more directly affecting and distressing. In Albacete, Jolly had met Ralph Fox, a left-wing writer and friend of Tom Wintringham's, and found him "a splendid fellow."[42] Jolly later learned that both Fox and the young poet John Cornford were among the many International Brigaders killed during a disastrous late-December engagement on the Córdoba front. "I continue to think so much about [Fox]," he told Irene Grant. "I was so deeply impressed by my short contact with him."[43]

At the end of January, another rumour circulated: The mobile surgical team would be posted to a new front in a week's time. This time the information proved accurate. Franco's forces were preparing a major offensive on the lines protecting the main road between Madrid and Valencia, a crucial supply route for the capital's defenders. If that road could be cut, Madrid would be isolated from reinforcements and almost certain to fall to the Nationalists. The ensuing battle was one of the most grueling and costly of the entire civil war. For Jolly's colleague Archie Cochrane, its most unpleasant feature was its duration. "It lasted far longer than anything we had previously experienced, taking up most of February 1937, a month which at times seemed as though it would never end."[44] The field of battle was a river valley called Jarama, a name that would become synonymous with "slaughter" for the International Brigaders.

"We wait the next move," Jolly wrote in a letter shortly before the battle began. "Probably we rush to another front for that is the habit in this Brigade. We always arrive where the danger is greatest and depart when the front is again stabilised."[45] This time he was ordered to locate his field hospital in the town of Campo Real, twenty kilometers southeast of Madrid. Passing on the news to Irene Grant, he sounded eager to return to the fray yet regretful that his team's hard-won expertise and resources might be lost in the move. "I would prefer to stay here as we have accumulated many adjuncts towards the running of a field hospital which are not transportable with our limited transport facilities and which may not be procurable elsewhere."[46] Some original members of his equipo had already been transferred to another unit, but he retained his now very experienced theater nurse Anna-Mária Basch, who had "worked like a slave" throughout the recent Las Rozas battle.[47]

During the battle of Jarama, only the most critical cases—those requiring an immediate operation—were treated, and all others, even if severely wounded, were merely stabilized before their transportation to more distant and larger hospitals. Wounds that penetrated the abdomen were Jolly's special responsibility since he had already acquired expertise at this exceptionally demanding branch of emergency surgery. "This type of injury is extremely serious," another authority has written, "because of the dangers of perforation of part of the intestine . . . the whole gut had to be inspected really closely."[48]

By the first days of the Jarama offensive, Jolly was evidently already an outstandingly accomplished and resilient frontline surgeon—rapid, expert, and seemingly tireless. Although his field hospital was at times utterly overwhelmed by the torrent of casualties, he appears to have spent almost the entire month-long Jarama assault at his operating table. This extraordinary degree of commitment, driven both by his Christian socialist values and his anti-fascist views, extended several times to operating on troops of the opposing force. "A thing that has impressed me" at Jarama, he wrote, "is the deep hatred of Fascism but not the Fascists. . . . I know that wounded Moors [Franco's Moroccan mercenary troops] have been brought to this Hospital by the Spanish Ambulances. I've operated on them."[49]

This hospital and Jolly's subsequent improvised field hospitals contended with daunting medical challenges imposed by the local environment and infrastructure. Keeping patients adequately cool in summer and warm in winter was almost impossible in the climatic extremes of the central Spanish plateau. The country in general was then poor and largely rural, with few sealed roads, sewerage systems that were either minimal or nonexistent, and scarce sources of running water.

By late February 1937, after horrifying casualty figures and with both sides exhausted, the fighting at Jarama subsided, and the front line stabilized. As with the attacks on the north of Madrid two months earlier, the Republicans repulsed the Nationalist offensive to smash their defenses at Jarama, and Franco was again forced to concede failure in his attempt to encircle and conquer the city.[50] Jolly's team was not immediately relieved once the worst of the fighting was over; instead, it was relocated fifty kilometers southeast to the town of Tarancón. The Republican medical services designated its red-brick Hospital de Santa Emilia and four other buildings as No. 2 base hospitals—that is, for treating less serious or less urgent cases evacuated from the frontline hospitals. In the days immediately following the Jarama campaign, the small town had become overrun with wounded, and Jolly's field hospital was stationed there to reinforce the permanent hospitals. His equipo set up in a school building in Castilla–La Mancha Square, near a Republican Army logistics depot that drew periodic air raids on both facilities.[51]

The team was assisted by new arrivals including an English nurse named Penny Phelps, who later gave detailed recollections of her work that deserve to be quoted at length: "We took charge of an empty school and at once set to, preparing a theatre, unloading our equipment and scrubbing and disinfecting floors and walls. . . . We had no running water in the building but we fixed up big chromium containers for boiling water and we fixed up our electricity."[52]

They set up three operating tables in a room on the ground floor and filled the corridors with rows of stretchers to accommodate the flood of casualties expected to arrive at any time.[53] "Before we were half ready, the first ambulance drew up outside, unloading its wounded. At the door, a doctor classified and sorted the wounded—only the worst cases were dealt with by us."[54]

Most of the wounded men already wore bandages applied by first aid dressing posts at the front line. Those who had been given injections of morphine and anti-tetanus serum had their foreheads marked with a large "M+."[55] According to Nurse Phelps,

> The wounded arrived in ambulances, on open lorries or any other available transport. They must have had a very hard time because the roads in this region are rough and it is mountainous. We were quite near the front . . . and the small hospital became overcrowded. Many of the wounded were left out in the yard from lack of space inside the school building, which must have been extremely stressful because it was very cold and there was often snow on the ground.
>
> The fighting went on continuously day and night and when the electric lights failed we had to resort to torches. There was no heating except from a small gasoline stove and sometimes it was so cold you would be glad to be in the operating theatre full of people.
>
> . . . When one went out for fresh air there was a tendency to stumble over bodies, some dead and others wounded, the latter crying out for *agua* [water].[56]
>
> Already after the first case I realised Doctor Jolly was one of the best surgeons I had ever worked with—and certainly one of the quickest. Long before he had finished with the first case, a second ambulance drew up, and a third, and quite soon they seemed to come in droves, while the faint rumble of guns never left off. Operating as fast as was possible for a surgeon, Jolly worked the whole afternoon, right through the night, the next day and most of the following night as well, practically without a break. He never seemed to tire or lose his concentration, and most of the time I worked with him.
>
> It was terrible on the front line—and we were right in the midst of it. As they were coming off the ambulance, picking them up and dropping

> them off, we were taking on laparotomies, stomach wounds, amputations and head injuries.[57]

"We used morphine and drips," nurse Phelps recalled, "but we were always running out. It was very, very difficult. Most of the cases were too far gone to give them anything to put them out, and there were terrible, terrible losses. People died who should never have died."[58]

> My own duties kept on mounting. Soon I was anaesthetising the wounded with ether or chloroform (in England I had seen so many anaesthetics given that I was quite familiar with the techniques) and handing over the face mask to an orderly as soon as the patient was under. . . . Sometimes I found myself assisting all three tables when my two nurse colleagues required rest pauses. . . . For five days and nights we had only brief snatches of sleep and that on blood-soaked stretchers not occupied by the wounded. We were sustained by mugs of black coffee, bully-beef sandwiches and cigarettes. I had begun to smoke, as did all other colleagues, male and female.[59]

As she told one interviewer,

> Once, just as we were thinking of finishing, but still had several cases to deal with, we heard the loud drone of planes and at once our lights, including the emergency light, went out. Before we could move, there were shattering crashes quite close, and the sound of falling glass. The next minute there were unearthly shrieks from outside and the sound of people running. Our doors were open, and before we knew what was going on, there was a wild stampede in the darkness. Civilians were rushing into our hospital, which was already full of our own wounded. The air was full of shrieking and moaning.[60]

After three weeks of this hellish ordeal, the field hospital was ordered to transfer to a new front, and on the morning of 5 March 1937, its trucks were fully loaded. Twenty-seven-year-old Penny Phelps was "taking a moment's rest by the roadside between Madrid and Valencia" when she heard again the drone of approaching aircraft. "There were children playing in front of me and I was thinking, what lovely brown eyes they have—such a pretty scene. Then there was a crash; my chair went from under me; things flew through the air. I reached for one of the children and held onto her. Dr Jolly emerged from the dust and took the child from me. I don't know if she was alive or dead."[61] Thirty-three people were killed in this daylight attack; the little girl survived, although she was severely injured with a shattered leg. "I stumbled with her in my arms to our hospital where Dr Jolly amputated the damaged limb," wrote Penny Fyvel (as she later became). "It was an incident I can never forget."[62]

Unsurprisingly, given the pressure of work he faced, Jolly wrote no letters in this period, and his heroic efforts at Jarama and Tarancón are known mainly through the recollections of those who worked alongside him such as Penny. It is not until later in March 1937 that his own letter writing resumed, with much the same hearty, imperturbable tone as before the battle. "The news that you have had of the situation here will be sufficient explanation of the lack of opportunity for writing. We've had a hectic time and are glad of this period of comparative tranquillity. . . . Except for the fact I have acquired a slightly septic finger, I am very fit—this life agrees with me. Before coming to Spain I felt badly done by if I did not get my seven or eight hours sleep—now I can manage passably well with one or two."[63]

Only the occasional phrase ("one can't keep going day and night indefinitely") suggests the immense strain the Jarama battle and its immediate aftermath must have cost him.[64] Many of his medical colleagues proved less physically and psychologically robust. A New Zealand nurse, Una Wilson, worked at another hospital in the village of Colmenar de Oreja, about forty kilometers northwest of Tarancón. Her diary from this period reads like the transcript of a nightmare.

> In my bed a dead man. I turned the bedclothes and found that he had been shot through the stomach. My bed was filled with blood. I had him removed, turned my mattress over and flopped on it . . . Never in my life have I been so utterly tired, miserable and unhappy. I would be grateful to be caught by one of the machine-guns which play about in the air. We seem to wade about in a river of blood without a break. . . . I'm off duty. Have lost my memory. At least I cannot remember clearly what happens from day to day and everything is very tangled. . . . My hands shake like a leaf and I cannot sit still for more than two or three minutes.[65]

Una Wilson recovered remarkably quickly from this state of severe nervous exhaustion and immediately returned to her duties in the operating theater.

Like Jolly, she worked at a frontline field hospital and was required to move to wherever the fighting was fiercest. Both she and Jolly now learned that the accelerating pace of the war made those moves ever more frequent. A month-long lull had followed the attacks on Madrid in December. After the blood-drenched battle of Jarama, a new offensive began in just a few days.

8 Urgent Need of Salvation

> The treatment of a war wound is the greatest test of the ability of a surgeon.
>
> —BRIG. SIR IAN FRASER

Writing for a left-wing Toronto newspaper in March 1937, Norman Bethune exuded zest and optimism as he described his journey to Jolly's latest hospital, an hour's drive northwest of Madrid:

> The hospital stood at the top of the hill on the right as we crossed the bridge coming into the town of Guadalajara.... In the back we had a refrigerator and ten pint bottles of preserved blood packed in a wire basket. We had left Madrid at ten and had made the 54 kilometres in less than an hour, rolling along the fine paved Zaragoza road at well over seventy most of the time.... Sharp turn left at the top of the hill and there was the 500-bed hospital. No more red crosses now. Last week the fascist planes tried to bomb it so down came the cross.... The sure sign of an engagement were [*sic*] the long rows of blood-drenched stretchers, propped up on end, leaning against the walls, waiting to be washed. All was bustle and hurry.
>
> ... Up we go to the operating room. Here three tables are at work, the close air heavy with the fumes of ether. Casting a glance, a nod, to the chief surgeon as we cross the room to the white enamelled refrigerator standing against the wall. The row of empty blood bottles on the top tells the story—three, five, seven empties and inside, only three unused....
>
> Out the door, down the long corridor filled with stretcher-men, doctors, nurses and walking wounded to Dr Jolly's department. His fine, open New Zealand face breaks into a smile as he sees us. We are old friends from early days in Madrid.... The room is packed with wounded. They sit on the floor with bloodstained bandages on head, arms and legs, waiting to be dressed.[1]

Guadalajara would ultimately prove a fortuitous battle site for the Republican forces, but when Jolly's equipo was posted there in the first week of March 1937, its advantages were not apparent. The Republicans were again on the defensive, resisting a Nationalist attempt to capture the town and then drive southward to take Madrid. The assault was headed by thirty-five thousand Italian troops reinforced by Fiat fighter planes, tanks, and artillery—all supplied by Mussolini's fascist state. The Republican forces opposing them were both outnumbered and outgunned.

Jolly, after just four months' service in Spain, now held the post of chief surgeon in the Eleventh International Brigade and had been promoted to captain, the same rank his father held in World War I. His hospital, in a large villa on the Madrid–Valencia highway, was shared with two other surgical teams and included veterans of the British Medical Volunteer Unit based at Grañén the year before. One of them, Archie Cochrane, believed that Bethune's blood delivery service from Madrid represented "perhaps the most significant advance" to frontline medical services since those early days.[2] Just as Jolly and other surgeons were siting their operating theaters as close as possible to the front line, Bethune had found a system for providing them with vital supplies of tested and classified blood. Recently renamed the Canadian-Spanish Blood Transfusion Institute, it could deliver blood to a hundred hospitals and smaller casualty clearing stations along a battlefront extending a thousand kilometers east of Madrid.[3] The Guadalajara field hospital had a refrigerator specifically for storing donated blood, and another of its doctors, Reg Saxton, had developed expertise in administering transfusions and was recruiting local donors.[4] Up to a hundred transfusions would be given daily during the forthcoming battle.[5]

The Guadalajara region was still subject to Madrid's dire "nine months of winter," and the Nationalist advance was made through snow and sleet, conditions that proved greatly to the advantage of the Republican defenders. Frozen roads and poor visibility caused the fleets of Fiat armored vehicles to stall in an immovable bloc, making them easy targets for fighter planes and bombers. For once, the Republican forces enjoyed superiority in the air, since by good fortune their aircraft could take off from an all-weather concrete runway while the Nationalists' air support sat on the drenched grass airfields. In addition, almost three hundred light and maneuverable T-26 tanks arrived from the Soviet Union in time for the Republican forces to use them with great success.

Mussolini's troops were soon forced into a chaotic and humiliating retreat, and for the first time in the civil war, the Republican government and its supporters could realistically envisage a final victory.

Nevertheless, huge numbers of wounded continued to arrive at the front-line hospitals, often beyond saving after spending agonizing days in subzero conditions. Of the more than three thousand casualties brought into Jolly's field hospital, many were suffering from frostbite. They included large numbers of Italian prisoners and deserters.[6] To the surprise of nurse Penny Phelps, they were "not Fascist bully-boys, but young conscripts from the Italian country-side."[7] "Don't believe the stories that are current that all Fascists, prisoners or wounded, are shot forthwith," Jolly told his friends by mail. "I have operated on a number of Italian Fascists."[8] His insistence, at Guadalajara and other battlefronts, on treating enemy wounded on the same basis as other patients brought him into fierce conflict with more ideologically purist colleagues. On one occasion, a Czech doctor, František "Franz" Kriegel, noticed Jolly labeling arriving casualties in order of the urgency of their condition and operating on them accordingly. First in line was a prisoner of war. Kriegel was outraged that this enemy combatant was given precedence over severely wounded Republican troops, but Jolly stood his ground. "The reasons that brought me here are the same reasons which will make me operate on that prisoner first; because he is in the most urgent need of salvation. And you can say what you like, and if you continue, I'm going home." Kriegel outranked Jolly but apparently tolerated this serious act of insubordination and made no further objection to his fixed practice of treating patients regardless of their uniform, insignia, and politics.[9]

Jolly questioned some of these wounded prisoners in the hope of learning a little about field medical services on the other side. "I spoke with an Italian prisoner who was a stretcher-bearer in the Italian Army. . . . He told me that their hospitals were far behind the lines, and that many abdominal cases died without operation."[10] This specific observation is borne out when comparing the organization of the opposing armies' medical services. The Nationalists relied on older, World War I–era models of treatment provision that proved less effective than the more innovative and improvisatory Republican systems at dealing with vast numbers of injured along a poorly roaded battlefront.

However, the equipment supplied to the Nationalist hospitals, as with the weaponry available to their troops, generally surpassed anything available to the Republicans. Among the very large quantities of war matériel captured from the retreating Italians at Guadalajara, and immediately put to use by their victors, was an entire tented field hospital whose heat-retaining double walls and other advanced features greatly impressed Jolly. In the cruder, single-walled tents available to him, "it was wholly impossible to subdue the slight glow at night which might attract the attention of a prowling aeroplane."[11] Furthermore, in the Republican tented hospitals, heating could not be controlled, and "the tragic plight of the wounded during the winter months can be imagined; in the summer it was almost impossible to work inside such tents or to maintain the progress of the wounded after operation." The exhaust steam from the autoclaves installed in trucks could be directed through pipes and radiators to heat tented operating theaters in winter, but more dangerous methods using highly flammable fuels were employed if necessary. "The best method of initially heating an operating room," Jolly found, "is to burn alcohol in a large flat dish, but the temperature should be maintained by some cheaper method."[12] The equipo's mechanic, John Kozar—a tough and swarthy former seaman of mixed Czech and Lakota Native American heritage from Canada—installed these improvised heating systems. Jolly knew him as "Topsy" and remembered him as "indefatigable and well beloved by us all. . . . Brave as a lion."[13]

At the end of March 1937, after "the furious, unbelievable rush of the recent campaign," Jolly found time to roam about on foot in the hill country behind the lines, "tramping through olive groves—peach and pear trees in blossom." The contrast between the recent gory scenes of mechanized warfare, he wrote, and the peaceful sight of "peasants working in the fields . . . is incredible." Although he shared in the general high spirits and soaring morale that followed the Republican victory at Guadalajara, occasionally his letters reveal depths of war weariness and depression that he was careful to conceal from his colleagues in Spain.

> You can't imagine the life here during a big attack. The terrible sights of war exist only as a grim reality. I don't believe they exist in the imagination of anyone who has not had the experience of war. When twenty or thirty big Caproni bombers come over one of these small towns behind our lines and drop a hundred or so large bombs on the streets where children and women go about their daily work—I can't describe the terrible horrors.

> When a dozen or so kids are brought in ripped to pieces, legs blown off, bellies and heads ripped open, it's almost the end of everything for me.[14]

Such passages, which somehow eluded the scrutiny of military censors, echo the most desperate of nurse Una Wilson's diary entries from the Jarama front, and soon after she wrote them, she suffered a major emotional and physical collapse. Even during his baptism by fire in the earlier battle of Madrid, Jolly had managed to sound consistently robust and optimistic in his letters home. The striking contrast provided by the passage quoted above suggests that even this sturdy Antipodean, driven by deep commitments to his medical calling, to those under his command, and to the political goals of the Republican war effort, could become overwhelmed by the daily horrors entailed by those commitments. "Dr Jolly is working under very great pressure," the Christian Left *News Sheet* reported in April 1937, "and it is hoped that some one may soon be found who will relieve him for two or three months."[15] No such relief was provided.

Like almost all those on the Republican side, Jolly continued to harbor hopes that the democratic nations of Europe might intervene militarily to bring a swift end to the war and that volunteers like himself needed only to persevere until that formal intervention occurred. "This must stop *soon*, and England can play a great part in the stopping," he reminded his friends in London.[16] Within a few weeks, however, his earlier tone of energetic optimism reappeared, and his letters rejoiced in a new reason to be cheerful. "My best friend in Spain is a Hungarian who has been living in emigration in Belgium for some time. A supremely grand person. We have to talk in French—Hungarian is such a terrible language that I could not begin to tackle it."[17] Although carefully coy about this friend's identity, and even gender, there can be no doubt he is referring to his highly competent theater nurse, Anna-Mária Basch, and that their friendship had become more than platonic. Like Irene Grant, Basch was married and some ten years older than Jolly, but she also had an impressive background as an anti-fascist activist in her native Hungary before gaining nursing experience in Belgium.[18]

Basch evidently reciprocated Jolly's affection and admiration, writing later of his "discipline and selfless dedication. . . . He himself did not belong to any political party, he was simply a doctor who was anti-fascist through extraordinarily high ethics. That is what brought him to Spain. He expected that everyone in his unit should forget the word 'me' and think only in terms of 'we' or 'they.' We often worked day and night without rest, helping the wounded and the sick with all our strength."[19]

Working at the limits of their capacity in this way, surrounded daily by evidence of the ephemerality of human life (Basch had herself come under fire at Fuencarral and in an ambulance on the Jarama front), and craving the solace of companionship, ardent affairs without regard for marital status flourished among many of the medical volunteers on the Republican front. The love affair between Jolly and Basch ended when they were eventually forced to return to different countries, but they remained intimate friends and correspondents for much of their lives.

"Spring is really coming here at last!" Jolly reported cheerily in April 1937. "Not before time—we've been nearly frozen for weeks; have had sleet and snow and the wounded were desperately shocked with exposure. Now that things are quieter the weather is warmer."[20] He was then regularly driving the several hundred kilometers between Madrid and Valencia on the Mediterranean coast, transporting war refugees eastward and bringing back food and medical supplies on the return trip. He continued to perform emergency operations in both cities and on one occasion, in Valencia, removed a bullet from a patient's hip without anesthetic.[21]

On another trip from Valencia he transported twenty-five thousand oranges, "which we picked ourselves aided by 50 people from a village known as Little Russia near here. The Socorro Rojo in Madrid were delighted with the oranges and danced on them until orangeade ran out of the bottom of the truck." His V8 Ford took "a terrible hammering over indifferent roads" on these long journeys, and he wrote to England in the hope of obtaining a new vehicle. "A covered truck would really be much more use out here than an ambulance, because it is an ambulance if occasion demands. . . . With this vehicle I could do a trip a day, and evacuate Madrid myself." The prospect of such an emergency evacuation, he admitted with rare candor, was ever more imminent. "Things are bad here [in Madrid]. The people are beginning to get demoralised under the continuous shelling which is becoming more indiscriminate every day. The Government definitely fear gas attacks and they have made what preparations they can—only by gas will Madrid fall."[22]

The Republican medical services greatly feared the threat of a poison gas attack like those carried out twenty years earlier on the western front, and the biologist Professor Haldane led efforts to develop protection against such an attack. His commitment to the survival of the Republic derived from personal as well as political motives. Haldane's wife Charlotte organized the recruitment of British volunteers from an office in Paris, and her son, Ronnie, had been severely injured while serving with the International Brigades at Jarama. The wound forced Ronnie to return to England, but Professor Haldane remained in Madrid, providing advice and training on dealing with the effects of toxic gas. Ultimately, those precautions proved unnecessary, but in the brief lull that followed the victory at Guadalajara, other steps were taken that greatly advanced the medical services provided to the Republican forces.

After the fearfully grueling but relatively static defensive actions around Madrid and at Jarama, the war had become increasingly mobile with the arrival in the country of more aviation and high-powered weaponry. In the dispersed and mountainous battlefront around Guadalajara, these developments had meant much longer delays in transporting critically injured men to the field hospitals. For the most severe injuries, including open fractures and the abdominal wounds that were Jolly's speciality, the death rates were horrifying. In the month following that battle, when the most active fighting was taking place on the northern front at Bilbao, Col. Oscar Telge—the International Brigades' chief medical officer—and his senior doctors inspected the Guadalajara battlefield. One of them, the young Catalan surgeon Moisès Broggi, defended the work performed by the surgical teams that he, Jolly, and others had headed. Injured men who had been transported for long distances, often by steep mountain tracks and through frozen terrain, said Broggi, typically arrived at the hospital in a condition that made it impossible to save them. In the future, he proposed, the operating theaters must be moved even closer to the battle lines. He continued, "It would be convenient to have a special truck with all the necessary objects and equipment, starting with the sterilization stoves, the operating table and plasters, a light and a group generator. Furthermore, the instruments should be prepared in metal boxes duly classified for different types of intervention (abdomen, extremities, skull, etc.) repeated a few times; [*sic*] With this, the instruments, previously sterilised, could be used without wasting time cleaning and sterilising them after each intervention."[23]

Telge, to his great credit, accepted this suggestion from a junior officer and arranged with the Renault automotive plant in Paris to build suitable vehicles to his surgeons' specifications. This remarkable collaboration between the army hierarchy and clinicians with expertise in emergency surgery "represented an indisputable advance in war surgery," Broggi wrote later. "It was probably the first case in the entire history of military health in which a hierarchical superior consulted on a problem of such importance with subordinates who were not military."[24]

During his training in civilian surgery in New Zealand and the United Kingdom, Jolly had never encountered or even imagined such medical advances as the military blood transfusion service or the *autochir* (as the mobile operating theaters were known, from the abbreviated French terms for "vehicle" and "surgery").[25] Their unorthodox introduction during the Spanish Civil War was due largely to the fervor of enforced improvisation that inevitably disrupted traditional ideas and lines of authority. Long-established routines and practices were thrown aside, and this combination of the demand and opportunity for medical innovation proved immensely productive. The lessons learned at Guadalajara brought a sharp reduction in amputations and in deaths from abdominal injury during the battle fought the following month in similar mountainous terrain at Guadarrama.[26] Broggi claimed, "The improvement in the results was spectacular and was manifested in all the wounded, but was most evident in abdominal cases which . . . reached a survival rate close to 50%, something never seen before."[27]

In the same month as Dr. Telge's surgical conference, John Macmurray, one of Jolly's close friends from London and an editor of *Christianity and the Social Revolution*, arrived in Spain as part of a nine-person religious delegation that included the dean of Canterbury. The Spanish government had invited them to investigate charges that the Republic encouraged persecution of the Catholic Church, one of the most compelling arguments used in Britain to oppose its formal military involvement in the war. During its brief visit, the delegation was able to witness from a distance an instance of such religious persecution, although it was carried out not by the Republicans but by their Nationalist opponents, who paradoxically enjoyed the backing of the Catholic Church worldwide: German and Italian aircraft working in relays bombed and strafed the small and undefended town of Durango in the Basque country.[28]

Two churches were hit during the celebration of Mass, killing an officiating priest, fourteen nuns, and most of the congregation.[29]

Macmurray returned to Britain apparently convinced that the Republic's fortitude in the face of such atrocities would ensure its victory. He told Irene Grant, "I've seen the rebirth of a nation . . . something is happening that is pure gain, and that cannot be undone."[30] A new edition of *Christianity and the Social Revolution* was rushed out to reinforce the timeliness of the book's central premise. In a preface to that 1937 edition, editor John Lewis appealed "for a closing of ranks and a new spirit of tolerance and comradeship between Christians and Socialists in the face of a common enemy." The Spanish Civil War, he wrote, had demonstrated beyond doubt the need for Christians and the Left to make a common stand against fascist aggression.[31] The British government remained unmoved, however, and continued to assert the necessity to uphold the Non-Intervention Pact, by then honored more in the breach than in the observance.

Macmurray's delegation traveled mainly in the north of Spain, so Jolly had no opportunity for a reunion with his friend even though he was then enjoying a period of "comparative tranquillity" following the latest offensive and swimming in the swift Henares River that flowed through Guadalajara. It may have been in this brief respite that a peculiar photograph was taken, possibly by his nurse Anna-Mária Basch since the print is now held by her descendants. Standing against a tree, an anxious-looking Jolly in his underwear has an apple on his head, and the slim and shirtless Peter de Sarigny takes aim at it with a crude bow and arrow. Apparently they were performing the Swiss folk legend of William Tell for the entertainment of the troops.[32]

Jolly was delighted when a box of new surgical instruments arrived from London but told his friends that he still greatly needed the drug Evipan sodium as an intravenous anesthetic and the equipment for treating laryngeal diphtheria.[33] The same equipment proved equally vital for patients with severe facial injuries who might otherwise inhale their own blood while on their stretchers awaiting surgery, and Allied surgeons later used it during World War II.[34]

The opportunity for rest and recuperation was brief since "there is talk of our quitting this Hospital and moving a few kilometers towards the front, there to set up another independent Hospital for our division."[35] As the shock troops of the Republican Army's medical services, field hospital teams were required to move constantly to the most active areas of the vast and shifting battlefront. Their next destination was kept secret for as long as possible to prevent the information from reaching the enemy, and often their convoy of vehicles was already underway by the time a dispatch rider arrived and handed the lead driver a sealed envelope with final orders.[36] Kenneth Sinclair-Loutit supplied a description of this mode of operation, which applied equally to both his and Jolly's equipos:

> We usually arrive at the village that has been chosen for us—some 14 or 15 kilometres behind the firing-line—in the small hours of the morning. Large convoys by day are too vulnerable to aerial attack. . . . We are usually housed in large villas of fascist ownership which, with a little initiative, can be converted into excellent first-line hospitals. . . . We attempt to follow the same plan in all our hospitals. We start with a large reception room which can hold about 15 stretchers and the same number of ambulant cases. Here, as the cases arrive, a rapid sorting is performed by the reception officer and the wounded are dispatched to major or minor operating theatres, or in cases of great shock, to the wards. He, too, is responsible for evacuations, dispatching those who can stand further transport farther back from the line. Here, also, any first aid treatment is given. . . . Next comes the operating theatre or theatres. . . . In the last two hospitals we have had to put all five tables in the one large room—this has proved an admirable arrangement and an economy in both material and staff. . . .
>
> The contrast between this and our former work on the Aragon front strikes one from every angle. At Grañen we were permanently established behind a stationary defence line . . . now, eight months later, we find ourselves behind a determined and disciplined army engaged in an offensive which stretches from the borders to the seas against a foreign fascist invasion.[37]

The transformation of the Republic's initial raggle-taggle forces into a "determined and disciplined army" was mirrored by the simultaneous reorganization of the International Brigades' medical services. The mainly German-speaking Eleventh Brigade, to which Jolly's equipo had been attached, was now part of the much larger Thirty-Fifth Division. All medical personnel serving with the International Brigades were also formally incorporated, with military rank, into the Republican Army. Some of Jolly's colleagues, who regarded their work as fundamentally noncombatant, found this an unwelcome development.[38] Jolly himself, however, with a family tradition of military service, is likely to have found it a proud and emotionally charged moment when he was issued his khaki uniform with its Republican Army five-pointed red star and his captain's twin bars. He kept these insignia with him for the rest of his life.

The medical service of the International Brigades eventually numbered more than two hundred foreign and Spanish doctors.[39] Apart from the Spanish, the largest and best organized group was North American, fielding fourteen surgical teams from May 1937.[40] About one in five of all the foreign doctors were women, an exceptionally high proportion for that period.[41] The great majority of the medical volunteers, including Jolly, averred no specific party or other political affiliation beyond their anti-fascist convictions.[42]

The first autochirs arrived in June 1937, funded by donations from Swiss trade unions. Built on a truck chassis and "the size of a moving van," they were designed to convert into fully functioning operating theaters in a matter of minutes.[43] While their design and gear varied, the first supplied to Jolly's equipo was equipped with an autoclave and copper oven for dry-sterilizing instruments, two operating tables, suitable lighting and heating systems, storage for supplies, and adequate facilities for scrubbing up. Sterilized surgical instruments were stored in separate metal containers according to their specific use. A refrigerator for storing conserved blood and even a small sewing machine and washing machine were included, plus a small electricity generator, making the vehicle entirely self-contained. Broggi found to his delight that these self-contained operating theaters incorporated "all the features we had hoped for."[44]

Jolly greatly valued the autochir for its capability to bring surgical services closer to the wounded soldiers his team served, but he found it too cramped for carrying out any but the most minor operations. Even the small, one-roomed stone shelters typically found in Spanish olive groves, he felt, were more suitable for performing complex emergency surgery.[45] Some of his colleagues disagreed. American surgeon Edward Barsky described the autochir as "a surgery on wheels. In it a surgeon, if he trains himself to stand still, can operate in perfect comfort under the most adverse conditions. . . . It revolutionizes our previous conception of frontline surgery."[46]

These purpose-designed vehicles became vital to, and symbolic of, the principle of providing an emergency surgical service as close as possible to the front line. Wounded soldiers were carried from the battlefield by *camilleros* (as stretcher-bearers were called in Spain), who sometimes used mules to carry two men at a time through steep terrain. They were brought first to the battalion first aid post, where they were typically given injections for pain and tetanus, torniquets if bleeding heavily, and splints for broken limbs. They could then be transported farther behind the lines in autochirs, in which surgeons provided further life-saving treatment, sometimes while under fire themselves. The injuries caused by modern weaponry were frequently contaminated with debris, and their treatment was further complicated by the patients' shock and blood loss. The most critically injured were driven to a No. 1 field hospital (also known, aptly, as a *hospital de sangre*, or "bloody hospital") about ten kilometers from the front and therefore out of range of artillery fire. In these temporary facilities for emergency surgery, wrote Colonel Telge in stirring, propagandist terms, "you will find the great and tireless English [*sic*] surgeon Dr. Jolly with the nurse operator Anne-Marie [Basch], or the well-known New York surgeon Dr. Barsky. . . . These comrades operate even when the house is shaking from the explosions of the bombs, but the scalpel and the needle do not shake in their hands."[47]

In addition to its autochir, each surgical team—a surgeon and assistant, two anesthetists, and nurses and orderlies—was assigned several ambulances and trucks for transport.[48] By extremely hard work, they could establish an emergency hospital in a suitably sited building such as a school, a convent, or a dung-strewn abandoned farmhouse within hours. Everyone pitched in without regard for rank, role, or social status, since "the traditional hierarchical divisions in British medicine disappeared, to some extent, in the grim realities of war."[49] Nurses performed minor operations such as removing pieces of shrapnel, acted as administrators, and took critical decisions about treatment, including euthanizing those beyond help.[50] At least one orderly, Jolly found, should preferably have professional experience as a barber so that patients could be shaved before an operation in the shortest time possible.[51] Anyone with knowledge of motor maintenance, plumbing, or other trades was called upon to use it, and Jolly paid tribute to the vital skills of his British mechanic, Harry Evans, for his work on repairing damaged vehicles and constructing other mechanical equipment from salvaged parts.[52]

After their rout at Guadalajara, the Nationalists turned their attention to the isolated and mainly Basque Republican stronghold in the north. It was during this campaign that the town of Durango was bombed, followed soon afterward by the near-total destruction of the Basques' spiritual capital of Guernica, in a calculated test by Franco's German and Italian allies of their latest aircraft and aerial destruction strategies. The clinical and sustained bombing of the town produced a civilian massacre and represented an entirely new and terrible form of warfare.

By late May 1937, the region's capital, Bilbao, was surrounded and facing heavy bombardment from both air and sea. In a desperate attempt to divert some of Franco's forces to another front, the Republicans launched an attack on the Roman-walled town of Segovia, about a hundred kilometers northwest of Madrid in the densely pine-forested Sierra de Guadarrama that was later the setting for Hemingway's civil war novel, *For Whom the Bell Tolls*.[53] A ski resort—the Club Alpino in a mountain pass at an altitude of fifteen hundred meters—was chosen for a field hospital. Its bar became an operating theater for Jolly, the Englishman Alex Tudor-Hart, and the highly competent young Catalan Moisès Broggi, who became one of Jolly's lifelong friends.[54] The injured were received and classified on the ground floor, where beds equipped to provide traction for fractures were installed.[55] For the four days of the attack on Segovia, wrote Broggi, "we could not close our eyes."[56]

Jolly himself was now acquiring a reputation throughout Republican Spain as a tireless and gifted clinician, and he was therefore a popular subject for wartime propaganda purposes. In late May, he was joined on a trip to this new hospital by the Czech polyglot Augustina "Gusti" Jirku. Born into privilege in the old Hapsburg empire, she took a remarkable career turn and worked for Moscow's foreign-language publishing service. She was sent to Spain to direct the press and promotional arm of the International Brigades' health service and wrote a booklet, *We Fight Death: The Work of the Medical Service of the International Brigades in Spain*, with a preface by "Dr. Jolly, Division Commandant-Surgeon."

Jirku also launched a multilingual periodical titled *AMI* (*Ayuda Médica Internacional* [International medical aid]) and evidently felt that the journey to Guadarrama might make good copy for it.

> It was a pleasant, sunny May day and the trenches looked like peaceful furrows in the red Spanish earth. Occasionally a khaki beret popped up among the rocks and the prickly scrub, with a tanned forehead and black

eyes below. . . . "Where is the front line?" I asked. "All around us: on the ground and in the air," the Brigade's chief surgeon, Mr Jolly, told me. He was driving his camouflaged car himself because his Spanish chauffeur regarded every car ahead as a rival to be overtaken at any price. Mr Jolly preferred to take the wheel himself on dangerous stretches.

We were driving towards a newly captured village. The Fascists had fled, the Republican troops had advanced and occupied the place, and the medical transports, doctors and nurses had followed almost at once. Mr Jolly wanted to make quite sure that everything was running smoothly. We raced over the bumpy Guadarrama road. During the last few days it had drunk a great deal of blood; Fascist bombers and artillery had tried, again and again, to cut this vital Republican artery. To the left, I saw cornfields pitted with black craters, and peasants harvesting what little of the crop had escaped the flames. To the right, under high cliffs, wandered herds of goats, and far in the background lay the dark chain of the Sierra de Guadarrama, crowned with snow.

The car climbed steep, narrow, hairpin bends in a cloud of dust. We overtook ambulances and heavily laden lorries, with only a few inches to spare. Then, quite suddenly, we saw a squadron of Fascist bombers break through the clouds. A second squadron followed and then a third, but that was ours; a handful of Loyalist fighters, all we possessed. They were faster than the enemy's heavy bombers and soon we heard the rattling of machine-guns and saw little white puffs in the sky. The driver made the sign of the cross. "Our field hospital will be one of their targets," Mr Jolly said in his calm, very English voice. "There are some more coming," the chauffeur said.

Above the plain ahead of us, four Junkers appeared; bright little dots that quickly disappeared in geysers of black smoke. At the side of the road, our ack-ack [antiaircraft] guns opened up. A tank came towards us and took cover behind a group of high cacti. A motorcyclist threw himself into the ditch. The Junkers were right above our heads. We kept racing over the bumpy road, and the car bounced furiously over corrugations, potholes and loose stones. Then there was a dull crash; the earth shook and we all missed a heartbeat. On the side of the road, thirty yards behind us, rose a pillar of smoke. "What lousy shots," Mr Jolly said without turning his head. We drove into the village street past scores of smoking ruins. . . .

> Scarcely an hour after we arrived, there was a second air-raid. All the patients who could walk were taken to a cellar. Meanwhile, Mr Jolly performed a stomach operation in the improvised theatre on the first floor, with bombs falling no more than fifty yards away. The blast shattered the windows and there was a shower of broken glass, followed by a stream of dust and smoke. Mr Jolly worked on in complete silence and with perfectly steady hands, while the Czech doctor assisted and Anne-Marie [Basch], the white-haired Hungarian nurse, passed instruments with the precision of a machine.[57]

Even allowing for the exaggeration and selectivity that is said to be the first casualty of war, this eyewitness account indicates the now widely renowned New Zealand surgeon was capable of maintaining a remarkable composure in the face of imminent danger and that this nonchalance inspired his colleagues to do likewise.

The conduct of the battle of Guadarrama—an initial Republican advance followed by a much stronger Nationalist counterattack that outnumbered and ultimately overwhelmed the Republican forces—was, sadly, to be repeated elsewhere with only minor variations for much of the rest of the war. In each case, the frontline surgeons worked furiously during the height of the battle and, once a retreat was ordered, were generally withdrawn to base hospitals some distance behind the lines. At least three of these base hospitals were in the vicinity of the Club Alpino field hospital, and Jolly probably worked at more than one in the intensifying furnace of the Castilian plain's "three months of hell," his first Spanish summer.

In a letter to his mother, Jolly revealed that in mid-June he had taken a rare rest break on Spain's south coast to recover from an unspecified illness. Together with his anesthetist Peter de Sarigny and American driver Joe Coombes, he stayed in a hotel in the small fishing village of Calpe, about sixty kilometers north of Alicante. "It was glorious—hot, hot sun every day, bathing in the Mediterranean, not to be bettered anywhere." He returned to find orders to pack up and prepare to move to a new location. "Again the problems attendant upon the establishment of a new hospital—to find beds, personnel and all the necessary furniture and equipment. This moving and installing oneself afresh I find the least agreeable part of the life here." The Grant family, he told his mother, had invited him to spend a month in Scotland with them in August, "but it is a fond hope. The need here is none the less and it is likely to be even greater if a decisive offensive is at last launched by our or the other side. . . . The Spanish Army has grown tremendously, with the subsequent increased need for medical organisations."[58]

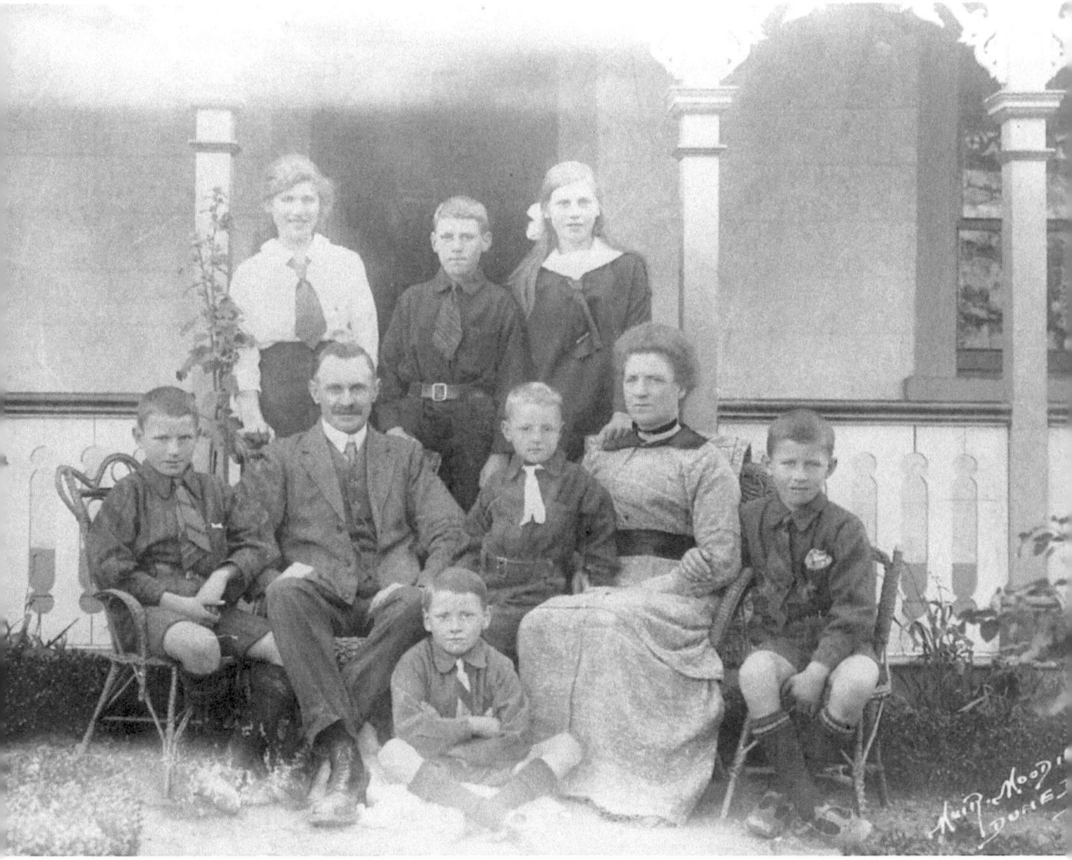

1. The close-knit and confident Jolly family, ca. 1914. Young Doug Jolly *at left*, and his unofficially adopted sister, Blanche Waddell, *standing left*. Photo: courtesy A. Ellison.

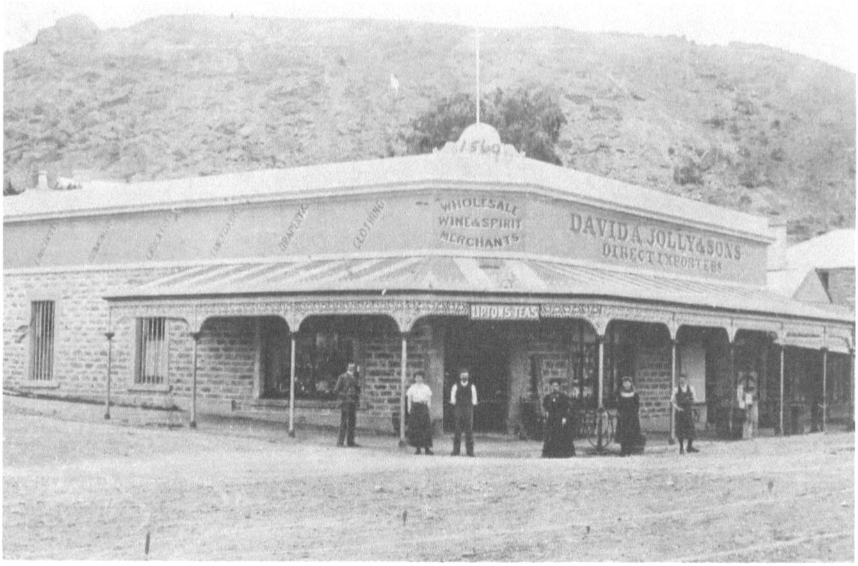

2. The Jolly general store, Cromwell, in 1903. Photo: Ron Murray collection, Hocken Collections Uare Taoka o Hākena, University of Otago.

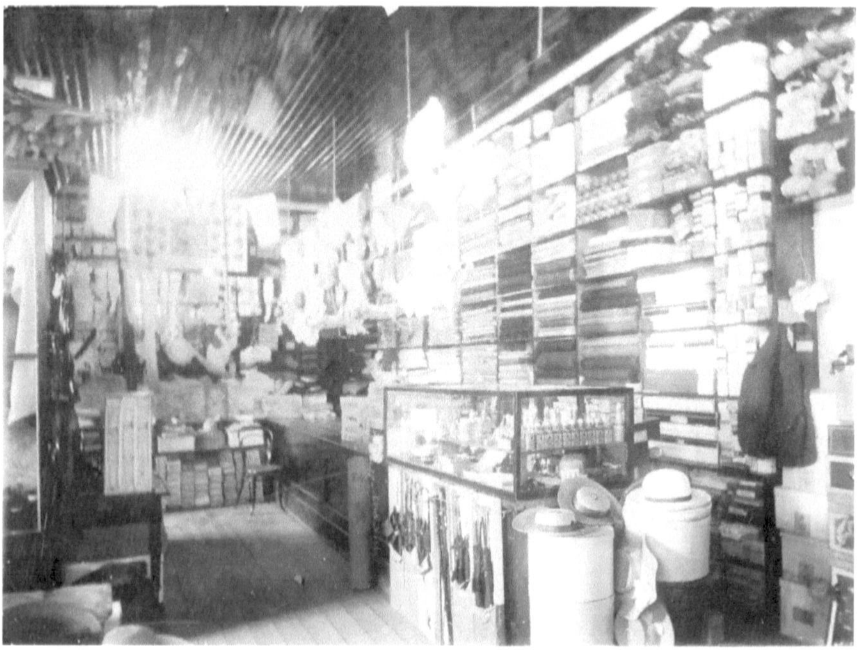

3. The Aladdin's cave that was the interior of the family's general store. Photo: Cromwell Museum.

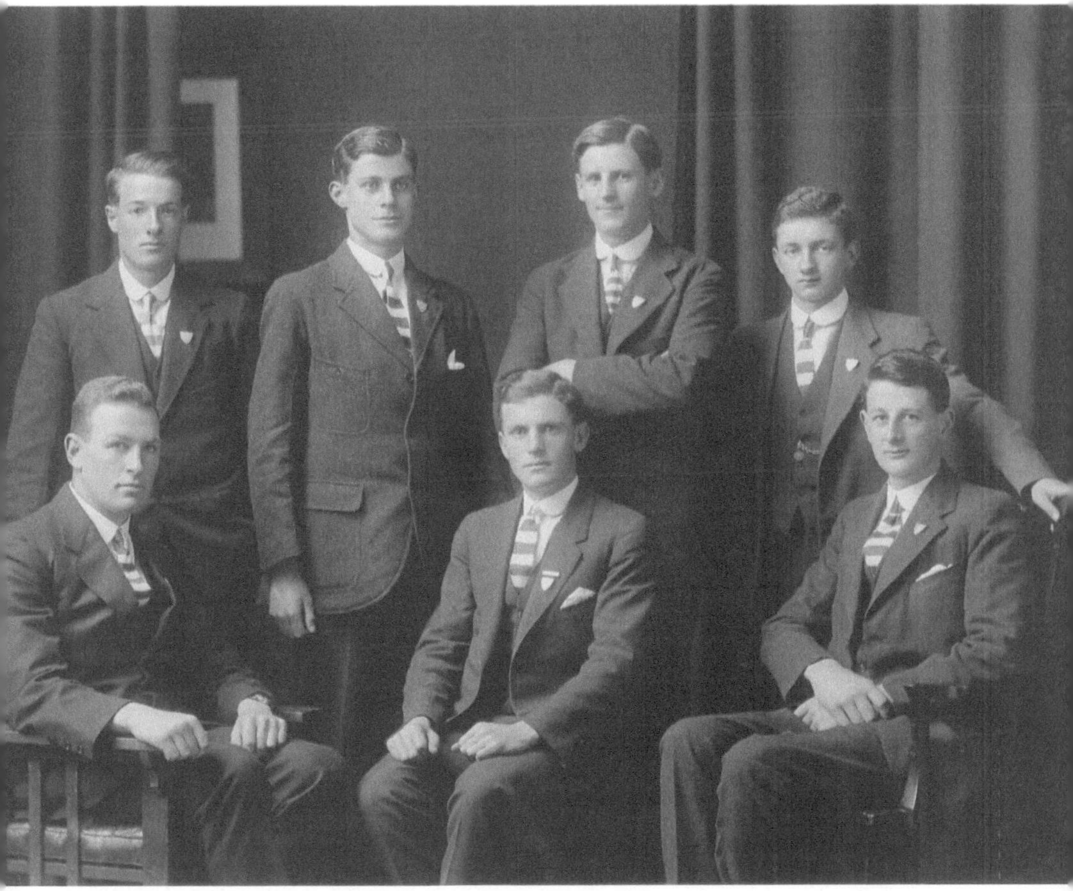

4. Champion athlete, indifferent scholar, popular role model—Jolly, *seated center*, was one of six prefects, or student leaders, in his final year at high school, 1923. Photo: Otago Boys' High School.

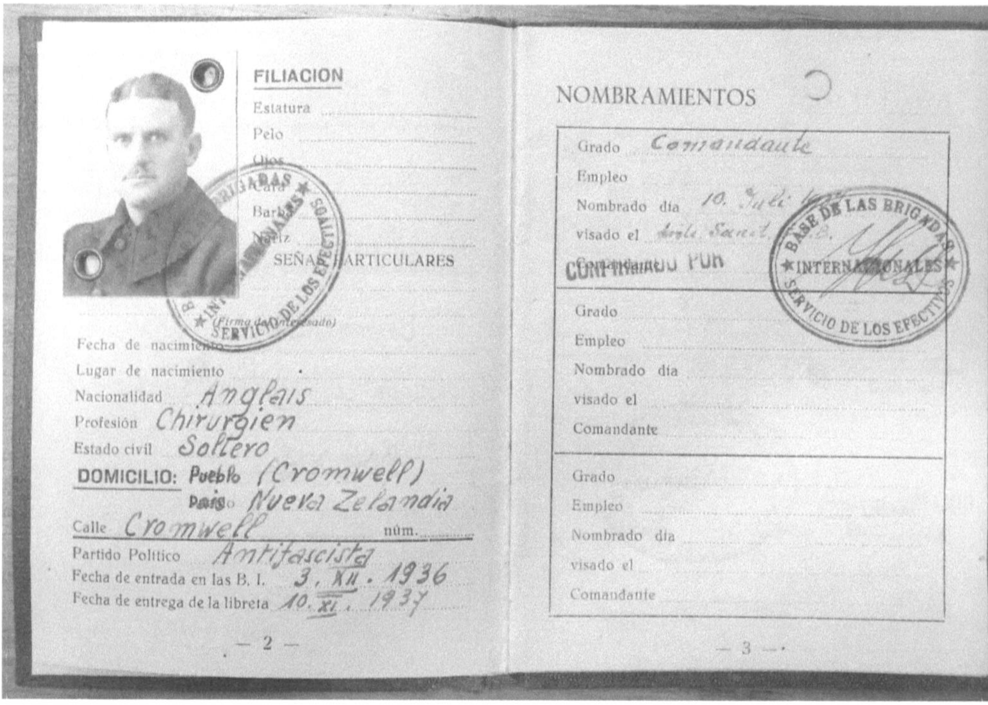

FILIACION

Estatura

Pelo

Ojos

Cara

Barba

Nariz

SEÑAS PARTICULARES

(Firma del interesado)

Fecha de nacimiento

Lugar de nacimiento

Nacionalidad Anglais

Profesión Chirurgien

Estado civil Soltero

DOMICILIO: Pueblo (Cromwell)

País Nueva Zelandia

Calle Cromwell núm.

Partido Politico Antifascista

Fecha de entrada en las B. I. 3. XII. 1936

Fecha de entrega de la libreta 10. XI. 1937

— 2 —

NOMBRAMIENTOS

Grado Comandante

Empleo

Nombrado día

visado el

Comandante

CONFIRMADO POR

BASE DE LAS BRIGADAS INTERNACIONALES SERVICIO DE LOS EFECTIVOS

Grado

Empleo

Nombrado día

visado el

Comandante

Grado

Empleo

Nombrado día

visado el

Comandante

— 3 —

5. In a mixture of French and Spanish, Jolly's Republican Army passbook gives his nationality as English, his profession as surgeon, and his political affiliation as anti-fascist, 1936. Photo: Bidda Jones Collection, Hocken Collections Uare Taoka o Hākena, University of Otago. Used with permission by Bidda Jones.

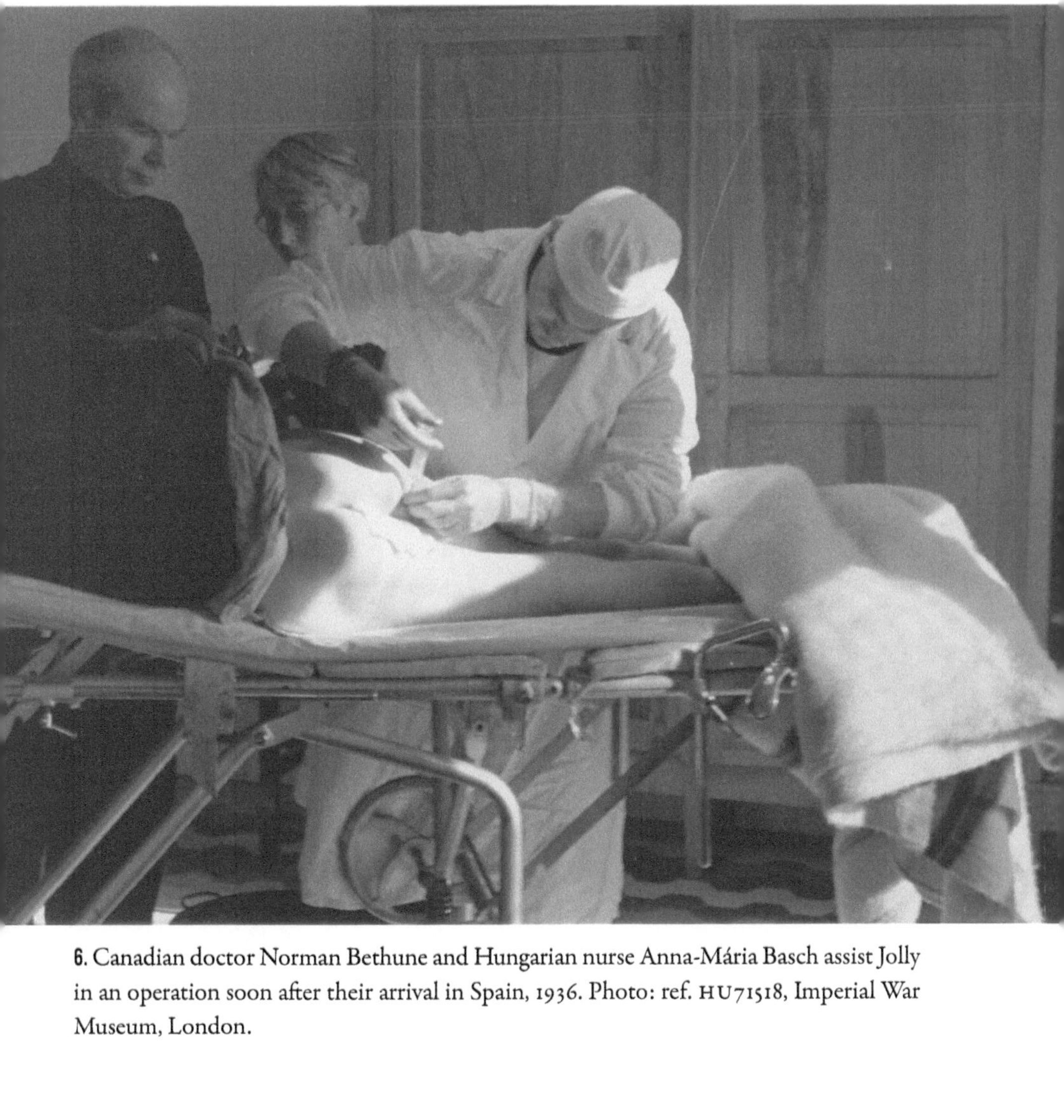

6. Canadian doctor Norman Bethune and Hungarian nurse Anna-Mária Basch assist Jolly in an operation soon after their arrival in Spain, 1936. Photo: ref. HU71518, Imperial War Museum, London.

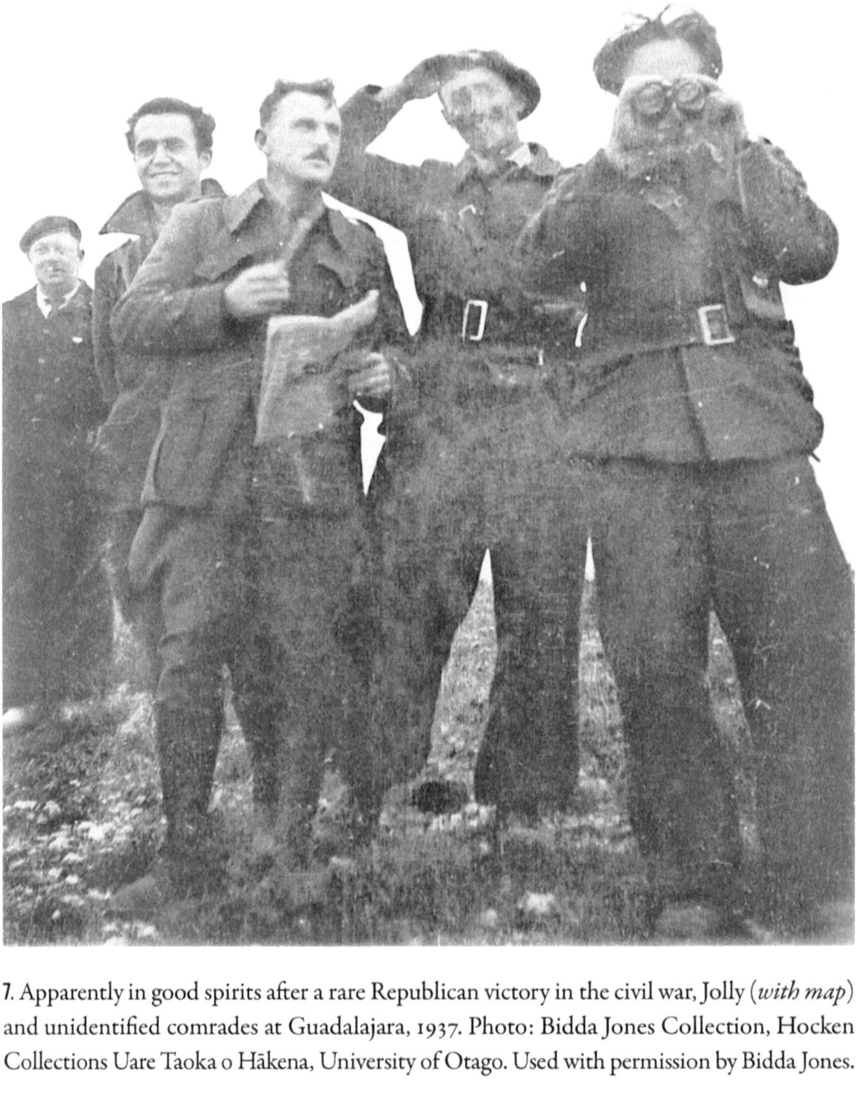

7. Apparently in good spirits after a rare Republican victory in the civil war, Jolly (*with map*) and unidentified comrades at Guadalajara, 1937. Photo: Bidda Jones Collection, Hocken Collections Uare Taoka o Hākena, University of Otago. Used with permission by Bidda Jones.

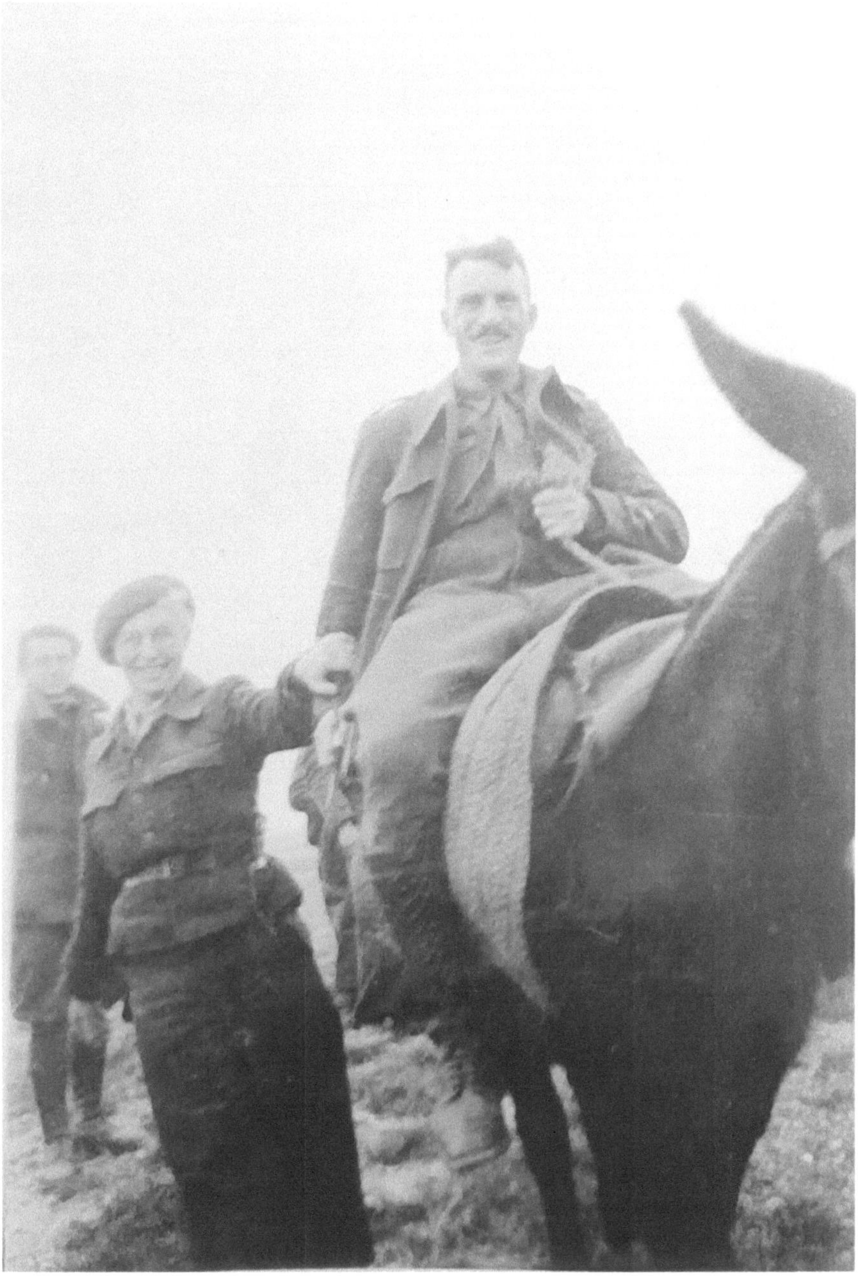

8. With his theater nurse and lover Anna-Mária Basch, Jolly enjoys an outing by *mula* (mule), the all-purpose means of transport in rural Spain. Photo: Basch family collection.

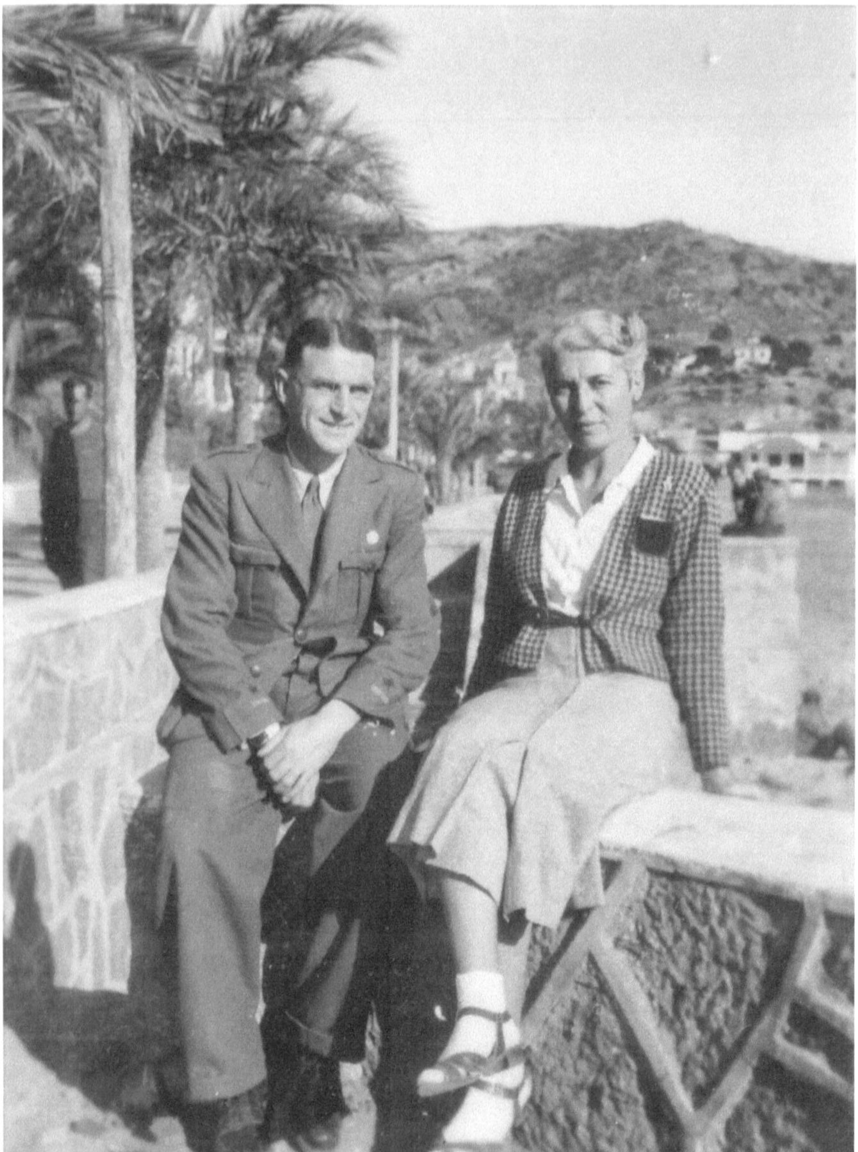

9. Recuperating from the horrors of Brunete, Jolly and Basch make a handsome couple in the restful Mediterranean resort town of Benicàssim, 1937. Photo: Basch family collection.

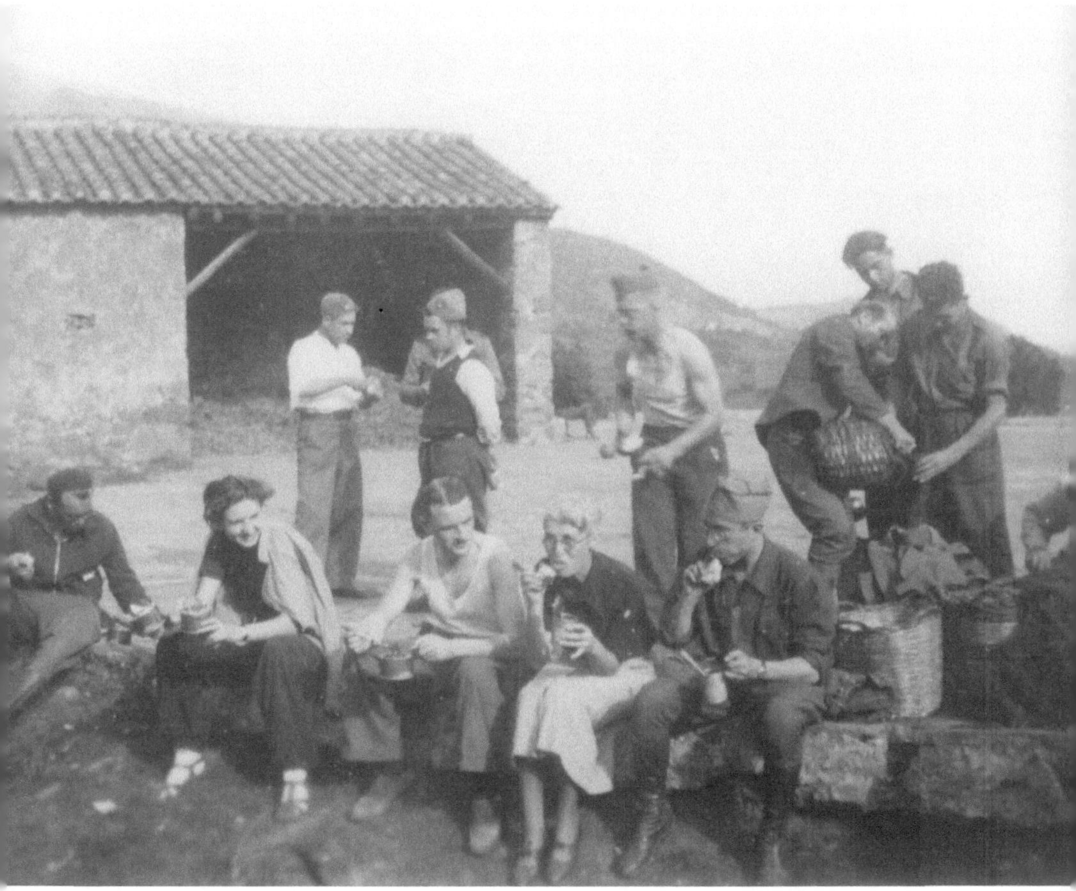

10. Filling wine bottles and spooning beans, Jolly, Basch, and other medical volunteers picnic in the courtyard of a farmhouse, probably in the Ebro Valley, summer 1938. Photo: ref. 81-338, Hungarian National Museum.

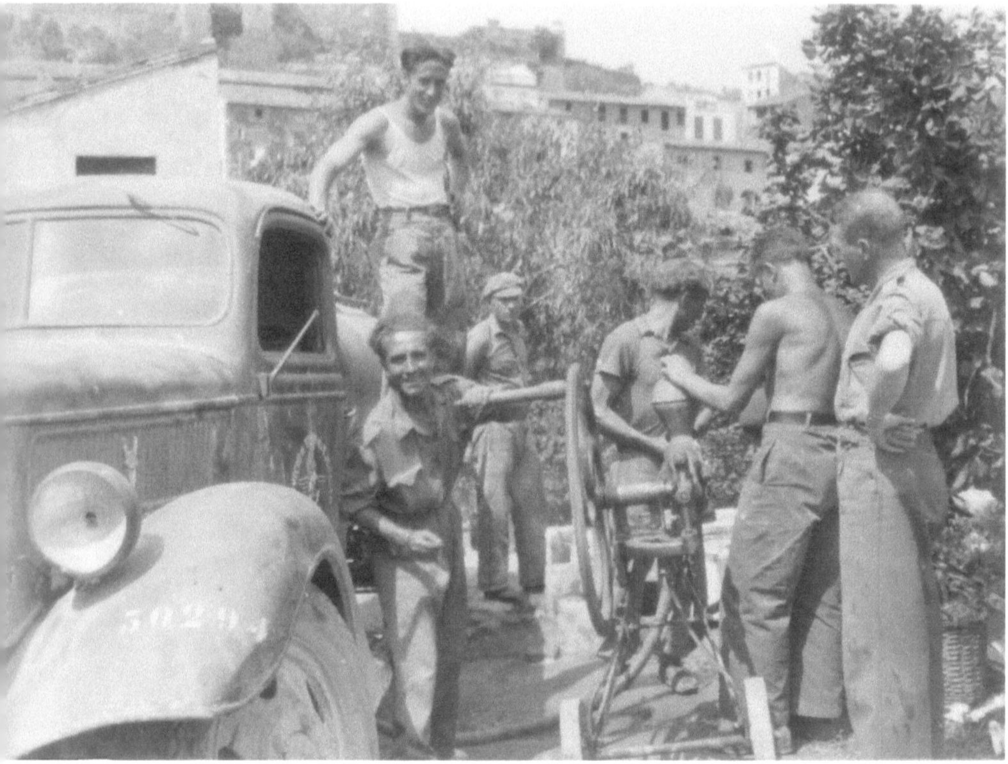

11. *Standing at right*, Jolly watches Hungarian International Brigaders fill a tanker truck from a mobile pump in Ebro Valley, summer 1938. Photo: ref. 81-317, Hungarian National Museum.

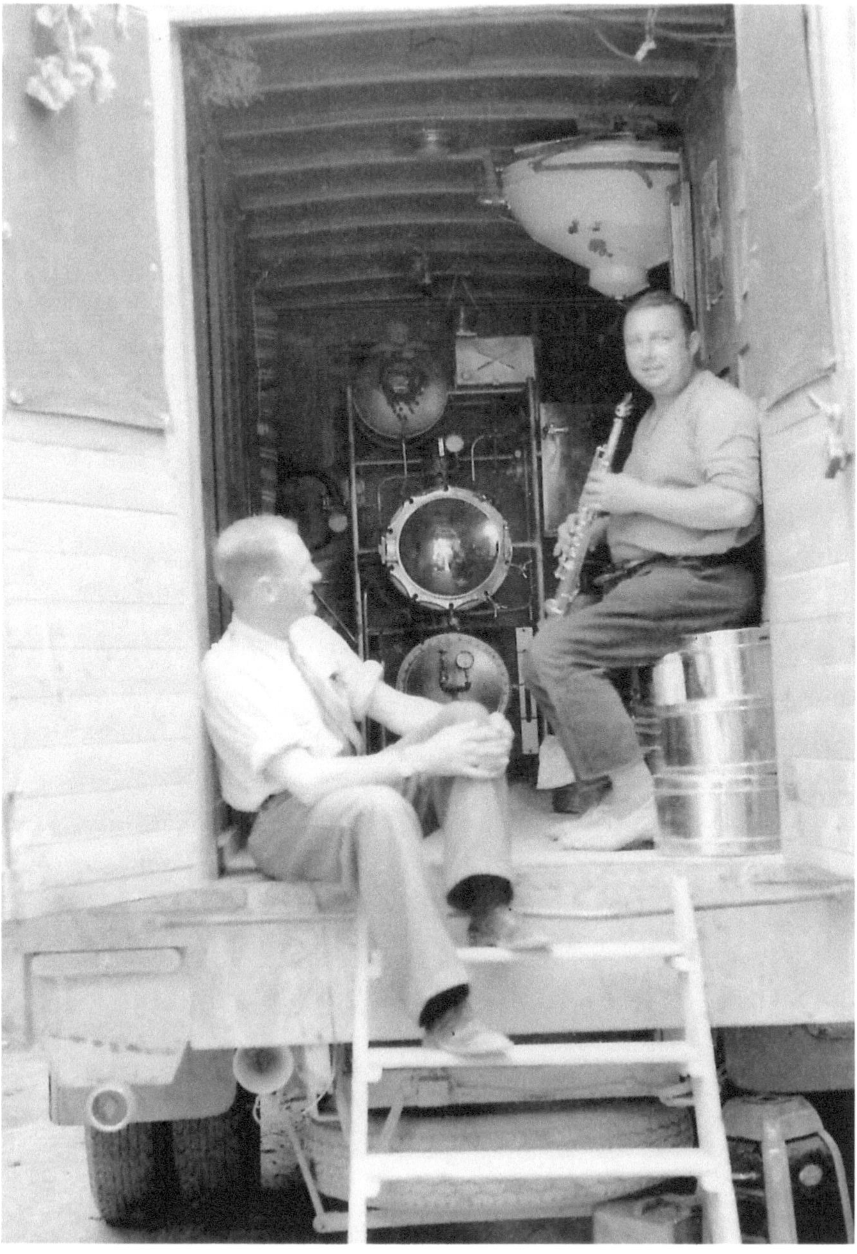

12. A fine singer whose voice was in demand at parties, Jolly appears to be practicing with an unidentified musician in the back of a sterilizer truck used for cleaning hospital bedding. Field hospital at Mas d'en Magrinyà, near Marça, 1938. Photo: Fernando Iaffa, Maximo Iaffa collection.

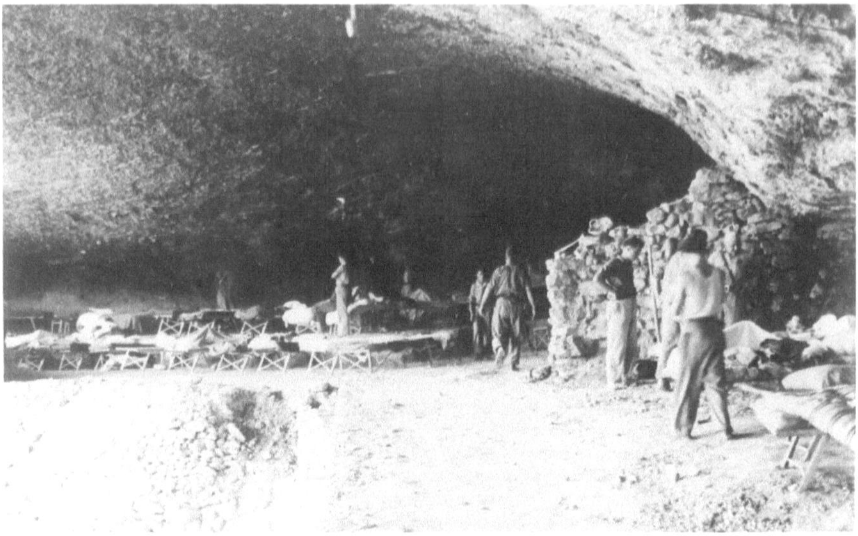

13. "The safest place in Spain," the field hospital built inside the Cova de Santa Llúcia near La Bisbal de Falset, Ebro Valley, 1938. Photo: HU33108, Imperial War Museum, London.

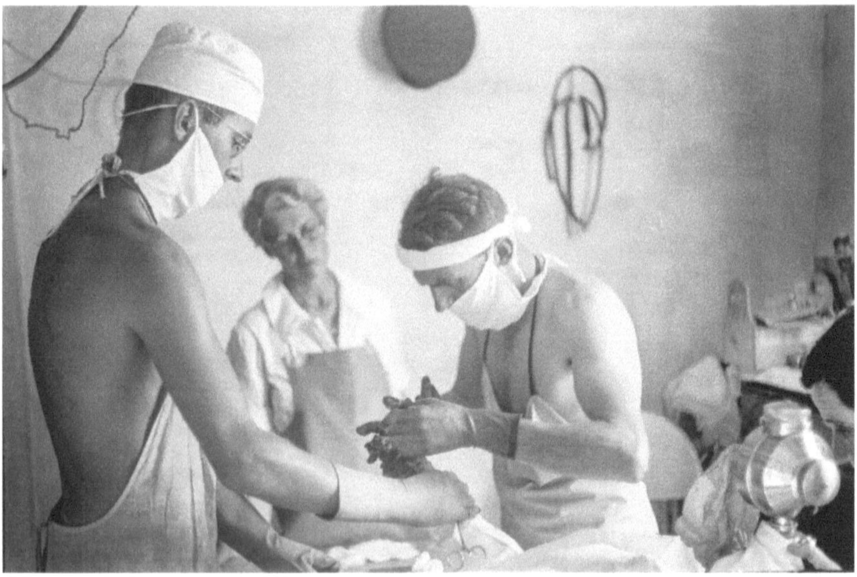

14. Shirtless in the stifling midsummer heat, American surgeon Franklin Bissell and Jolly, with nurse Anna-Mária Basch, at work in the field hospital in the Ermita (Hermitage) Santa Magdalena, Ebro Valley, 1938. Photo: #55-20 taken by Alec Wainman, © The Estate of Alexander Wheeler Wainman, John Alexander Wainman.

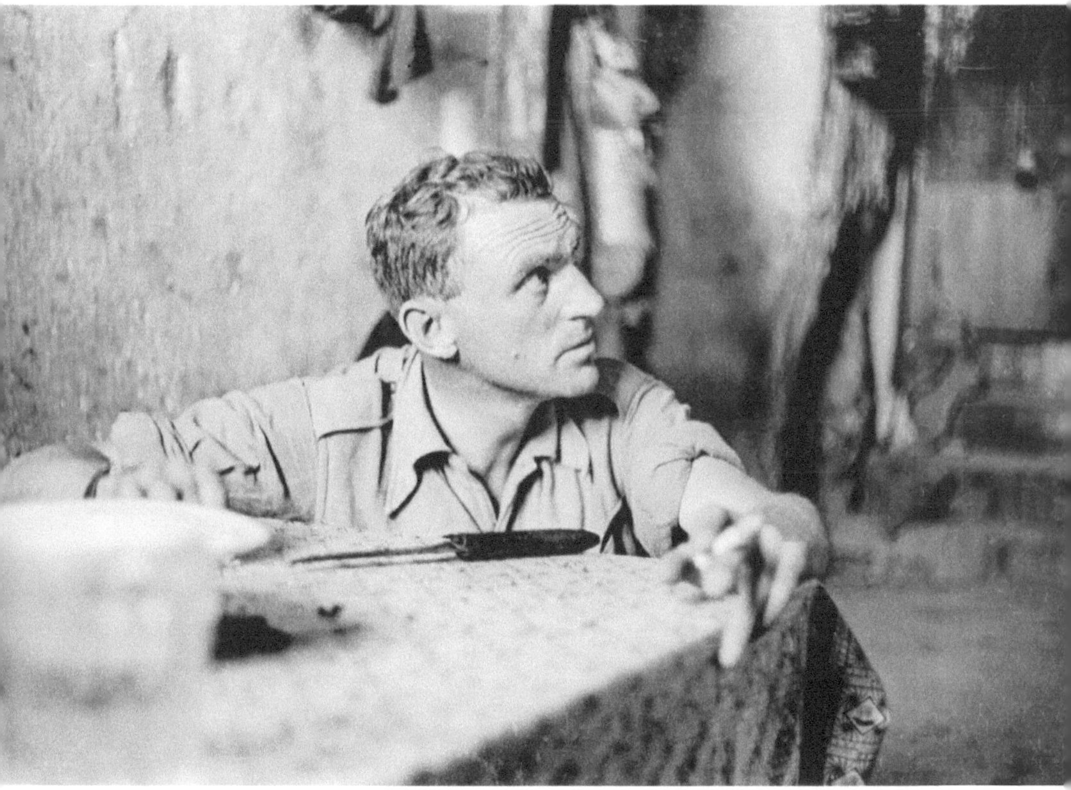

15. Cigarette in hand, and perhaps listening for enemy bombers, Doug Jolly takes a break from his operating table at the field hospital in the Ermita (Hermitage) Santa Magdalena, Ebro Valley, 1938. Photo: #54-19 taken by Alec Wainman, © The Estate of Alexander Wheeler Wainman, John Alexander Wainman.

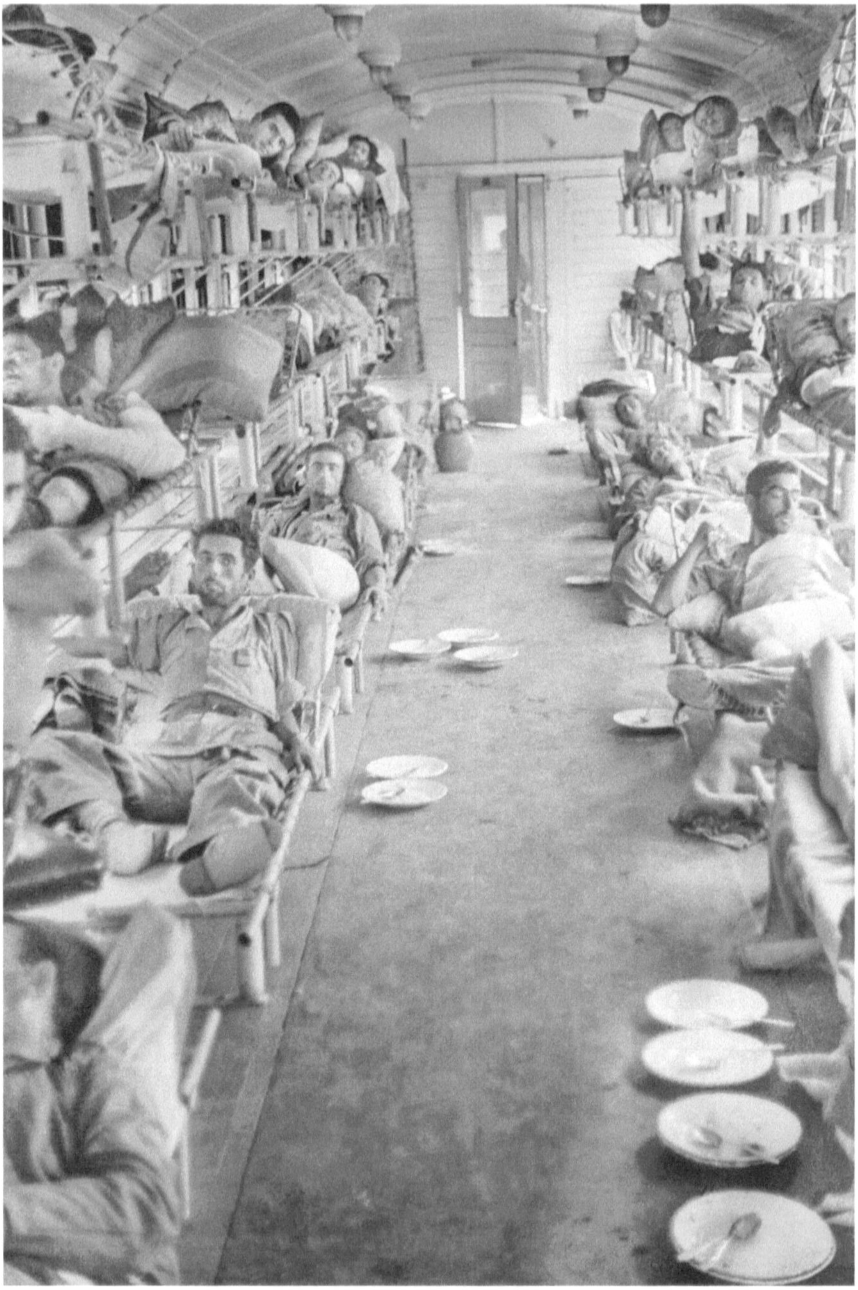

16. Mealtime for the patients of this three-level hospital train standing in the railway tunnel of l'Argentera, Ebro, 1938. Photo: #56-34 taken by Alec Wainman, © The Estate of Alexander Wheeler Wainman, John Alexander Wainman.

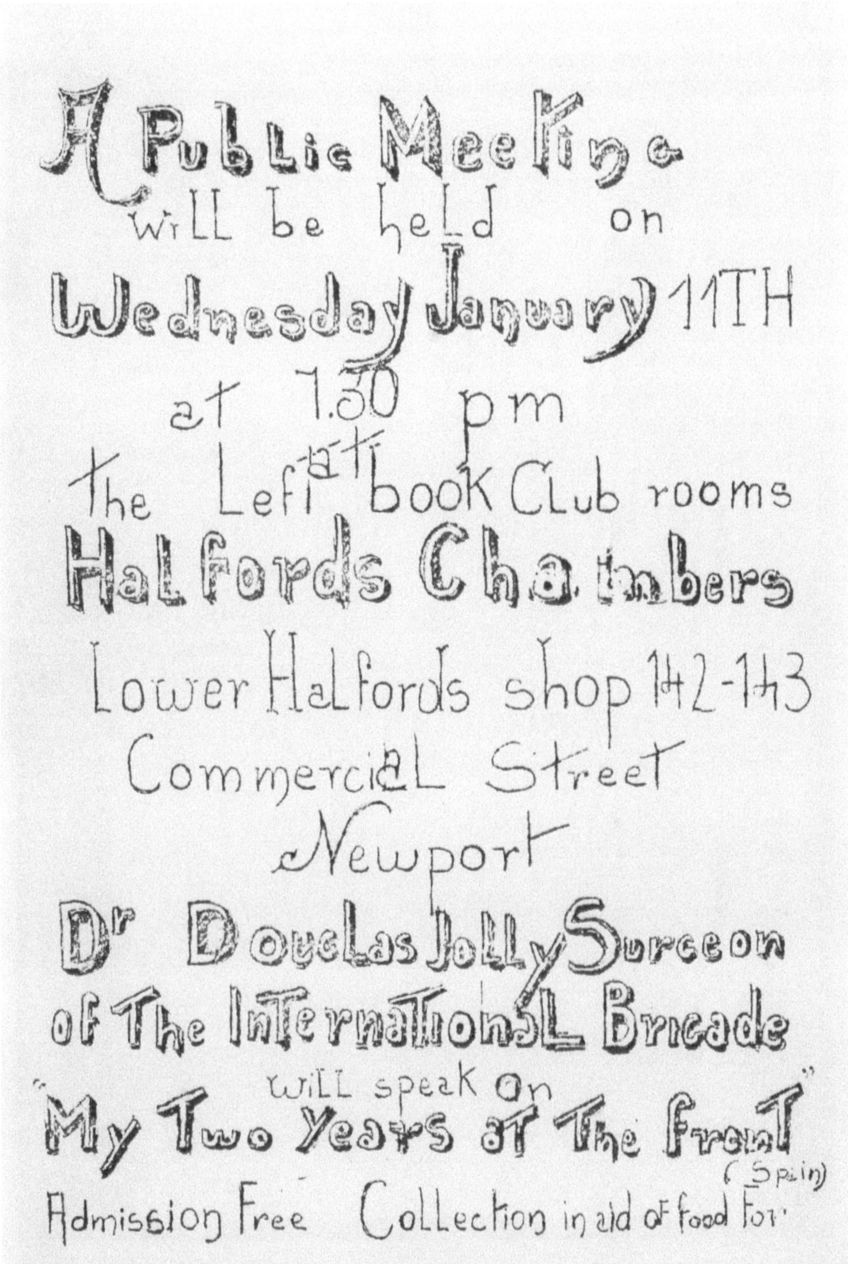
A Public Meeting
will be held on
Wednesday January 11TH
at 7.30 pm
the Left at book Club rooms
Halfords Chambers
Lower Halfords shop 142-143
Commercial Street
Newport
Dr Douglas Jolly Surgeon
of The International Brigade
will speak on
"My Two Years at The Front"
(Spain)
Admission Free Collection in aid of food for

17. On his return from Spain in late 1938, Jolly gave many public talks around Britain. This hand-lettered notice advertises one in Newport, south Wales. Photo: Núala Grant papers, Hocken Collections Uare Taoka o Hākena, University of Otago.

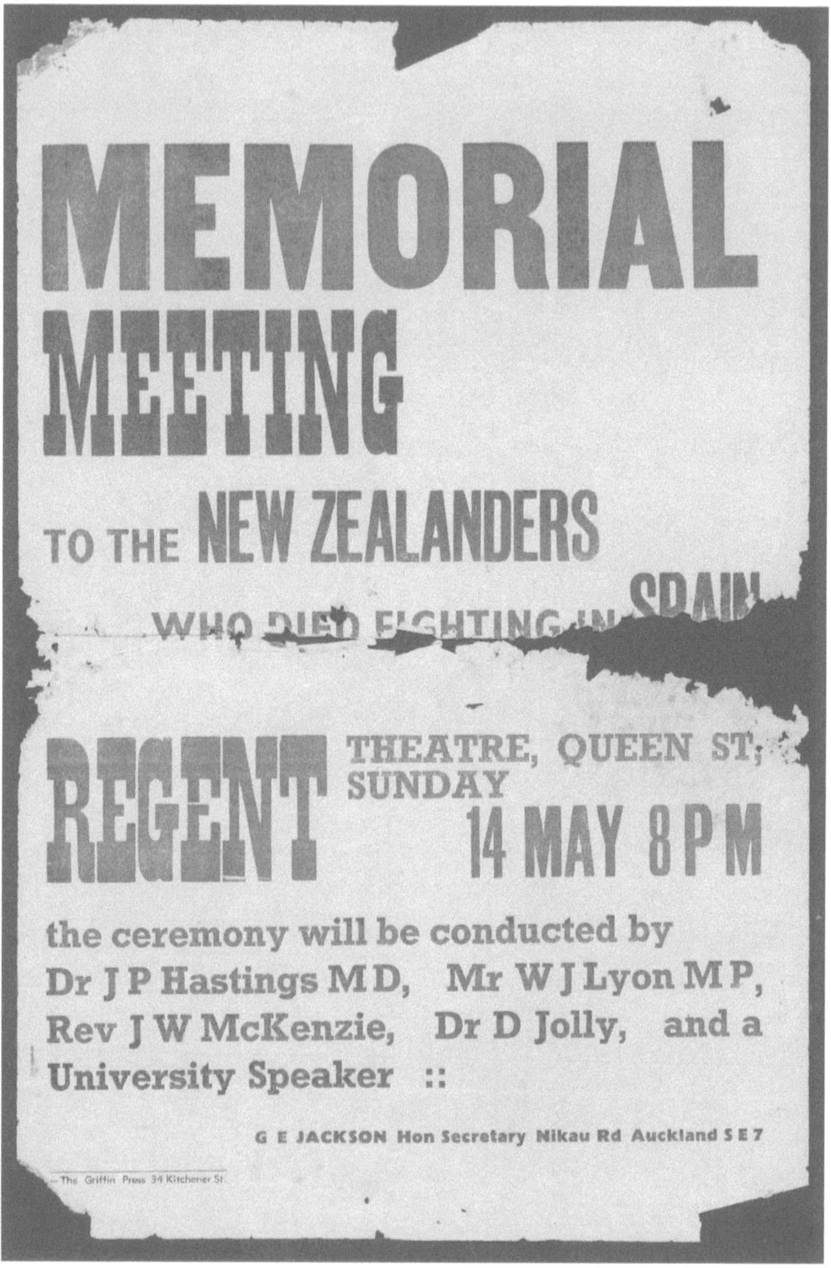
MEMORIAL
MEETING
TO THE NEW ZEALANDERS
WHO DIED FIGHTING IN SPAIN
REGENT
THEATRE, QUEEN ST,
SUNDAY
14 MAY 8 P M
the ceremony will be conducted by
Dr J P Hastings M D, Mr W J Lyon M P,
Rev J W McKenzie, Dr D Jolly, and a
University Speaker ::
G E JACKSON Hon Secretary Nikau Rd Auckland S E 7
The Griffin Press 34 Kitchener St

18. Returning to his homeland after more than seven years, Jolly toured the country, speaking in support of the Spanish Republic. This May 1939 meeting in Auckland commemorated five New Zealanders who died fighting in Spain. Photo: ref. 90-234-05/2-02, Alexander Turnbull Library, Wellington, New Zealand.

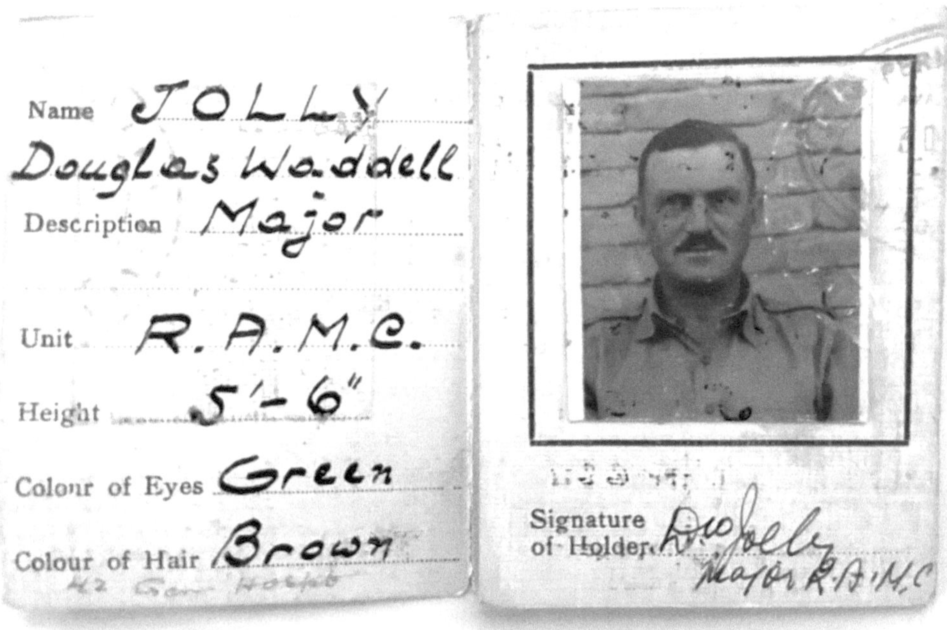
Name JOLLY
Douglas Waddell
Description Major
Unit R.A.M.C.
Height 5'-6"
Colour of Eyes Green
Colour of Hair Brown
Signature of Holder
Major R.A.M.C

19. With the rank of major, Jolly enlisted in Britain's Royal Army Medical Corps in 1940. Photo: Bidda Jones collection, Jolly papers, Hocken Collections Uare Taoka o Hākena, University of Otago. Used with permission by Bidda Jones.

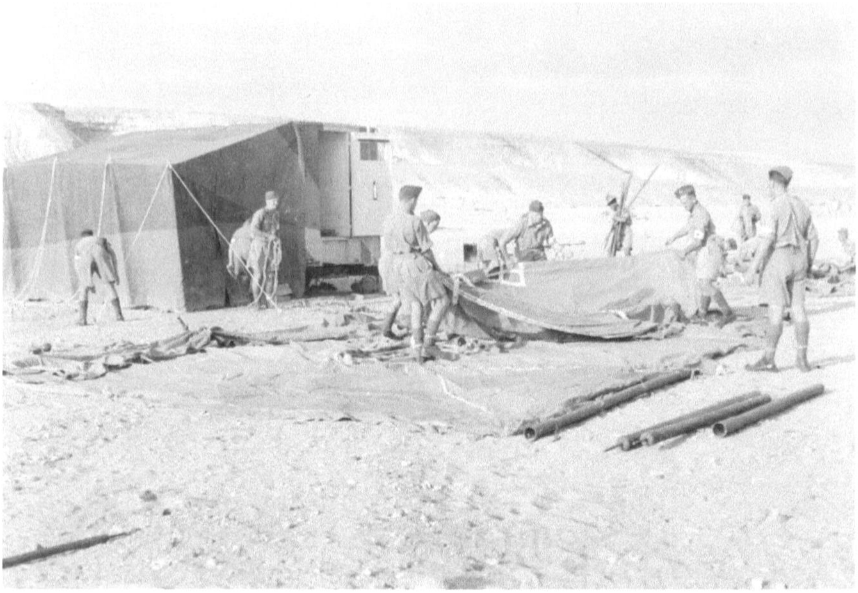

20. The NZ Army's Mobile Surgical Unit, seen here setting up a field hospital in Maadi, Egypt, in 1941, was modeled on the "three-points-forward" system Jolly developed in Spain. Photo: ref. DA 1943, National Army Museum, New Zealand.

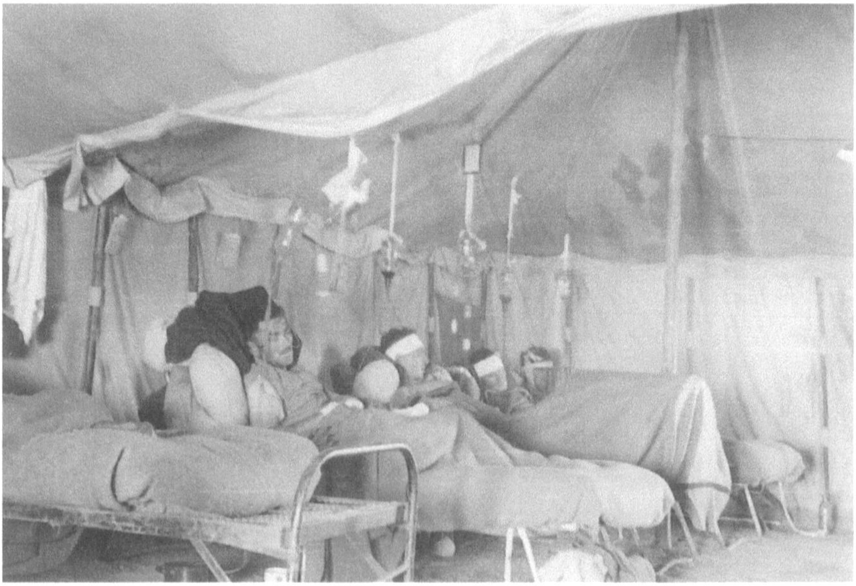

21. Injured troops in the NZ Mobile Surgical Unit's postoperative recovery tent, 1941. Photo: Stanley Wilson, Anna Hunt collection.

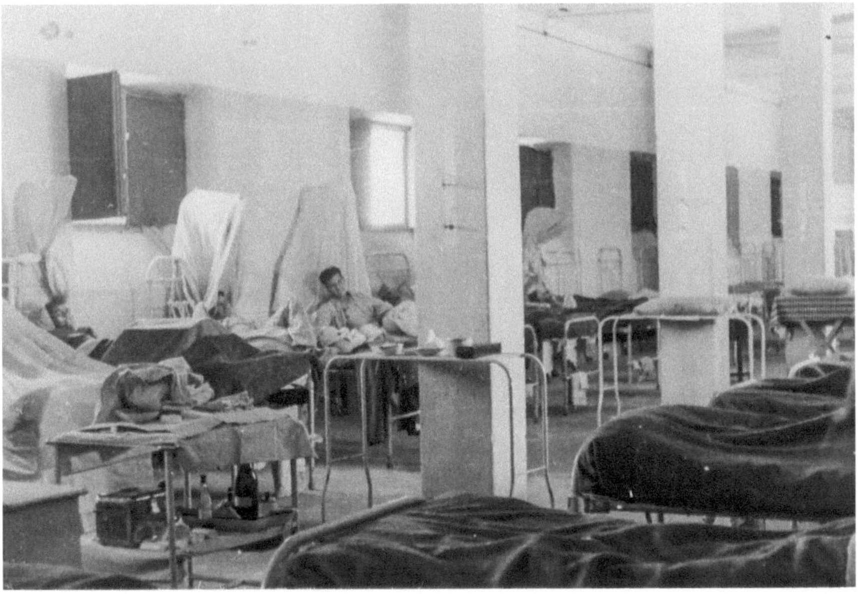

22. No. 62 General Hospital in Tobruk, Libya, where Jolly served as chief surgeon in 1941, was based in a former school building that still displayed pro-Mussolini slogans. Photo: ref. RAMC/1302, Wellcome Collection. Image courtesy of the Board of Trustees of the Museum of Military Medicine Trust.

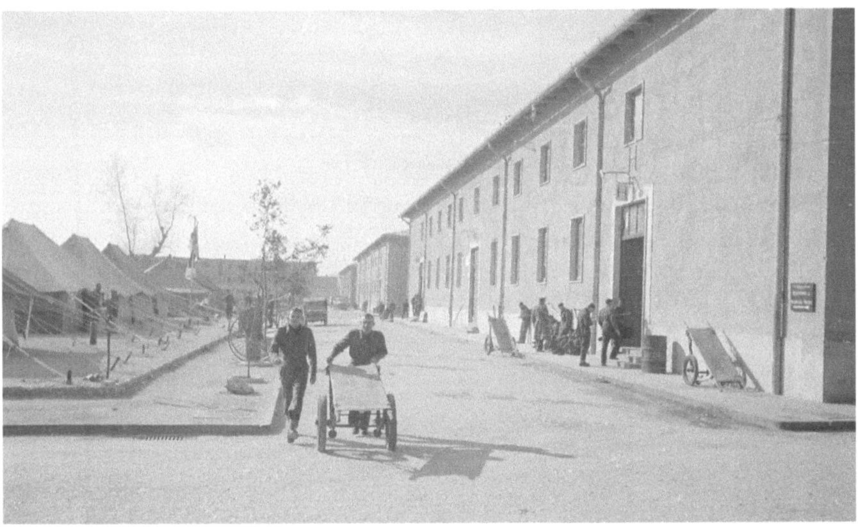

23. Wheeling a stretcher through the courtyard at the No. 2 New Zealand General Hospital in Caserta, Italy, 1944. Photo: ref. DA-05239-F, Alexander Turnbull Library, Wellington, New Zealand.

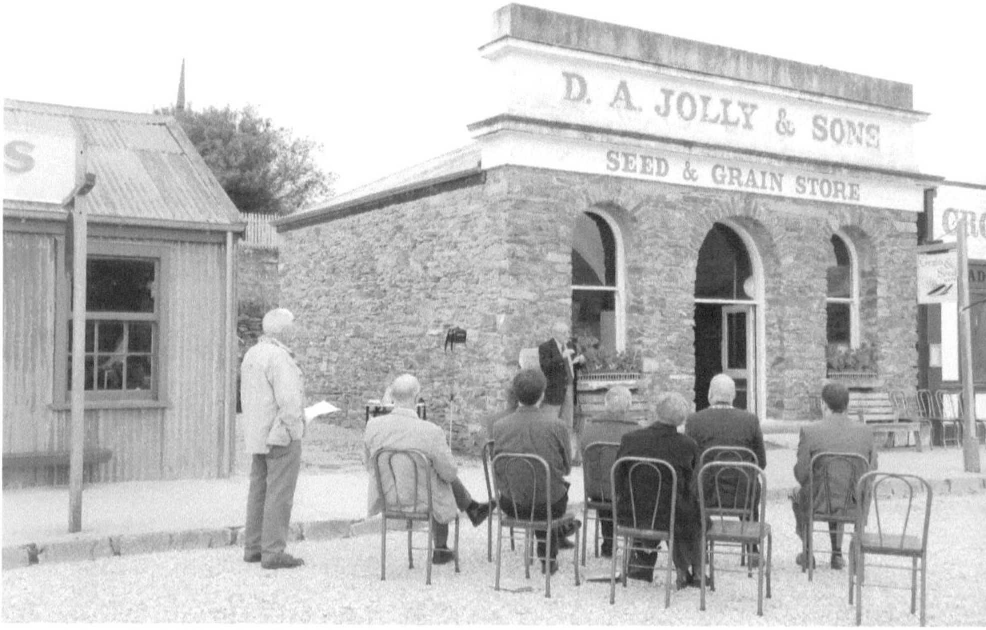

24. The stone-built general store founded by Doug Jolly's grandfather in 1870 still stands in Cromwell, central Otago, although now relocated above an artificial lake. In 2018 a plaque to Jolly was unveiled at the store. Photo: Jo McKenzie-McLean, Stuff Limited.

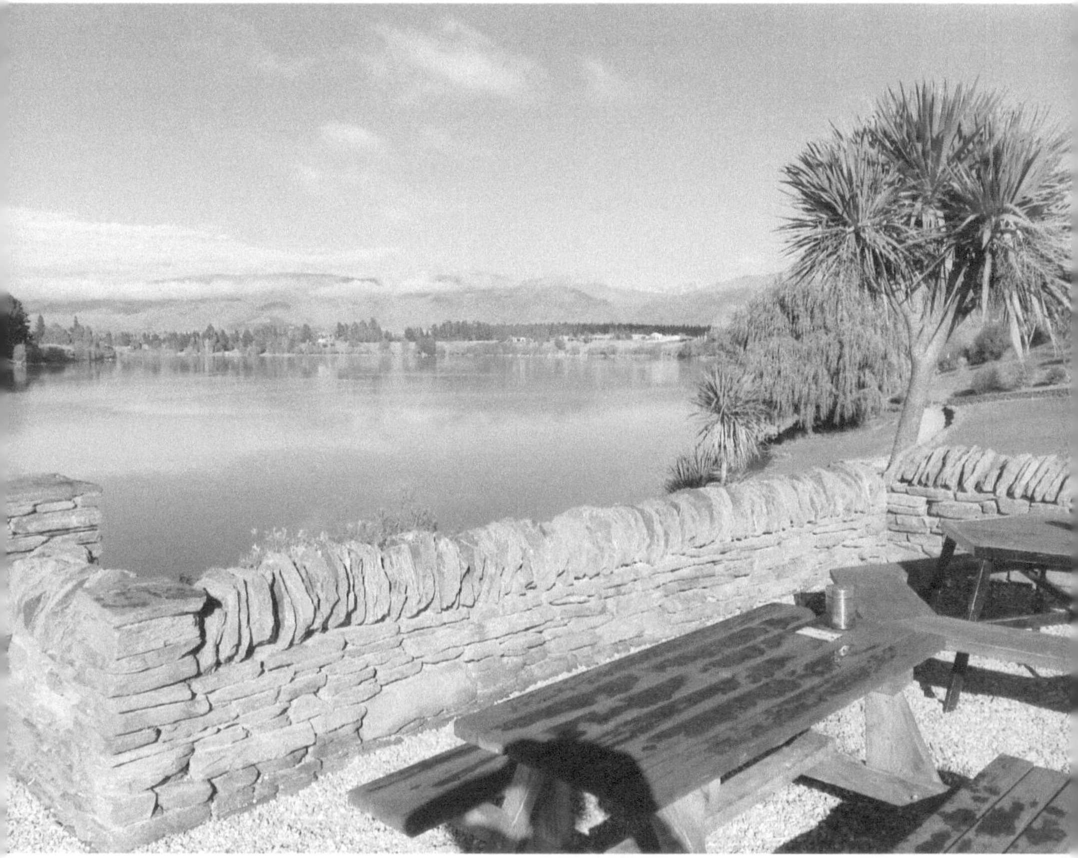

25. The magnificent setting of Lake Dunstan, Cromwell, where the Jolly family's general store now stands. Photo: Mark Derby.

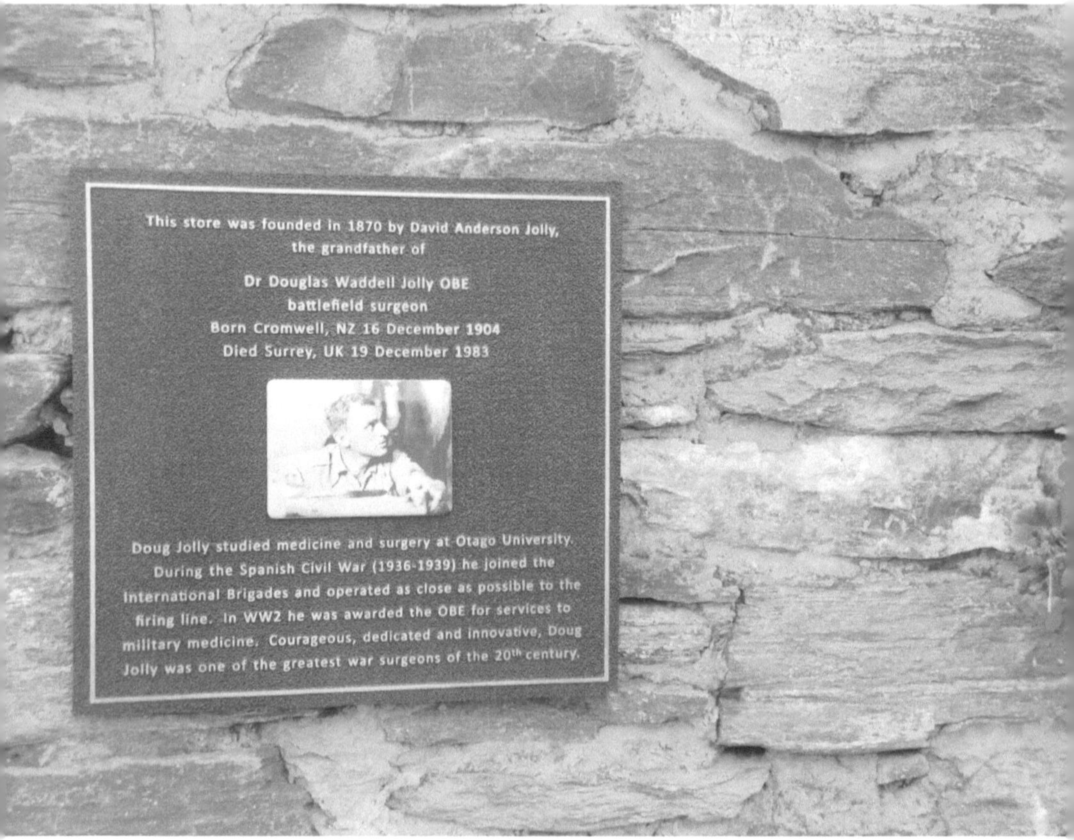
This store was founded in 1870 by David Anderson Jolly,
the grandfather of
Dr Douglas Waddell Jolly OBE
battlefield surgeon
Born Cromwell, NZ 16 December 1904
Died Surrey, UK 19 December 1983
Doug Jolly studied medicine and surgery at Otago University.
During the Spanish Civil War (1936-1939) he joined the
International Brigades and operated as close as possible to the
firing line. In WW2 he was awarded the OBE for services to
military medicine. Courageous, dedicated and innovative, Doug
Jolly was one of the greatest war surgeons of the 20th century.

26. The small and isolated community of Cromwell acknowledges the internationally significant achievements of an expatriate former resident. Photo: Mark Derby.

9 He Does Honor to His Name

As Jolly's latest instructions indicated, in the summer of 1937 the Republican Army launched an attack with the greatest concentration of troops and matériel it had yet assembled in the war: more than seventy thousand troops and all of the precious tanks, other armored vehicles, field guns, and aircraft that could be spared from other fronts. This massive force was directed at a tiny, hitherto barely noticeable village called Brunete, about twenty-five kilometers west of Madrid. The dual aim of the offensive was to shatter the Nationalist cordon around the capital by cutting off its supplies and reinforcements from the west and to relieve pressure on the northern front, where the provincial capital of Bilbao had recently fallen but the stubborn Basques elsewhere in the province had refused to surrender. A clear Republican victory at this critical point in the civil war might prove to the world that its army could do more than conduct doomed holding actions and could seize new territory from the Nationalists. Brunete, one historian of the civil war has written, "was an important step forward in the evolution of the Republican Army. At Madrid and Jarama, in previous months, it had been on the defensive. At Guadalajara it achieved a victorious counter-offensive. At Brunete, taking the initiative, it passed over to the offensive."[1]

The Republican Army's medical services were required to expand in size and capability to match this growth. Jolly's and the other international units were no longer assigned to specific brigades but rather to the much larger and newly formed Thirty-Fifth Division, which incorporated all the International Brigades and expected to serve as a spearhead of the forthcoming Republican assault.[2] At Jarama, Jolly and his colleagues dealt with hundreds of casualties; at Guadalajara, with thousands; and at Brunete, they could anticipate treating tens of thousands while also planning to move forward in support of the army's advance.[3]

Jolly had recently been promoted to major, the highest rank for which foreigners in the Republican Army were eligible. He and his battle-hardened team were instructed to set up the largest and best-equipped hospital they had worked in yet. All five International Brigades were to take part in this assault, and the frontline hospital for their wounded was scaled in keeping with the forthcoming battle. It was sited ten kilometers behind the lines and about forty-five kilometers northwest of Madrid in the historic seminary of San José de los Sagrados Corazones, just below the sixteenth-century El Escorial, one of the largest royal palaces in Europe and where centuries of Spanish royalty lay in their ornate tombs. Spread throughout the ancient seminary's four floors, as many as four surgeons could work simultaneously, each with his own operating room and with access to larger wards and more beds than they had previously seen in the war.[4]

Noel Carritt, a British volunteer with the International Brigades, had transferred to driving an ambulance after suffering a hand injury at Jarama. He considered the seminary "a magnificent place for a hospital and almost for the first time we had plenty of room, plenty of space."[5] The Scottish doctor Archie Cochrane was equally pleased to find that ambulances could safely maneuver within the grounds of this huge building and, once their cargoes were unloaded, that it had a large area suitable for triage, his special responsibility. "Reggie Saxton was there with his blood transfusion service and there was even a small X-ray unit which did occasionally locate odd bullets."[6] Cochrane noted, however, that "the stairs up to the wards were steep and difficult for the stretcher-bearers." English ambulance driver George Green thought likewise, writing to his wife, Nan, of the strain placed on "the local boys whom we co-opt as *camilleros* with no time to train them properly. . . . We work dourly, saying hardly a word, cleaning out rooms, scrubbing, wiring, fixing lights in the theatres and in the triage downstairs . . . where the first clean-up takes place, bloody trousers are ripped from quivering thighs, and the wounded are sorted into severe, not so severe—and dead."[7]

At first all went promisingly on the battlefront. The attack was launched in the early morning of 6 July, and the village of Brunete was taken, albeit at great cost, the following day. The Republicans initially dominated the skies, but Franco's generals soon brought up extra divisions and faster aircraft, including the Condor Legion's newly introduced Messerschmitts, which were far faster and more numerous than the Republican air force's aging machines. Aileen Palmer, an Australian working as an administrator to the medical teams, described the conditions in a letter to her mother:

> Every night the aeroplanes were over us, usually the electricity was switched off at the main and the theatres had to operate with candles and torches, until we established our own emergency lighting. In any case most of the hospital was in darkness, and the large classification room, where most of the wounded were brought, had to work with only one light. . . . Incendiary bombs were a new feature that we had not come across yet. We were used to the thud of bombs in the distance, sometimes close to us, but this time you would not hear the bombs falling, only going out in the small hours of the morning you would see a glow as of bushfires all round the horizon: fire-bombs dropped among the forests and crops. To the personnel in the hospital, though, the risk was of the slightest: the people who suffer are the drivers, going up to the first-aid station at Brunete and driving back, sometimes the planes would follow the ambulances, swooping down and machine-gunning them. Two of our ambulances were put out of commission by bombs.[8]

A left-wing Hungarian-language newspaper from this period describes Jolly operating on a severely injured Italian fighter named Bolo who had "suffered a dumdum [exploding] bullet, and his thighs are full of metal splinters. His legs need to be saved. . . . The windows rattle, the walls shake: long-range guns around the hospital. In the makeshift operating theatre a gigantic fight is going on." An incision in the abdomen reveals "a part of the intestine pierced through and through. The bullets whistle." Jolly decided that a further blood transfusion was needed, "but Bolo's blood type is out of stock and it would take a few hours to get it from the central blood bank." Archie Cochrane proposed to give a direct transfusion himself. "Be careful," said his colleague, Alex Tudor-Hart. "If you give blood you won't be allowed to work for 24 hours, and we're waiting for another shipment." Cochrane insisted, and the transfusion went ahead.[9]

The toll of casualties strewn across the parched and treeless Castilian plain mounted steeply, and the stretcher-bearers who carried them to safety were injured or killed at a rate even higher than that of the Republican infantry.[10] Jolly wrote later of these extraordinarily self-sacrificing men: "I did not know that such epic bravery existed until I saw it. Never imagine that the most important person in a military medical service is the surgeon. Without the courage of the stretcher-bearers who bring the wounded from the lines to the First Aid Post, the surgeon in the comparative safety of the First Emergency Hospital would be useless."[11]

Convoys of ambulances stacked with wounded began streaming into the monastery hospital, and their stretchers were carried into a large waiting room where emergency transfusions were given, if necessary, and the triage process was carried out. Less urgent cases were evacuated directly to base hospitals in Madrid. Those considered beyond saving were taken outside again to a large marquee, where they lay "waiting to die. Covered in flies and dust and all that, not even cleaned up properly." French doctors were known to prowl the tent at night, giving lethal injections to "those that were absolutely beyond salvation."[12] Those deemed suitable for immediate surgery were carried to the operating rooms in order of their severity. Their injuries were worsened by a lack of fresh water and the pitiless heat at forty degrees Celsius (104 degrees Fahrenheit). "In the theatre it brought millions of flies," remembered nurse Penny Phelps. "They settled on the wounds and instruments and everything!"[13] Saxton recalled that the staff and patients were plagued by various other pests: "mosquitoes, flies (many of which sting), fleas, ants, and at least two kinds of body lice; but worse than all, aviation."[14] At night the drone of approaching Caproni bombers meant that all the hospital's lights were immediately extinguished, and the theaters continued their work by candlelight and handheld torch.[15]

Although stored blood for transfusions was among the most desperately needed of all medical supplies, the Madrid-based blood donor service was no longer capable of providing it. In the months before the Brunete battle, Bethune's increasingly erratic behavior, heavy drinking, and frequent absences to secure new equipment in France led to his resignation.[16] Fortunately, Saxton found that the original service established by Frederic Duran i Jordà in Barcelona was "so perfectly organised that after a couple of days . . . a refrigerated truck arrived from there ready to supply all the blood required." The truck's paintwork—white with red rays—represented its vital function of transporting blood from the Barcelona center to every battlefront where it was needed.[17] Even with this service, said Saxton, "we gave transfusions so often, and sometimes in such quantity, that the supply often ran out, and I was obliged to take blood from the already overworked staff."[18]

Soon other medical supplies also ran short. When nurse Phelps had no more ether or chloroform for general anesthetics, she was forced to administer a local or provide spinal anesthesia. "When we were without gowns," she wrote, "I draped the surgeon in sheets given to us by the civilians."[19] Taking two hours at most for sleep in each twenty-four, the teams toiled to stabilize only the most critically injured. The Australian Aileen Palmer described how she and other staff would "fall asleep on a patch of floor" during their rare and fleeting breaks.[20] "We were all put under real strain," Cochrane remembered. He had worked previously with Broggi and Hart but never before with Jolly, and Cochrane found him to be "a man of the highest competence for whom I developed a great admiration. . . . He ran a remarkably efficient ward for abdominal cases."[21] Into this ward, some two weeks after the battle began, was carried the shattered and dying photographer Gerda Taro (as described in chapter 1).

Under these physically and emotionally exhausting conditions, the hospital staff maintained a routine that they had developed and refined to a high degree of efficiency. Nurses supplied each surgeon with a specific set of sterilized instruments for the operation required, and they treated three thousand men within a few days. "Throughout those days we could perform remarkable work with great results," recalled Broggi with evident pride.[22] One injured International Brigader from California, Robert Colodny, was not expected to survive when he was carried into Jolly's operating theater. He had been shot between the eyes and contracted gangrene of the brain. Jolly and a Spanish surgeon named Gregorio Marañón gave him what treatment they could, including, it is said, implanting a metal plate in his skull. To their own surprise, after forty days in a coma, he recovered with only slight paralysis in one hand and returned to combat at the battle of Teruel.[23] There he relapsed and was invalided home to the United States, eventually becoming a distinguished professor of history at the University of Pittsburgh.[24]

"The day the [Brunete] battle finished," wrote Broggi, "we felt that the world had stopped. We could no longer hear the infernal noise, until then an uninterrupted cacophony of explosions from bombs, cannons and aeroplanes moving through that great plain. At the same time ambulances were arriving continually, carrying young men in the prime of life with their bodies destroyed. After almost a month, all this suddenly ceased and we felt that we had woken up from a nightmare."[25] In that sudden stillness, he said, "we perceived with terrible clarity the real hatred and repugnance that war always has. In all those days of the battle and afterwards, living together in those dramatic moments with so many problems that we resolved together served to establish and strengthen between all of us relations of brotherhood that have endured ever since, as if we formed part of a great and close family."[26]

Franco's forces had recaptured most of the territory they lost at the outset of the battle, including the village of Brunete. Republican casualties eventually numbered twenty-five thousand, along with 80 percent of their armored vehicles and a third of the fighter aircraft deployed.[27] For a fortnight after this searing battle, the surgeons dealt with the small number of remaining injured, especially those with fractures who needed casts prepared for them. The medical staff also had time to explore the historic monastery where they worked and to exchange impressions of the experience they had undergone. During this period, Jolly became convinced that through innovations such as autochirs and the blood transfusion service, a momentous improvement in traditional systems of wartime surgery was evolving. In discussions with his fellow doctors and nurses, he appears to have begun developing ideas that he later crystallized in a highly influential manual of field surgery.[28]

In the aftermath of Brunete, this seemingly indefatigable figure also confessed to feeling

> a bit too thin and a bit nerveux. This last "do" was rather gruelling from the surgical point of view. I find that I can't stand the strain to the same extent as I could nine months ago. Long hours and little sleep take their toll. . . . Many of our ambulances were almost total wrecks after the last offensive—shot through and through with machine gun bullets and bombs from the Junkers. You don't know and you can't imagine under what conditions our ambulance drivers continue to work, bringing in wounded under the most intensive aerial bombardments that have yet been seen in this world.[29]

Among the ambulance drivers killed in this battle was Noel Carritt's brother Anthony, newly arrived in Spain.[30] Noel himself was injured by shrapnel in the leg and was then transferred to work as a driver behind the lines at the base hospital of Huete. "I remember meeting Dr Jolly . . . and him suggesting (perhaps because I had a degree in Biology; I can think of no other reason) that I might like to train as his anaesthetist. I was interested in this idea and agreed to sit in beside the acting anaesthetist during a minor operation. A man, a soldier, was having some shrapnel removed from his knee. My experience of this convinced me that I was quite unsuitable as an anaesthetist and was much better as an ambulance driver."[31]

Jolly's original anesthetist, Peter de Sarigny, had returned to the United Kingdom and was finally replaced by a *practicante* (second-year medical student) from Madrid named Florinda Pérez.[32] The role of frontline anesthetist had become rather more sophisticated with the introduction by mid-1937 of nitrous oxide gas.[33] The highly regarded local anesthetic Evipan was now often used only in the preliminary stage of an operation, "with anaesthesia then most commonly maintained with ether."[34]

In late August, Jolly wrote to his friends in London: "We had to pack and move again. This time a long, long way."[35] Wartime secrecy prevented him from revealing that his new destination was the landlocked rural region of Aragón in the northeast. A 120-kilometer battlefront ran through the province from north to south, with the Nationalists controlling the larger area to the west, including the regional capital, Zaragoza. This city was the main objective of the new Republican offensive, although the front was to be penetrated at several points to prevent a concentrated counterattack, which had proved so disastrous at Brunete.

Jolly's hospital was therefore set up well south of Zaragoza but still close to the front line, near the small village of La Puebla de Híjar. It had no great and historic structures like those he had occupied at Brunete. Instead, with the help of young boys from the village, the operating tables, beds, and other equipment were hastily set up in four wooden huts that lacked running water or electricity. Within twelve hours of the first advance, the wounded began arriving, and the team performed 160 operations in a theater that was "little more than a shed."[36] Jolly's Spanish theater nurse, Aurora Fernández, who had been educated at an elite Madrid institute and spoke English well, found that many of the wounded were so terrified by the sound of enemy aviation passing overhead that they had to be comforted by the local helpers "so the poor boys would not jump out of bed and hurt themselves more."[37] The hospital staff had no accommodations of their own and simply rested in the patients' beds so they could be available at a moment's notice.

As previously, the initial advance progressed rapidly, with the promise of a complete victory. The nearby town of Quinto was one of the first to fall, and Jolly's field hospital was moved up behind the troops to occupy the cellar of a badly damaged flour mill. The advance was so rapid that this hospital was installed while still within range of the retreating Nationalists' artillery, although the presence of a number of "very dead mules" in a stable alongside was a more pressing hazard. "As I look out of the window," wrote Jolly cheerfully, "I see a Camion [truck] coming to drag them one by one into the country. Perhaps the flies and the mosquitoes will also go into the country. Here's hoping."[38] His friend Tom Wintringham, by then a staff officer with the Fifteenth Brigade, was brought to this hospital with a shoulder wound that ended his service in Spain. Although the injury proved slow to heal, Wintringham commended Jolly's surgical skills. "I have to thank him (and a clean bullet) for much the neatest among my scars."[39]

Moving behind the advancing forces to one Aragónese village after another, Jolly saw at close hand how these country people responded to the arrival of the Spanish Republican Army. "How glad the women and children were to see our troops! They have now all been sent further back out of danger. . . . It is grand to be behind troops that are victorious, the morale is so much higher and everyone better-tempered. Big things are happening in this part of Spain—good and I hope important for the ultimate outcome."[40]

In this exhilarating phase of the war, he urged the Grants, and by implication the British people generally, in somewhat high-flown terms not to take for granted the peaceful existence they still enjoyed:

> In the world today there are people fighting and dying that such freedom to live may be the recognised privilege of *all* men. That's what this war in Spain is about. The Spanish people don't *like* war. . . . But having won by the vote the beginning of the freedom of life which has been denied them by the King, the Nobles and the Church in Spain for centuries, they are willing to fight and die rather than give up to the Fascists of Spain, Italy and Germany these hopes of a greater and increasing joy in life which have been so long delayed in coming to them.[41]

These hard-fought political gains were fragile, he recognized, and utterly dependent on foreign support if they were to be maintained. "How terribly important the voice of the English working-class seems when 'not heard' from Spain at this juncture in European politics. You don't know how we here all long for the rising voice of Labour in England. I really believe it's the only thing that can save the peace. Poor Spain, heavily laden and struggling, and always silence in England."[42]

The town of Quinto stands in a fertile valley beside Spain's largest river, the Ebro, and in that strange and violent summer, as bombers and tanks roared around them, the peasants continued to till and harvest their crops by methods that had barely changed in centuries. The food they produced was critically important for sustaining both the army and the wider population. Jolly, who had grown up in a small rural community but one in which horse-drawn implements were rapidly giving way to mechanised farming, was astonished at the immemorial tools and practices he saw from his hospital window. "Agriculture in Spain is primitive in the extreme," he told New Zealand audiences after the war.

> Ploughing is done by the mule or ox-drawn single-furrow wooden plough, threshing, on the baked-clay village threshing floors by driving over the spread grain with a sledge or stone roller, winnowing by repeatedly tossing the shaken grain in the wind with a wooden spade. . . . It was strange to see the Spanish peasants in villages a few miles behind the front, threshing with their Biblical methods, one eye on the mule and the other on the approaching bombing squadron, then a quick dive into a handily dug open trench beside the threshing floor, then quickly out again; a laughing, dusting, jabbering in musical Spanish, and so on with the threshing. We came greatly to love these peasants with their childish gaiety, adult seriousness and deep, clear understanding of what the war was about.[43]

The last of Jolly's field hospitals in this campaign was established in the small but well-fortified town of Belchite, which was defended by the Nationalists at great cost to both sides and surrendered only after the Republican attackers cut off its water supply in the intense midsummer heat.[44] It cannot have been easy to find a suitable building to use for a new field hospital since much of the town was by then reduced to rubble, a state it remains in today as a memorial to the devastation of the war.

After this pyrrhic victory, the entire Aragón offensive ground to a halt. The earlier Republican advances had ended largely with the arrival, from mid-July, of

Germany's latest high-speed monoplane, the Messerschmitt Bf 109. From this point, the Nationalist dominance of the air became absolute. The Republicans failed to take the city of Zaragoza, their ultimate objective, while farther to the north the Nationalists continued their advance through the Basque country toward the crucial Republican center of Barcelona.

Jolly's next posting was therefore to the port city of Tarragona, directly behind the northern front on Spain's northeast coast and about a hundred kilometers south of Barcelona. There a base hospital had been set up in a former tuberculosis sanitorium called La Sabinosa that had been built on a rocky headland directly above the ocean, since fresh air was thought to promote recovery from that disease. His staff now included the Dutch nurse Nora "Noor" or "Noortje" Diamant from a progressive Jewish family in Amsterdam. The equipo spent only a short time at La Sabinosa before moving to a succession of Catalonian villages, typically spending just a week or two in each one. They were given the use of schools, convents, or other suitably large buildings for their makeshift hospitals, although in the town of Lérida they were able to occupy "a beautiful house." Each building first had to be scrupulously cleaned, and the staff carried out most of this work themselves, sometimes with the help of local girls and women. A town crier might also go through the village calling for extra hands to carry out duties such as washing laundry. By this stage of the war, the staff faced critical shortages of all kinds—from water, furniture, firewood, and soap to disinfectant, dressings, and syringes—and had to exercise great ingenuity to overcome them. Even so, here as elsewhere, the foreign medical staff made additional efforts to overcome the illiteracy of their Spanish colleagues with, according to Diamant, "astonishing results."[45]

At this time, Jolly finally took his first overseas leave after more than ten months of near-constant work, most of it within earshot, and frequently within range, of bombing and artillery fire. Even his remarkably robust constitution, he learned, could not maintain such a pace of activity without a break. He had informed his friends in August that "after a few months more I think I will have to apply for permission to go to England for a week or two. There is much that I could do there in the way of propaganda, looking for surgical material that I find it impossible to get here in Spain. Spare parts for our motor transport is also always a pressing problem."[46]

As that letter suggests, even this well-earned spell of leave was spent on various missions related to the war effort. During the month Jolly spent in England and France from early October 1937, and in addition to the important tasks listed above, he spoke with "military surgeons who had seen service with the British and French armies in the Great War," discussing the promising developments in military medicine that were emerging in Republican Spain.[47] It was a subject of keen interest for the remaining democratic countries in Europe, where the geopolitical landscape was sharply deteriorating. Even high-ranked army officers who may have disagreed with Jolly's staunch support for the Spanish Republic are likely to have welcomed the opportunity to exchange ideas with him. His reputation for physical endurance and surgical skill now extended throughout the Republican zone and even beyond it to his homeland. Within days of his return to Spain in early November, Jolly visited an International Brigades base hospital in an abandoned monastery in the small Castilian town of Huete, halfway between Valencia and Madrid. This twelfth-century building with meter-thick stone walls was known as the English Hospital.[48] Two of its nurses came from Jolly's own distant country, and one of them, Isobel Dodds, wrote about his visit in a letter home that the local newspaper of his hometown of Cromwell proudly reprinted: "We met a New Zealand doctor the other day, Dr Jolly. He is quite a 'big noise' out here, and what is more important, a thoroughly good surgeon. He specialises in abdominal surgery and has had unbelievable success repeatedly. . . . We were thrilled to see him. He made a special visit to Huete to see us."[49]

Latvian-born, Edinburgh-trained surgeon Len Crome, who was several years younger than Jolly and had "a devastating irreverence for authority," and Jolly now served as the chief medical officers for the entire Thirty-Fifth Division, comprising two International Brigades and a third mixed (i.e., Spanish and international) brigade.[50] Jolly's great friend and fellow surgeon, the Catalan Moisès Broggi, encountered him at work in the village of Alfambra, and they had a convivial afternoon tea together with members of the U.S. medical unit headed by Ed Barsky. Alfambra lay in the isolated, mountainous, and impoverished province of Teruel, and Barsky explained to the other surgeons that the next major military operation by the Republican Army would be an all-out attempt to capture the province's main city, also named Teruel. He had great hopes for this latest assault, noting that if the Republican forces could demonstrate their capability of taking a city from the enemy, then the multinational

Committee of Non-Intervention might well change its hidebound attitude and provide material support to the Republican cause. His colleague, San Francisco surgeon Leo Eloesser, thought the Thirty-Fifth Division, and therefore their own medical units, were certain to be called in for the attack, since this division was always ordered into battle "when things were desperate."[51]

As predicted, in the harsh winter of December 1937, the Thirty-Fifth was ordered to join a Republican offensive to forestall an anticipated Nationalist assault on Teruel's vital road link between Zaragoza and Madrid. Even today, Teruel is a bleak and isolated city, sited on a harsh plain and bordered by a precipitous gorge. Several members of Jolly's team had remained with him from their first days together in Madrid, including his very dedicated theater orderly Joe Edenhoffer, a Czechoslovak-born Englishman, and his Spanish nurse Aurora Fernández. Shortly after the civil war ended, these two married and later lived in Edenhoffer's home city of Prague. Remembering those she had worked with in the medical services during the war, Aurora said, "I owe them all I have been in my life."[52]

At Teruel, she recalled, "after much travelling and many hairpin bends and the snowbound roads sometimes blocked for days, our lorries and trucks got to a small mountain village." In this poverty-stricken hamlet, named Cuevas Labradas (Carved Caves) for its distinctive topography, Jolly, Broggi, and Tudor-Hart set up yet another field hospital in an old woolen mill. It was a large, draughty building with no electricity. The operating theater lighting was generated by car batteries, and elsewhere the staff used lamps made from condensed milk tins filled with oil and wicks.[53] In this remote terrain, with no possibility of receiving stored blood from the blood banks, the already overstretched hospital staff sat on the floor alongside the stretchers holding their wounded patients and donated their blood directly. "It is true we all gave blood in direct blood transfusions," said Fernández, "nurses, even doctors, and stretcher-bearers."[54]

The high-altitude town experiences the coldest temperatures in all of Spain, and the winter of 1937–38 was the worst in a century. Temperatures dropped to minus twenty degrees Celsius (minus four degrees Fahrenheit), and telephone poles, as the only fuel available, were felled for firewood.[55] In their now ragged and inadequate uniforms, more men died from the effects of the cold than were killed in battle. In the deep snow and implacable cold, the hospital's ambulances and other vehicles became barely usable. Radiators were drained overnight, requiring their drivers to undertake a frantic search the next morning for thawed water to refill them. The injured arrived so badly frostbitten that amputation was often the only possible treatment. Rats ran everywhere and had to be prevented from gnawing at living bodies, while the daily drone of enemy aviation strained tempers to a breaking point.[56]

Aurora Fernández recalled, "We had another great torture; lice. It is true lice had bothered us in the summer and autumn, but now the chance of having a wash was very small due to the cold weather so we scratched and scratched day and night. . . . I had the idea to pinch a little ether for anaesthetics and pour a little on so the lice slept and also myself." Another nurse, the Englishwoman Lillian Urmston, gently warned Fernández against the practice of sprinkling herself with highly flammable ether. "Everyone is smoking and you could go up in flames."[57]

Urmston herself found that the harsh and frozen terrain produced wounds of a different type than she was used to treating. "It was snowbound, hard, rocky and no-one could dig trenches deep enough, so instead of just getting head and chest wounds which were typical of the Spanish war, we were also getting abdominal wounds galore and also what was terribly sad, wounds in the groin."[58]

Late one night in early January 1937, an American ambulance driver pulled up outside the hospital. "Two operating tables were going full blast. A door would open, with a vision of silent figures dressed in white, and naked bare skin and the bandaged stumps of arms and legs, rags floating in slop jars of reddish liquid. Stretchers went up and down the stairs, even while pickaxes were chipping at the plaster walls to make turning easier. Why was it that nothing was being done to ease the occasional low whimpers that came from the figures under the blankets?"[59]

In a letter later published in the *Lancet*, Reginald Saxton admitted to the ordeals he and his colleagues were facing:

> We are having on the whole a much stiffer time than last winter. The cold has been more severe, and we have continual bursts of rain and very little sunshine. Also there is the constant strain and racket of the enemy air-raids and bombings which sometimes badly affect the morale and nerves of the staff. . . . Everybody has put his shoulder to the wheel with marvellous energy and goodwill, but all the same, the staff is having a pretty grim time.

> We sleep on floors, rough barrack room boards. The food consists largely of beans, macaroni and oil. We have not yet been able to do much in the way of adequate water supplies and sanitation, and have been up against influenza and other epidemics.[60]

In this desolating working environment, Jolly yet again showed his extraordinary capacity for leading his staff by example. To Aurora Fernández, it appeared that "he was never tired. Once, in the middle of the night an ambulance came with an urgent case. It was after a fortnight when no one slept. . . . Dr. Jolly got up as if nothing should happen and operated on the man. It was a case of appendicitis. It could have been evacuated but Dr. Jolly did not take the chance."[61] She later wrote that the New Zealand surgeon

> does honour to his name—a man more "Jolly" it would be difficult to find. I remember once, waiting an order to leave for the front, all of us nervous and tense, fearful that planes would arrive. . . . Dr Jolly began to tell jokes and seeing that the Spanish did not understand this, began to dance and sing in the style of the Maoris, and he inspired the group of spectators and all were smiling and the tension went down. The time passed so rapidly that before we noticed the train had arrived. We loaded ourselves on, nurses, doctors, stretcher bearers and in a freight car for merchandise we continued the journey, the rhythm of the Maori music interpreted by Dr Jolly still sounding in our ears.[62]

On this occasion Jolly seems to have reassured and distracted his colleagues with a haka, the exclamatory and vigorous Māori war dance that he had learned to perform at his Dunedin high school. Nurse Fernández was not alone in noting his ability to reenergize people at their lowest moments. When the English nurse Penny Phelps was transferred from the front line to work at an evacuation hospital with Spanish surgeons, she found that "they were not like Dr Jolly whose inspiration and boost to morale I missed very much."[63]

By Christmas 1937, morale along the entire Republican front soared briefly when the provincial capital of Teruel was captured after "the most horrific of all the battles of the civil war."[64] On Boxing Day, Jolly wrote a long letter to Donald and Irene Grant's medical student daughter Wendy that was later reprinted in the newsletter of the Christian Left:

Teruel was a name that one did not want to talk of before, even to think of very much, because it was potentially the most dangerous point in Spain. Now it is shouted in every village street throughout Government Spain. It is a tremendous thing!

We are having a Teruel fiesta this afternoon in our hospital here in this small village—a fiesta for the kids of the village, with a distribution of toys. They are lovely, black-eyed, friendly eager little things. . . .

I spent yesterday (Christmas Day) with a battalion of men from Karli's [Karl Polanyi's] country [i.e., Hungarians. It seems likely that Jolly's Hungarian nurse Anna-Mária Basch prompted this friendship with her compatriots, although Jolly's earlier friendship with Polanyi may have been a further bond.] In the evening we ate a wonderful paprikas [a paprika-based stew], and then the whole evening they sang songs as only Karli's people can sing. They are a grand people, gay, light-hearted and splendid fighters.

I am sitting in the best room of a peasant's cottage in the village where we have our hospital. A delightful, fine-looking old woman is my hostess and we get on splendidly together. She has just carried in and placed at my feet a large brass tray of wood embers, for it's bitterly cold away up here in the mountains.

"Hace muy frio, mi commandante?" [It's very cold, my commander?]

"Si, compañera, muy frio!" [Yes, comrade, very cold!]

"Espera un momento." [Hold on a moment.]

And so on. Now I can continue to write in comfort. They're a lovely, simple, friendly people. They've known terribly hard times for generations, and now know what they are fighting for. . . .

This victory at Teruel must have a great uplifting effect on the morale of the people here in Spain. It must have a unifying effect. It would not be strange if, after losing ground so steadily in North Spain (Bilbao, Santander etc) many of the less politically aware among the soldiers and civil population were becoming disheartened. We can sense the great uplift and new determination everywhere.[65]

The mood of triumph was tragically short-lived, as Franco once again brought up additional divisions and heavy artillery to retake this symbolically important prize. The subzero conditions stalled his tanks, but his dive-bombers and fighters were able to take off once the ice was chipped from their wings. The constant air barrage made it impossible to bring wounded into the Cuevas Labradas hospital by daylight, so the Republican ambulances were forced to crawl without lights along steep and icy mountain roads after dark. For the severely wounded and half-frozen men inside them, the accidents and delays this caused were often fatal. Hospital staff were similarly at risk from the bombing, and during night raids, Jolly and the other surgeons worked by candlelight or with pocket torches taped to their heads to avoid providing a target for the pilots.[66] At the most dangerous times, the hospital staff members were forced to shelter inside the large caves in the nearby hills for which the village was named.

The only safe means of evacuating patients under these conditions was by using railway wagons converted into train hospitals. Teruel lay on the railway line to Valencia, and a number of wagons were fitted with three tiers of bunk beds, a kitchen, and dining car. Some carriages even held operating tables so that further emergency treatment could be conducted en route. "Instruments were sterilised in fish kettles on primus stoves, and the only warmth for the patients was from alcohol burned in open pans, a dangerous practice with ether being used as an anaesthetic."[67] If enemy bombers appeared, "a hospital train with 60 to 100 beds would pull into the tunnel and be attached to the operating theatres until its beds were full. It would then steam off to the Sector Evacuation Hospital and its place would be taken by another hospital train. In the event of the line behind the train being demolished, evacuation could be effected by Evacuation Ambulance Groups."[68] These hospital trains represented the most ambitious and imaginative use to date of Jolly's evolving "three-points-forward" system—a graded succession of medical services for treating patients whose conditions were of decreasing urgency the farther back they were transported behind the front lines.

In subzero conditions that appeared interminable, New Year's Day passed in Cuevas Labradas with little cheer. By February 1938, the Nationalist counterattack succeeded in recapturing Teruel, leaving, it is said, thousands of frozen corpses strewn through its streets. The hospital was forced to withdraw rapidly northward, and for the next several months, despite a succession of brief stands, the entire Republican front was pushed back toward the Mediterranean coast in a campaign for survival known as the Great Retreat.

"Our front hospital is in tents now," administrator Aileen Palmer told her friends in Australia.

> It's not safe to work in villages any more. The tents are pitched in an olive field, surrounded by hills. The ambulances come down a rough track and disgorge the wounded into the first tent, which serves as a classification room. The worst wounded are sent to the second tent, which is an operating room, and the lightly wounded are dressed and evacuated rapidly. The third tent is set up as a ward [where patients could recover after their operations]. Most of the work is at night. Today the sky is alive with the continual menace of wings. The bombs fall close. We crouch or lie on the floor. Then one falls just outside the tent, shrapnel pierces the thin canvas, and the place is filled with dust. No-one hurt? Then get on with the evacuation, that ambulance shouldn't be standing there a moment longer. Tonight the hospital is to be moved further back.[69]

American surgeon Leo Eloesser headed a surgical team that "set up and dismantled ten different hospitals on ten consecutive days" in this period, with "the fascists pounding hard down the road on our heels."[70] The trauma and demoralization this experience produced caused his staff to become "fearful and hysterical." One of them, Dr. Ed Barsky, "was in deep depression . . . it broke your heart to see his sad, quiet dignity." Barsky and two of his most experienced nurses were finally evacuated to the United States, suffering from severe anxiety and exhaustion.[71]

Jolly's own state of mind in this period is not recorded. Perhaps he could not bring himself to write about it.

10 The Safest Place in Spain

Exhausted, demoralized, often without weapons or even boots, the fragmented Republican Army withdrew in disorder after the Nationalist recapture of Teruel, fleeing toward Catalonia and the coast under continuous attack from Franco's triumphant Army of Maneuver. Jolly wrote that the Nationalist pursuit was led by "armoured columns supported by massed aircraft, filtering through weak points without any immediate attempt to clear or occupy the territory. The Republican Army was split by these infiltrating columns into brigade and battalion groups, retreating independently, fighting a rearguard action and repeatedly surrounded by mobile sections of the invading force."[1]

"During the several days of this headlong retreat with complete absence of any defined line or zone of resistance," he later wrote, "it was quite impossible to establish any forward hospitals. Indeed, the retreat was so rapid that very few seriously wounded men could be retrieved and evacuated from the diffuse battle zone." At least one autochir and many ambulances were lost to aerial attack during this chaotic retreat, and some surgical teams were forced to destroy their equipment as they evaded enemy columns.[2]

Finally, in early March 1938, a stand of some sort was made in eastern Aragón near the town of Caspe. "Here reserve Republican divisions had established a line of resistance held in depth, forming a screen through which the retreating army fell back to the rear for reorganisation."[3] A tent hospital was created between the villages of Batea and Gandesa, and mobile surgical units brought up from the rear were "leapfrogged" over this hospital to establish field hospitals nearer the front. The equipos worked mainly from tents for speed of movement, operating in them as long as possible, then hastily packing all their equipment into trucks. The wounded were sent on ahead of the staff to the next point considered safe.

Now assigned to the army's Forty-Fifth Division with the rank of *comandante cirujano* (surgeon major), Jolly set up such a hospital together with the Spanish surgeon Luis Alonso and the Belgian René Dumont in the country town of Maella. His unit's report stated, "The team has an outpatient operating room with an operating table, five ambulances that are available to the division, sterilisers, a portable X-ray machine, a radiology technician and a complete set of instruments for amputation laparotomy."[4]

They treated more than a thousand wounded in fifteen days before this town also fell to the Nationalists in April 1938.[5] Once the region around Gandesa came under heavy bombing from enemy aircraft, the hospital at Maella was moved to a railway tunnel near Pinell. Boards were laid over the rails to create a bombproof two-hundred-bed hospital with six surgical units. As the Republican troops fell farther back toward the coast, their field hospitals withdrew to this tunnel. Eventually it was decided that even this hospital, now with fifteen surgical teams, would also withdraw northwest across the River Ebro into Catalonia, where a new hospital was set up in a disused lead mine at Mola. "During the whole of this phase," Jolly notes with evident pride, "no personnel or surgical equipment was lost."[6]

The war was reaching a fateful turning point, as the Nationalists threatened to break through the Republican lines to reach the Mediterranean and split the Republican-held territory in two. Anticipating that disaster, the International Brigades' base was transferred from Albacete to Barcelona. American surgeon Edward Barsky replaced Oscar Telge as the head of the brigades' medical services.[7] Soon afterward, the advancing Nationalists reached the coast at the town of Vinaròs, midway between Barcelona and Valencia, the last remaining Republican-held centers.

With the arrival of spring, the Spanish Republic appeared to face almost certain and imminent defeat. Its troops were in poor shape physically and militarily, and Barcelona, its new capital, lay vulnerable and poorly defended. Yet instead of deploying his Army of Maneuver northward to take that city and rapidly end the war, Franco made the curious decision to push southwest along the coast toward Valencia. That move is explicable only by his determination to crush his opponents entirely and eliminate any future resistance to his political rule. The Republic had already been negotiating for some months to sue for peace, but Franco refused all proposals for a settlement that would leave any of the country's assets in his enemies' hands. The only acceptable outcome of the war, he insisted to his generals, was total victory followed by the reconstruction of a royalist, Catholic-run, archconservative Spain.[8]

The immediate impact of this calculated extenuation of the war, however, was the loss of the momentum of the recent Aragón campaign. The unexpected interlude enabled the shattered Republican forces to reorganize and rearm. New armaments had just become available to them following the French government's decision to reopen its Spanish frontier and permit troops and munitions to enter the Republican-held territory of Catalonia.

Jolly recalled that the frail but resilient Republican front was divided in two, with one half swinging north toward Barcelona and the other south to defend Valencia.[9] Both cities then suffered intense ground and air attacks, but withstood them and even achieved tactical victories that exceeded those at Guadalajara a year earlier.[10] Although at times outnumbered four to one, the troops defending Valencia held strong positions and suffered relatively few casualties. Barcelona, however, experienced the heaviest aerial bombing raids of the entire war, with fleets of Italian bombers sweeping over the harbor day and night.[11] The blood bank established in the city before the war by the Catalan hematologist Federico Duran i Jordà proved a crucial factor in treating thousands of civilian as well as military casualties. It was a more sophisticated system than Bethune's in Madrid, with some thirty thousand donors giving blood monthly. Their blood was typed and tested for syphilis and malaria, and, if necessary, the donors themselves were X-rayed for tuberculosis.[12]

Jolly spent part of this defensive campaign behind the battlefront at a six-hundred-bed base hospital in the Catalan town of Valls, southwest of Barcelona. Here Saxton had set up his blood transfusion laboratory and a local donor system among the civilian population with the aim of creating a supply of stored blood of every type required. "We also investigated as blood donors most of the staff of the medical and surgical units with whom we worked in case blood transfusion from these people would be required."[13] The American medical services in Spain developed a further transfusion laboratory. Hank Rubin, a former medical student from California, served as an infantryman in the International Brigades until invalided out of the lines with hepatitis. He then helped modify a large ambulance into a laboratory equipped with a small oven, an incubator for growing cultures, a refrigerator for storing blood, and bunks for two lab technicians.[14]

South of Valls, toward Valencia, the once-luxurious beach resort of Benicàssim stood among orange orchards and palm trees beside a sea of intense Mediterranean blue. In late 1936 Dr. Oscar Telge had selected this paradisical location as the site for a complex of hospitals that became "the most desired hospital rest center for all the wounded of the International Brigades." Catalan surgeon Josep Maria Massons thought it "the closest thing to Eden" after the tribulations of frontline service. Eventually comprising a hospital, a convalescent center, and a dental surgery, the Benicàssim complex had a total of twelve hundred beds, all under the direction of the Austrian doctor Fritz Jensen.[15] It also served as an administrative center for the outlying field hospitals.

Jolly and his nurse and faithful companion Anna-Mária Basch spent a relatively blissful period working there that coincided with a visit to the hospital by the internationally renowned anti-fascist journalist Egon Kisch, popularly known as the "Raging Reporter." Kisch was adamant that while visiting injured International Brigaders, he repeatedly saw a phenomenon he had not encountered in any other field of war: Wounded combatants convalescing from their injuries made desperate efforts to return to the front, often escaping from their hospital beds "with their wounds still open, the bandages not removed or with crutches under their arms." His brother Frederick, formerly a well-known Prague surgeon, was chief of the Czechoslovak surgical unit in Spain and confirmed he had seen patients "deserting to the front" from every hospital where he had worked in the war.[16] So, too, had the German Rudolf Neumann, the International Brigades' first chief medical officer. "One of the tasks of military doctors in other countries has always been to discover those who pretend to be sick to escape service. It happened to us the other way around. We had to confront those who wanted to go and fight at all costs, and hid their wounds for fear that we would not let them return to the front."[17]

In this period, the journal of the army's international medical services, *AMI* (*Ayuda Médica Internacional*), published a lengthy article by Jolly (translated into German, French, and Spanish in the following issue) on the treatment of the injuries in which he had come to specialize—those of the abdomen. It is a discursive and, under the circumstances, surprisingly iconoclastic contribution. Jolly had found that in Spain, although abdominal wounds made up no more than 6 percent of all battlefield injuries,

> the organisation of front line hospitals is regulated very largely by the necessity of dealing adequately with abdominal cases. These are the cases, above all others . . . where the timelag between the moment of being wounded and the moment of operation is of vital importance. With every hour that passes, the possibility of recovery falls in geometrical progression. So this question of dealing with the abdominal case is the most important factor in the determination of the placing of the frontline hospitals . . . smaller ambulances are always held in readiness at our classification post to obviate the necessity of keeping abdominal cases until the larger evacuation ambulances are ready to move off with their full complement of wounded. So the tempo of the evacuation service from the front line is largely regulated by the most serious cases, the abdominal cases.

A system for reducing the time lag between sustaining and treating abdominal wounds had dramatically improved outcomes since World War I, when "20% to 30% of all abdominal cases brought to Casualty Clearing Stations were diagnosed as hopeless and no operative effort to save them was made." In Spain, by contrast, "over 95% of all abdominal cases arriving at front line hospitals receive operative attention—only those obviously in extremis on arrival and who fail to respond to such restoratives as blood transfusions do not reach the operating theatre."[18]

This transformation in the survival rate for abdominal operations was achieved under the most challenging conditions imaginable. Although based in another field hospital high in the Pyrenees, Welsh nurse Margaret Powell's account of her work applies as well to Jolly's unit:

> We had no electricity but worked with primus lamps and candles and when all the mantles broke, just candles. Imagine if you can, a surgeon performing a laparotomy, finding and suturing a liver wound, or maybe 24 or more intestinal perforations . . . all by candlelight. Meanwhile we grope around the table for instruments, thread needles, break catgut capsules all in the flickering light. . . . Blood transfusions were given whenever possible, but we could not employ the tubes of blood because we had no refrigerator in which to store them, so the direct method was always used. There were times when it was impossible to find a donor, for everyone within reach had given as much as they could.[19]

Another medical volunteer, New Orleans–born ambulance driver James Neugass, also noted this sharp and significant reordering of priorities in the treatment of the severely wounded. "I understand that during the [First] World War all of the magnificent equipment and technical skill of the Medical Corps were concentrated on giving the maximum and the most quick treatment to the light wounded, so that these might be soon cured and sent back to the lines, and that the proportion of deaths among the heavy wounded was therefore very great. With us, the heavy wounded come first. We seem unable to adopt the careless attitude towards life which might help us strengthen the lines."[20]

Abdominal operations, Jolly calculated, took up about 30 percent of the time and effort of frontline surgeons. Despite the massive reductions in mortality rates since World War I, the survival rate among these cases in Spain was still only about 50–60 percent. Therefore, a third of the surgeons' time was devoted to saving the lives of just 3 percent of the wounded, and of those, half would later be found unfit for further frontline combat roles. "Our whole front line hospital system," he concluded, "has been built up on the knowledge that we must do everything humanly possible to save the lives of these men, few of whom will return to the front line to carry on the fight against Fascism."

From questioning the wounded prisoners he treated, wrote Jolly, he was confident that no such humane and compassionate equation was calculated on the other side of the lines. "In the Fascist mind . . . such sentimentality has no place. They preach that the greatest end of man is to die gloriously for his country and his Führer."

Here the earnest precepts of the Christian Left are given practical, concrete form: "The unassessable value of every member of these forces shall continue to regulate the medical service of our Army . . . figures and percentages have no meaning for us except as a means of checking our mistakes and remedying the inefficiencies of our Service."[21]

Invariably, after a major setback such as the collapse of the Aragón front, the Republican high command was riven by bitter mutual recrimination and attempts to attribute blame, such as allegations of incompetence or of spying for the enemy. In early 1938, Dr. Oscar Telge was summoned to Moscow to face accusations of this kind, and André Marty, the bizarrely paranoic inspector general of the International Brigade, called a meeting of its entire medical service in Barcelona. Three hundred people—surgeons, physicians, technicians, ambulance drivers, and nurses—attended and heard Marty attack Telge, without giving details or evidence, as "an unscrupulous traitor who would now have to answer to a People's Court in Moscow."

The publicist Gusti Jirku (later Stridsberg) was sufficiently rash and impolitic to publicly challenge the volatile Marty over this proposed show trial, blurting out that she and all her colleagues had willingly followed Dr. Telge's direction. "If what you are saying is true, all of us who have followed his line with conviction have made serious mistakes. Why not specify them? For myself, I ask nothing better than to be questioned by this 'court of the people' that you spoke about." For once, Marty was taken aback by the courageous public declaration of support for a persecuted "nonperson," and he clumsily attempted to placate Jirku. Although Jolly's limited French prevented him from taking an active part in this defense of a victimized colleague, he afterward praised Jirku for her stand.[22] His fellow surgeon Josep Maria Massons later learned that after Telge testified in his own defense in Moscow, he was banished to Siberia but managed to return to his native Bulgaria after World War II.[23]

Behind the natural barrier of the fast-flowing Ebro River, the weary, disheartened Republican forces regrouped and rebuilt in the Catalan-speaking north as spring arrived. Franco's single-minded focus on attacking Valencia had given them an unforeseen opportunity to rearm and train intensively for a renewed and possibly final assault. The International Brigaders were based in the Priorat region, near the picturesque villages of Marça and Falset. Their numbers had been so reduced by the Aragón campaign that recent Spanish conscripts now composed more than half of each brigade, which were no longer referred to as "international" but as "mixed."

The landscape around them ranged dramatically from fields of almond and cherry trees in the valleys to steeply terraced vineyards backed by sheer outcrops topped with pine and wild rosemary. As the weather warmed, training became more intense: target practice with both rifles and machine guns, lessons in stripping and reassembling the weapons blindfolded, forced marches through the olive groves and over the ridges, and mock attacks on lookout points, buildings, and railway tunnels. John Longstaff, a young foundry worker from the north of England, was trained as a runner, scout, and sniper, and learned to signal messages using a heliograph (mirror) and flags in daytime and lamps at night. Like his fellow fighters, he was lean and fit from the constant exercise and spartan diet, and deeply tanned from the Mediterranean sun.[24]

The Hungarian National Museum holds photographs of Jolly and Anna-Mária Basch enjoying the hospitality of Hungarian brigaders during this carefree period. The two are shown feasting at an outdoor table, inspecting a tanker truck with its crew, and picnicking in a farmyard among shirtless men and one unidentified woman, presumably a fellow medical worker.[25] These images tell a story of a sparsely equipped yet determined and high-spirited army, apparently recovered from the bitter retreats of the previous winter and steadily rebuilding their resources under the Catalonian sun.

The medical teams scouted locations for hospitals at several points along the planned front line. Beneath a steep bluff between the villages of Marça and Torre de Fontaubella stood a large farmhouse with outbuildings arrayed around a courtyard big enough for ambulances to enter and turn around. This local landmark, Mas d'en Magrinyà, became a well-equipped hospital with three surgical teams. Jolly's resourceful mechanic, John Kozar, wired it for electricity powered by a small generator, which he "nursed with immense skill and care" in one of the outbuildings.[26] There Kozar also lived in relative comfort. "He had a table spread with an embroidered cloth; he had vases of flowers, ashtrays, posters on the walls, a couple of comfortable chairs and every sort of cooking utensil, including a Primus stove."[27] About fifteen kilometers away in the village of El Molar, another hospital was set up in the offices of a lead mine, with operating theaters near the entrance and wards upstairs.[28] Railway tunnels that had been blasted through the mountains in the previous century were converted into other temporary hospitals, providing the dual advantages of shelter from aviation and ready-made transport for evacuating patients. The four-thousand-meter-long l'Argentera tunnel, still one of the longest in Spain, had double tracks, so one train could be used for surgical operations while another evacuated the wounded.[29]

The largest and most remarkable of the improvised hospitals on the Ebro was sited some distance from the river itself, in the mountains near the village of La Bisbal de Falset. The road to this village winds steeply upward in a series of hairpin bends. Nearby stands a broad-mouthed yet shallow cave, with a spring of fresh water rising within its walls, known in this Catalan-speaking region as Cova de Santa Llúcia.[30] Inhabited periodically since prehistoric times, screened by pines, and topped by a massive rock lintel overhanging its entrance, the cave offered near-perfect protection against bombing. Jolly described it as "ideally safe and cool" for a frontline hospital.[31] However, its distance from the battlefield meant that once the wounded were brought back across the dangerous river, they still faced a grueling ambulance ride along rutted mountain roads.[32] The formed road ended in the valley below the cave, and ambulances could drive no farther. To give stretcher-bearers foot access to the cave, a pathway was blasted out of the hill below it. Reg Saxton's mobile blood transfusion unit was based in an olive grove nearby, which provided cover from aerial attacks.[33]

The cave floor was roughly flattened to make two usable levels—an operating theater and main ward above, and a separate ward for prisoners, who were mainly Italian, below. "After a hundred sappers had spent a day levelling the floor," wrote Jolly, "the cave was adequate for the installation of 150 beds and an operating theatre. In the cave were pure water springs which saved us the trouble of carrying water by motor tank from a pure water source a great distance away."[34] A car engine was modified to power the electric lighting. Leah Manning, a visiting British Labour MP and secretary of the Spanish Medical Aid Committee, thought that "in all the history of modern warfare there has never been such a hospital. It is the safest place in Spain, beautifully wired for electric lights and with every kind of modern equipment."[35] The cave hospital came to serve as a powerful visual symbol of a people with its back to the wall who yet retained both the will to resist and the capability to provide succor.[36]

As the sweltering summer days ripened their crops, the local people continued with their early harvesting, while these hospitals were readied for use and as the reinvigorated battalions trained in the fields around them. The area was Catalan speaking, so even Spanish troops could not always communicate easily with their hosts, yet the two populations interacted readily and warmly. The brigaders volunteered their help with the harvest and organized lectures and literacy classes for Spanish soldiers and staff. The locals received treatment at the military hospitals, including at least one childbirth, and everybody took part in the numerous festivals.[37] On one occasion, the cave hospital staff gave a picnic for the local children, long remembered by the youngest of them because it featured the best food they had ever eaten, including chocolate.[38]

"The Ebro battle was like a breath of fresh air to a dying man," thought the nurse Aurora Fernández.[39] It was a last desperate gamble by the Republican Army command to turn the tide of the war. A massive force of eighty thousand Republican troops was to assemble at several points on the eastern banks of the river and push inland with the aim of stalling a Nationalist advance on Valencia and reuniting the divided Republican zone. This battle would prove to be the most hard fought of the entire war.

By mid-July, the meticulously planned offensive was put in action. As the permanent bridges across the Ebro had all been bombed, a fleet of small rowing boats, built in secrecy at workshops some distance from the river, were hauled to its banks on trolleys.[40] Using these boats, barges, and twelve hastily assembled pontoon bridges, the advance units crossed the Ebro in the night and early morning of 24–25 July. According to Longstaff, "Everyone was silent and thinking about the fighting to come. The Spanish and International Brigaders had muffled even the oars. I had a lot of equipment, a rifle, about 100 rounds of ammunition and my blanket tied round my body."[41] The Nationalist guards on the far bank were caught by surprise, and for several days the Republicans pushed rapidly forward as planned until, forty kilometers from the river, their attack stalled at the town of Gandesa. Franco's mobile reinforcements by then had been brought up in strength and pounded the attackers with artillery and aerial bombardments. The Republicans could respond only with light weapons since, in a devastating and preemptive move, the Nationalists had opened the floodgates of hydroelectric dams in the Pyrenees upstream from the crossing points. A two-meter-high torrent of water was released down the river that washed away the pontoon bridges, preventing most of the Republican tanks, guns, and motorized infantry from making the crossing.[42]

As Republican engineers toiled overnight to repair bridges that were promptly bombed again the following day, their infantry dug in as best they could on the treeless hills of the Sierra de Pàndols, with little cover from Franco's artillery and dive bombers. Their corpses accumulated but could not be buried in the bare rock. Typhoid and dysentery, as well as enemy fire, took a terrible toll.[43] Each night water was hauled up the mountains to the parched fighters, and their wounded were carried away.[44]

Jolly wrote that the field hospital system put in place before the battle began "worked excellently during the first day of the advance, and the seriously wounded arrived within the five-hour period"—which he regarded as the maximum time for effective treatment of the most serious wounds—"but from the moment the bridges were carried away the casualty stream stopped. Boats rushed to the river on lorries were used to ferry the wounded across. . . . But the battalion ambulances which had followed the troops over the first pontoon bridges were insufficient to deal with the growing numbers of wounded as the journey back to the river grew longer and longer behind the rapidly advancing troops. The time-lag rose to twenty and sometimes thirty hours. During the next two days most of the seriously wounded died."[45]

In the harsh terrain of the Sierra de Pàndols, the stretcher-bearers frequently resorted to using *artolas* (litters hauled by mules) or to carrying the men on their own backs. At the first aid stations, the *heridos* (wounded) were given morphine and crude splints for broken limbs, and loaded in ambulances for the jolting journey to the riverbank. Only the worst cases were brought back across the river, often by local boatmen. They then faced a further excruciating drive to the nearest field hospital, frequently arriving there many hours after their injury and in severe shock.

At the well-protected but distant La Bisbal de Falset cave hospital, ambulances halted at the foot of the hill and unloaded their laden stretchers, which were then carried into two tents housing the reception and triage facilities.[46] The groaning figures were laid out on the ground in rows for triage, and those who qualified for immediate operation were carried by hand up the steep path to the cave. These cases soon proved so numerous that they were then graded again as either "serious," "medium," or "wait."[47] English nurse Patience Darton found this process especially distressing. "We got them sometimes hours after they'd been wounded and some of course, we couldn't save because of that—they were already too bad."[48] She also found the cave very uncomfortable to work in. "It was very dark, very low and all uneven. The metal beds were all higgledy-piggledy over the floor and you could barely see—we hadn't got lights. We had lights for the theatre, run off one of our ambulances, but we hadn't got [electric] lights in the cave, and we had to do our work by tiny little oil lamps, cans—ordinary tin cans—with a wick in them with oil."[49]

"The hospital served a double purpose," Jolly pointed out, "for it accommodated not only casualties from the front but also the worst of the [civilian] wounded from the villages in the rear, which were being subjected to intense bombardment from the air."[50] Curtains strung on wires demarcated the surgical ward, recovery room, patients' area, and sleeping quarters for the staff. Hank Rubin remembered working as an aide for three days and nights on end as the ambulances arrived without letup. When there was no more room for the wounded inside the cave itself, they were laid in front of its entrance without protection from enemy aircraft.[51]

Hank Rubin and the other staff subsisted on stale and moldy bread, gristly fragments of donkey meat, and tinned, sweetened condensed milk. The local wine, fortunately, was plentiful.[52] As usual, medical supplies ran critically short. Each morning a row of dead lay outside the cave awaiting burial, and Patience Darton battled fiercely with stretcher-bearers who tried to inter the corpses in precious hospital blankets, sometimes resorting to a tug-of-war with them.[53] As in every other field hospital Jolly had worked in, burying the corpses of the least fortunate patients was a daily task. At La Bisbal de Falset, the mayor organized teams of older men from the village to take the dead in lorries in the early morning to the municipal cemetery, where a trench had been dug as a common grave. The bodies were piled in four and five deep, and eventually the trench extended almost the entire length of the cemetery.[54] The identities of those buried in it were recorded in a carefully typed list that ran to more than sixty names, mostly Spanish and Catalan, but several were evidently foreign, including a Welshman, Harry Dobson; a Finn, Walter Forsman; and some listed only as *sin identificar* (unidentified).[55]

Despite this somber morning ritual, nurse Aurora Fernández thought the cave hospital was "where we worked in greatest harmony." Her Spanish patients, mainly very young and frightened men from the countryside, addressed her not as *enfermera* (nurse) but as *curandera* (healer), since the only health services they had known had been provided by village women with a knowledge of curative plants and folk medicine.[56] One of her patients was a young local boy, Manuel Álvarez, brought from the village of Corbera with multiple injuries after a Nationalist bombing.[57] In early August, the village of La Bisbal de Falset was itself heavily bombed, and several people, including two young girls, were killed.[58] Yet even in these desperate conditions, patients were treated regardless of their political loyalties. Patience Darton was called upon to donate her own blood to a Moorish prisoner who was convinced it would poison him, while a downed Italian airman also received life-saving attention.[59]

According to the English nurse Lillian Urmston, a few days after the Ebro battle began, rumors reached the hospital that "hundreds of wounded were lying on the other side of the river, and could not be brought across. . . . We were all sick with horror at the thought of this unnecessary suffering and begged with our chiefs to send us across the river." At one o'clock the next day, the most senior medical officer instructed Urmston and other staff to be ready in twenty minutes to make the crossing. "I hurriedly issued orders and in a very short time we were ready. I was to go, along with Dr Jolly, the Spanish doctors and *sanitarios* [medical auxiliaries], and set up as large a hospital as possible."[60]

Dawn was breaking as their convoy of vehicles, including an autochir and Saxton's mobile blood transfusion laboratory, drove across a newly repaired pontoon bridge. The truck carrying Jolly's team broke down midway and had to be towed across by another truck, no doubt to the great anxiety of its passengers.[61] "We had just reached the other side," Lillian Urmston said later,

> and our ambulances were toiling along the hastily prepared road when we heard the familiar cry "*Aviación!*" Ambulances were pulled up at the side of the road, under the shelter of the cliffs—and we lay in ditches, tense with expectation and apprehension. But it was only our usual early-morning caller, the observation plane. We continued our journey for exactly 25 minutes, and then twelve huge bombers came into sight. We all pulled into an olive grove, just off the road, and hastily camouflaged our ambulances and *autochir*. . . . We all lay down under trees and bushes. The planes bombed all along the river banks, and roads, and crossroads. Our anti-aircraft guns were going magnificently, and managed to bring down one bomber.
>
> Suddenly came the familiar rat-tat-tat of machine-guns—they were strafing the helpless people who happened to be anywhere in view. At last came a number, six I think, of our pursuit planes, and engaged in a glorious dogfight. . . . After an hour of this the bombers soared higher and disappeared. We were all relieved. And weren't we hungry! Rations of bully beef and bread were issued, then we again moved off.[62]

By early afternoon, they reached the huge white hermitage of Santa Magdalena, standing high on a summit and therefore a prominent landmark for enemy aircraft but nevertheless the only suitable building for a considerable distance. "We cheerfully acted as charwomen," Lillian Urmston remembered, then quickly set up a hospital. We were again interrupted by a heavy bombardment—luckily the bombs did not fall too near. By 11pm our hospital was complete and a steady stream of ambulances started to arrive. We only received the more severely wounded cases and our beds were quickly filled. Work was carried on for four days and nights with but slight respite, but conditions were satisfactory. All day long we had the enemy planes overhead. Bridges and roads were bombed daily, and many ambulances were smashed and rendered unfit for use. Work continued but under greater difficulties. Food and medical supplies could not be regularly brought across the river, so belts were tightened and brains racked to provide a solution to the problem of medical supplies.[63]

In the fierce midsummer weather, conditions inside the old building grew so uncomfortable that Jolly and his assistant worked bare chested beneath their theater gowns, and only their nurse, Anna-Mária Basch, remained in full uniform at the head of the operating table.

The wounded were evacuated from this hospital to either the pontoon bridge that the staff themselves had used or further downstream at Móra d'Ebre, where a motorboat ferry service was operating.[64] On the fifth day, shells began whistling overhead as Nationalist heavy artillery targeted the monastery. The shelling continued intermittently for three days; then the order came to evacuate. First the wounded were sent back to a safer hospital, and at 2:00 a.m., Jolly and his staff left to establish a new base. Without lights, they drove ten kilometers northward, noting the occasional flash of enemy guns, until they reached the town of Flix on a promontory above a bend in the Ebro River. The town was in ruins, but its double-tracked railway tunnel remained intact and could be rendered secure against further bombing.

An accumulation of many years' soot and grime enveloped the walls and roof. We stumbled along in the dark, continually falling over railway lines. Everyone was cold, tired and hungry—but the hospital had to be prepared. . . . We all worked furiously, digging, scraping and scrubbing, and soon we had ready another hospital complete with 65 beds. . . . No time for rest—a furtive dab with a powder puff, a meal of bread and black coffee, and again all ready for work. Wounded were already being brought in, so we must carry on. We had no satisfactory lighting system—one lamp for three operating tables, and a few candles in the huge ward. . . . Occasionally a bomb fell directly above us, and then we were all enveloped in soot.[65]

Jolly worked in this hospital for nearly two months, and it was gradually made more serviceable despite frequent bombing raids. "The whole of the forward area," he wrote later, "was subjected to attack by massed enemy bombers. For weeks and months flights of 50 to 80 heavy bombers at a time bombarded the Republican communication lines almost daily from daylight to dusk; yet by using caves, railway tunnels and deep bomb-proof shelters the forward surgical system continued to function in security. One autochir stationed just inside the mouth of the tunnel at Flix was partly wrecked by a 500-kilo bomb."[66] Both ends of the tunnel were sandbagged against such attacks, and Jolly's operating theater was set up fifteen meters inside one entrance. One of his Spanish colleagues described the conditions: "On the stretchers lie the worst mutilated, groaning in voices that don't seem to belong to human beings. . . . The floor becomes covered with cotton and gauze, soon soaked with pus and blood. The sharp smell of sweat, human filth, burnt oil and tobacco fills the dense, cold, atmosphere. The oil lamps only illuminate about a square meter and in this dark, suffocating, gloomy environment, people move laboriously, like ghosts."[67]

Among the gravely wounded men carried into the tunnel for treatment was nineteen-year-old Johnny Longstaff with a severe facial injury. A Nationalist bullet had entered his nose and lodged in the left cheekbone, blinding him temporarily in both eyes. He was evacuated from the battlefront by walking with his hands on another man's shoulders and eventually reached the hospital where Jolly carried out the sophisticated surgery required to repair as much as possible of the young man's face and restore his eyesight.[68] Later photographs of Longstaff show a handsome man without noticeable facial disfigurement.

Operations such as these relied heavily on Saxton's mobile blood transfusion laboratory, which was installed in a bombed-out ambulance that had been rebuilt and filled with basic equipment for blood storage, grouping, and testing. In this vehicle, Saxton traveled with Jolly's team and to other field hospitals, taking cover periodically against air attacks. On several occasions, he was forced to drive off the road into olive groves and use loose branches to camouflage his truck from the air.[69]

Two months after the offensive began, more than a third of the Republican force had been killed, injured, or captured.[70] Aurora Fernández overheard her English colleagues saying, "This is the end or very near," although they broke off their tense conversation when they noticed she was listening. "Apparently they did not want to frighten us young Spaniards."[71] Realizing that this last-ditch military maneuver had failed, Spanish prime minister Juan Negrín was reduced to a desperate diplomatic gamble. In late September 1938, in what Jolly later described as a "quixotic gesture," Negrín told the League of Nations that his government would unilaterally withdraw all its foreign troops in the faint hope that the league would then pressure Franco to order his Italian and German allies to do likewise. The order to withdraw left Jolly's English colleague Reggie Saxton feeling "like the rats running out of a sinking ship . . . we felt there was a chance that we could still come out victorious. . . . How could [the French government] let another Fascist government be established on their other flank?"[72]

Whether Jolly was aware that these forlorn international negotiations were underway, and how he felt at the prospect of an imminent Republican defeat, is unknown. He remained at his post in the Flix tunnel hospital, treating the endless flow of wounded from the merciless Nationalist counterattack driving the Republican troops back toward the banks of the Ebro. One Welsh medic described it as "twelve weeks of organised, unyielding, mass slaughter."[73] Those who could not reach the Flix hospital often had to be ferried back across the river at night in barges, tightly packed and in extreme discomfort. Jolly was later critical of the Republican medical command's slow response to the problem of moving the autochirs and other field transport across the Ebro after all the pontoon bridges were swept away. Apart from that delay, however, "the time-lag of under five hours for the most urgent casualties was maintained," and during the several brutal months of the Ebro offensive, "no wounded man in hospital and no member of the hospital staff was lost in air bombardment in the 156th Army Corps."[74]

By October 1938, the Republican Army held only a small strip of territory on the west bank of the Ebro.[75] In accordance with Prime Minister Negrín's undertaking to the League of Nations, all members of the International Brigades were then ordered to withdraw from the lines and assemble in Barcelona. After a poignantly defiant farewell parade through the Diagonal, the city's main street, in front of 300,000 people, they were formally disbanded and repatriated. Jolly does not appear to have taken part in this famous and undoubtedly moving ceremony; instead, he remained at his tunnel hospital. However, he and his medical service colleagues were presented with a simple printed acknowledgement of their work that reads, in part, "When life finds its way again, when the roads of Spain do not carry guns and soldiers but workers and agricultural machines, the Spanish people will still and always remember you. Legends will be woven around your heroic behavior. Some fighter of today, then old, will tell how someone from a distant country provided him with medical expertise and how he owes his life to those who came here out of a human impulse of solidarity."[76] Jolly's copy was countersigned by several Spanish colleagues who added affectionate messages testifying to his good-humored stoicism and the expert clinical practice that saved thousands of lives and limbs. He retained this testimonial throughout his life.

He remained at the tunnel hospital until, in early November, his equipo received the order to withdraw, and they moved downstream toward the crossing point at Móra d'Ebre. They spent the night beforehand in a whitewashed, stone-and-stucco farmhouse serving as the local army headquarters. Among its weary and disheartened occupants was a large, tweedy civilian with an American accent. Jolly finally met Ernest Hemingway, whose writing on Spain he had admired almost two years earlier during the battle of Madrid. The famous author was disgusted by the response of League of Nations members, including that of his own country, to the crisis in Spain and spoke of "the mess everything's in, and the sort of let-down and carnival of treachery and rotten-ness that's going on." What Jolly made of this bulky and blustering celebrity is unknown. More than thirty years later, he merely noted that "we spent the evening with Ernest Hemingway who was also 'in retreat.'"[77] Next morning, in the company of several others including the photographer Robert Capa, whose lover Gerda Taro had died at Brunete the year before, Hemingway crossed the turbulent and fast-flowing river in an overloaded rowing boat.[78] "A series of treacherous spikes had been sunk in the river to discourage all navigation on it," and after the boat almost struck one and capsized, Hemingway seized an oar and hauled them to shore.[79]

Jolly's equipo appears to have crossed without incident and joined another railway tunnel hospital in the town of Falset. "When no more casualties were filtering back across the river—after a few days—we were sent to the neighbouring village of Marsa where we set up a hospital in a farmhouse."[80] Yet again the wearily familiar routine of triage, surgery, recuperation, and evacuation carried on while Nationalist air raids and artillery bombardments drew steadily closer. His team, along with the other frontline units, sent daily casualty lists to the town of Flix, where a medical headquarters had been set up under Dr. Len Crome, commander of the Thirty-Fifth Divisional Medical Corps. Later studies have concluded that Crome's innovations "ensured that the wounded under his care received better treatment than they might have expected in the best teaching hospitals of the time in London."[81]

The highly competent and active English nursing administrator Nan Green typed and compiled the daily casualty lists. She had developed a system for classifying her patients by the category of wound suffered (head wounds, leg wounds, amputations, etc.), the type of weapon that had caused them (mortars, shells, bullets), and the treatment they received. "With the aid of a box of water-colours and some drawing instruments," she converted this data into hand-colored graphs to assist Crome and other medical staff to immediately identify the supplies most urgently needed and to prioritize treatment.[82] Jolly found this simple method of presenting daily case data in visual form hugely helpful, and he later employed it during the Second World War in hospitals in North Africa and Italy.[83]

Even after Nan Green heard that her musician husband, George, was missing while serving with the International Brigades' final defensive stand in the Sierra de Caballs (learning later that he had been killed in action), she maintained her calm demeanor and instinctive compassion. In the wreckage of the bombed-out Marça farmhouse, she discovered an English china teapot complete with tea cosy and managed to create a kind of living room, with armchairs and a table, in a corner of the shattered building. There she served cheering cups of tea around the clock.[84]

This site appears to be the last in the long series of field hospitals that Jolly headed in Spain. Barcelona did not fall to the enemy until January 1939 and Madrid, not until March, after putting up an extraordinary two and a half years of resistance. However, by late November 1938, following the longest and bloodiest battle of the entire war, Franco's forces overran the last opposition on the Ebro, and the fate of the Republic was thereafter sealed.

In that month, Jolly left Spain carrying demobilization papers recording his service on almost every major front of the civil war. A commendation from the army's chief of surgical services testifies that Jolly's role as chief surgeon "of the advanced shock brigade surgical team has been brilliant, as much with respect to his personal bravery and valor as to the high technical quality of his surgical work. In every moment he has greatly distinguished himself for his decision to work in dangerous places in order to save the lives of our injured without taking into account his personal risk nor the bodily fatigue. . . . For all of that, he deserves the recognition of the Republican government and all Spanish people."[85]

Jolly also had with him a highly regarded military decoration, the Medalla del Deber (Medal of Duty). Depicted on one side is an armed soldier and on the other, a young woman, the *niña bonita* (beautiful young girl) who symbolized Spain's Second Republic. This medal, for "notably outstanding merits or war services," was awarded only to those who had spent at least three consecutive months in a combat zone, figured in at least three armed clashes, and been active "in any phase of them from positions of great danger."[86] Under those conditions, the citation reads, Jolly had demonstrated "a great spirit of sacrifice and work, as well as excellent professional competence."[87]

Yet perhaps more effectively than any other document, his army discharge certificate, written in the terse and staccato language of such military communications, manages to convey the nature and extent of Jolly's distinctive contribution to the Republican struggle. It describes him as "an excellent surgeon, courageous and totally reliable. He has worked with great skill and enthusiasm. He has always wanted to operate as close as possible to the firing line. His relations with the comrades are magnificent. Although not affiliated to any organization, he is an excellent anti-fascist."[88] The last sentence may be a politically coy reference to Jolly's persistent refusal to join the Communist Party in either Spain or Britain. Members of the Spanish party, obediently subordinate to its Moscow parent, wrote or vetted the demobilization papers of every departing International Brigader, and few noncommunists earned such warm praise from them. Repatriated noncommunist British volunteers were ranked under five categories of political reliability in a list sent to the British party in December 1938. The assessors, all party members themselves, issued harsh judgments on most of these returning men ("drunkard and thief," "undisciplined and dull") and ranked most of them as either "bad" or "weak." Of the eighty-three names on the list, only Jolly earned the highest rating, that of "cadre."[89]

*

During the subsequent four bleak decades of Franco's postwar dictatorship, the cave of Santa Llúcia became an abandoned and rubbish-strewn site, and each year fewer local people knew of its significance. One of them, however, was Enric Masip Gorgori, who at the age of five went there with his uncle during an exceptionally dry summer to haul water from the spring. "He explained to me that there was a hospital here during the war that healed wounded soldiers." From the early 1980s, after the restoration of democracy in Spain, Masip Gorgori, by then a councillor (and later mayor) of the nearby village of La Bisbal de Falset, began the process of cleaning and restoring this historically redolent landmark. It stood on private land, and after the Spanish government declined to fund the project, the village council and its people raised 2 million pesetas (about $US13,000) to bring it into public ownership and preserve the memory of its use as a wartime hospital. It is now a carefully maintained museum and shrine to the days when the civil war overwhelmed this quiet corner of rural Catalonia. From that period, says Masip Gorgori, "along with its dead, two symbols have remained in the town for history—the Municipal Cemetery and the Hospital Cave of Santa Llúcia. Both today form an inseparable historical and sentimental ensemble."[90]

11 Changing the Front and the Weapons

> The four main areas in which medical science advanced during the Spanish Civil War are the treatment of wounds and injuries, the development of blood banks, medical diseases (especially in relation to malnutrition) and the organization of medical support to the armed forces.
>
> —NICHOLAS CONI

Jolly's departure from Spain was as brisk and frictionless as his arrival was two years earlier. "Having jealously guarded my fully visa-ed NZ passport," he later wrote, "[I] was able without any trouble to step on board a Spanish plane at Barcelona and be flown by LAPE [Spanish national airline Líneas Aéreas Postales Españolas] over the Pyrenees to Toulouse and thence by train to Paris and air to London, where I arrived just before Christmas."[1]

He was acutely aware that many others who had supported the Republic, whether in military or civilian roles, were less fortunate. They now felt imperiled by the prospect of Franco's victory and the retribution he had threatened. Traveling out of the battle zone to Barcelona, Jolly's former colleague Aileen Palmer saw

> all along the roads . . . the painful pilgrimages—peasants driven from their homes by the annihilating bombs, uprooted Spaniards trekking eastward to the coast with their flocks and herds if they have any, with their ramshackle mule-drawn carts piled up with mattresses, bits of furniture, bits of food, sometimes taking their hens and chickens which are all they have, sometimes people who have nothing at all to eat, women carrying children and making the long journey on foot. . . . They are mostly people who have never moved from the villages where they were born and have grown up, and who have suddenly seen the whole world they knew turned into a heap of dust and crumbled shards.[2]

Franco's forces did indeed exact reprisals on Spanish citizens in forms ranging from the merely vindictive to the near genocidal. The Nationalists occupied La Bisbal de Falset on the final day of 1938. The cave hospital had been evacuated beforehand, and those remaining in the village were ordered to speak only Spanish, not Catalan, thereafter.[3] Several of Jolly's colleagues from the International Brigades health services, including Anna-Mária Basch, were in double jeopardy as they could neither remain in Spain nor return to their homelands for fear of Nazi terror. Before his departure from Spain, Jolly circulated a letter to friends overseas seeking financial help for these desperate and displaced medical refugees from eastern Europe. One who responded was his former high school teacher Alexander Aitken, now a professor of mathematics at Edinburgh University. He sent a guinea, saying it was "little enough but it is all I can spare," since he was also supporting "many exiled Jews and other non-Aryans, of whom there are many about the university here, and a few in the Mathematical Department."[4]

While in France en route to London, Jolly detoured to Perpignan, near the Spanish border. There he found that the desperate torrent of Republican refugees who had fled for safety across the Pyrenees were now confined on windswept beaches in vast concentration camps originally built to contain German prisoners of war during the Great War. The latest inmates included many of his former colleagues, such as the surgeon František Kriegel, whom Jolly regarded as "the finest doctor I knew in Spain."[5] Kriegel managed to send Jolly a letter in faulty Spanish expressing "muchissmo interes" in the prospect of starting a new life in New Zealand, and in accordance with his country's immigration requirements, Jolly lodged a guarantee with the New Zealand government to support Franz until he found regular work there. Nevertheless, the highly skilled and dedicated Czechoslovak doctor was not granted entry; instead, along with some twenty other former Republican medical volunteers, he eventually traveled to China and gave his services to Mao Zedong's Red Army.[6] Jolly then transferred his immigration guarantee to Anna-Mária Basch, telling a New Zealand friend, "I feel pretty sure that we could eventually get her work in this country even though it might take a little time." She was likewise denied entry. His former senior officer in the international medical service, Dr. Rudolf Neumann, then sought to join him in London but, as a German national, was also refused.[7] With the help of an expatriate New Zealand lawyer named John Platts-Mills,

Jolly later lobbied New Zealand's Labour prime minister, Walter Nash, to allow entry to his homeland for imprisoned International Brigaders. Nash and his cabinet remained unmoved, and none were permitted to immigrate.

Predictably, Jolly's first home address in London after his two-year absence was the Grant family's reliably welcoming household at 25 Pyecombe Corner. The temptation to rest and recuperate there must have been almost overwhelming, yet he did not succumb to it. Upon his return to civilian life, he continued almost without pause to support the now-reeling Spanish Republic by other means—"merely changing the front and the weapons," as Nan Green put it.[8] She and other British medical volunteers had founded a relief organization, the British Medical Unit from Spain, to support victims of the war, including the refugees and the thousands of former combatants now held in Franco's prisons.[9] Within a week of Jolly's return, he and several other British doctors who had also recently returned from Spain—including Archie Cochrane, Reg Saxton, Len Crome, and Alex Tudor-Hart—published a letter in the *Lancet* appealing for support for "a number of our colleagues, who are by nationality German or Austrian [who] have been moved to French territory." Their financial situation was desperate, the signatories said, and "they cannot return to their homes."[10]

The Christian Left group still functioned, Jolly found, but in a greatly reduced state. Its newsletter was no longer professionally printed but instead reproduced cheaply on a hand-cranked duplicator. Through this humble means, Jolly made another attempt to raise funds to assist "doctors and nurses who had been serving under the Spanish Government, who were now to be repatriated but who, in many cases, would not be admitted to their own country on account of their political associations." Donations were to be sent care of Irene Grant at her Pyecombe Corner address. At the sparsely attended 1938 annual meeting of the Christian Left, "the Treasurer contrived to acquire a surplus of one guinea, which was handed over to Douglas Jolly."[11]

Nan Green's group encouraged its members to speak to meetings throughout Britain on the conditions in Spain, and during early 1939, Jolly threw himself into this work, sharing his experience of the war with all who would listen.[12] In mid-January, the British Medical Association hosted a reception at its central London premises for "ten British medical men who have recently returned from service in Republican Spain." Some 250 people attended, and afterward "questions and discussion continued until a late hour." Saxton spoke on blood transfusion, Tudor-Hart discussed limb surgery, and Jolly described the organization of field hospitals. "While the fighting was going on," he told the audience, "there was no pause between operations. The next patient was being prepared while the operation was taking place on the first." One of the many vital lessons learned from this experience, he said, was the need for a foolproof and speedy method for identifying triaged patients, such as color coding, so that orderlies assisting the surgeon could immediately tell what degree of urgency each patient had been assigned. "A rule-of-thumb method and one obvious to the untrained person was required." He then spoke of the continuous improvement in the Republican health services during the past two years. "The formless embryo became adult. It earned the gratitude of the Spanish people who would crowd in with food and wood and offers of service."[13]

At a meeting in Newport in Wales organized by the local chapter of the Left Book Club, Jolly spoke on "my two years at the front."[14] He told this audience that he admired the spirit of the Spaniards who continued to fight against the Italians, Germans, and Moors. "He felt that if they were allowed to buy arms they could hold out, but that if they continued to be stopped, under international law, then a Franco victory might ultimately be expected."[15]

In February, little more than a month after he arrived in the United Kingdom, Jolly departed for his own country. As he had done on the outward journey from New Zealand, he worked his passage, this time as the assistant ship's surgeon aboard the Shaw Saville passenger liner *Arawa*.[16] He had spent almost a decade away from his country of birth, and immediately on his return, he made the long journey to the family home in Cromwell, finding his mother ailing but overjoyed to see him. In a curious footnote to this homecoming, just days after his arrival, the press announced his engagement to a Miss Frances Farmer of Diamond Harbour, Christchurch.[17] Given the timing of this whirlwind romance, which echoes his earlier engagement in 1931, the couple may have met on board the ship. For whatever reason, their marriage plans did not proceed.

Throughout the Spanish Civil War, New Zealand's trade union movement had ranked among the staunchest and most dependable local sources of support for the Spanish Republic. Among the many messages of goodwill on Jolly's arrival was a telegram from the Miners' Union branch in the tiny and remote coal-mining settlement of Ngākawau on the South Island's remote west coast: "Union congratulates you on your services in Spain and welcomes you back to NZ."[18]

As in Britain, the returned veteran permitted himself just a short time with his family and friends before embarking on a further nationwide speaking tour to bring attention to the increasingly desperate plight of Republican refugees and International Brigade prisoners following Franco's imminent victory. The portly generalissimo was refusing all peace terms and insisting on an unconditional surrender as he prepared to take Madrid.[19] For five weeks, under the sponsorship of the Spanish Medical Aid Committee, Jolly stumped New Zealand from end to end, speaking in every major city and in many small towns. One newspaper described him as "a forceful platform speaker."[20] He was often joined on stage by two former International Brigaders. Charlie Riley, ten years older than Jolly, was a tough little Cockney Londoner who had immigrated to New Zealand as a young man. He served in World War I, attaining the rank of sergeant, and was working as a miner in Australia when he learned of the civil war in Spain and arrived there in time to take part in the battle of Brunete. His experience with explosives led him to the exceptionally dangerous work of close-quarter anti-tank warfare, and he was severely wounded during the retreat across the Ebro River.[21] Bert Bryan had worked for Communist Party publications in New Zealand before leaving for Spain, where he also took part in the final battle of the Ebro.[22]

Both of these former fighters were able to enthrall local audiences with their accounts of battlefield valor, but it was the less ideologically purist, decorated, noncombatant commissioned officer who made the strongest impression on New Zealand audiences. Many who came to these meetings had been inclined, through reading local newspaper reports of the conflict, to regard the civil war in Spain as a proxy battle between communist and noncommunist forces, and were wary of siding with the Republic. At every speaking venue, however, Jolly attacked the farce of nonintervention, described the Spanish government as a coalition of various progressive forces, and maintained that Franco's victory was due entirely to the support he received from Hitler and Mussolini. The evidently upright and humanitarian doctor, with direct knowledge of all the major battles, proved an authoritative and persuasive speaker, capable of reaching elements of New Zealand society that had not previously taken a stance on the civil war.[23] "Dr Jolly's explanation of the situation prior to the war," reported the local paper of one rural district, "was vastly different to the distorted views forced upon the people of the Dominion by scanty messages published in the Press."[24]

Jolly apparently delivered much the same speech wherever he appeared, probably reading from notes, which were later found among his personal papers. He described Spain as geographically and socially distinct from the rest of Europe, with a population that was largely illiterate and socially dominated by the church. He emphasized the abject poverty of the rural peasantry, who worked under primitive conditions on estates controlled by their titled absentee landlords. "I remember with gratitude and admiration," he said, night after night,

> a people living under the stress and privations of war, never knowing at what moment enemy bombers might appear over their villages, yet almost gay and cheerful—anxious to do all they could for the streams of wounded men arriving daily from the front. In the Government part of Spain were some 16 million of the 24 million inhabitants of Spain. The food problem was acute. Spain had always been deficient in motorised transport, and military requirements made things worse. Had it not been for the whole-hearted co-operation of the peasants with their strange carts drawn by long strings of mules and donkeys, the problems of food distribution would have been insoluble.[25]

Jolly downplayed the communists' influence on the Republican government and recounted the occasions when he had operated on Franco's troops as well as their sworn opponents. In one counterattack during the battle of Madrid, he said, more than a hundred of Mussolini's men were brought to his hospital, all fully equipped with their Italian-made uniforms and equipment. Nevertheless, he also made it clear that he was no neutral who provided his medical services untinged by political partisanship. "My sympathies were completely with the Government; that was why I went to Spain and I saw nothing there which altered my mind." He lost no opportunity to denounce Franco's intentions for ruling the country he had conquered, and Jolly warned his New Zealand audiences that fascist ideologies could soon reach as far as their own shores. Buoyed by the effectiveness of their display of military might in Spain, he said, Germany and Italy now held a much stronger strategic position in Europe, with grave implications for maintaining peace in the wider region.

As he had done in Britain, this mild-mannered yet unquestionably authoritative figure urged the immediate creation of a new model of military medical organization to manage the anticipated casualties from a future war that would be dominated by intensive aerial bombing. He also offered hope for the ultimate outcome of such a war. Despite the grim future the Spanish people now faced under Franco, Jolly maintained that their recent conflict had reawakened among other Europeans, especially in Britain and France, an awareness of the need for collective security, which he considered the chief means of achieving a lasting international peace. His New Zealand listeners showed great interest in Russia's role in the recent conflict, and they frequently questioned Jolly about the strength and dependability of Russia as a potential military ally of Britain and its commonwealth. "From what I have seen of Russian arms, aeroplanes, and transport in Spain," he replied, "I would say that as an ally, Russia would give us no cause for fear."[26]

Communities large and small turned out in surprising numbers to hear Jolly and his fellow speakers. The left-wing journalist Elsie Freeman (later Locke) reported on a meeting in the placid South Island town of Nelson in July. "Next time anyone tells you that Nelson people are too comfortable to be progressive, don't you believe it. Seven hundred of them rolled up to hear Dr Jolly and Bert Bryan, from Spain, a few weeks ago."[27] A collection was taken up at each meeting to support Republican refugees. The remote southern township of Hokitika collectively subscribed the not inconsiderable sum of three pounds, and the entire amount, Jolly promised, would be allocated to relief services. "Not one penny would be used for the purpose of the lecture tour, or any other purpose except the comfort and feeding of the refugees."[28]

Early in his tour, Jolly revisited his old high school in Dunedin and addressed the entire student body. The school magazine recorded the event in its customary stolid tone: "At the close of his address Dr Jolly referred to the courage and endurance of the people of Spain, who had fought for what they believed to be right. It was a truly interesting and enlightening talk, and we showed our appreciation by cheers and a haka."[29] He also turned out for the school, along with other former pupils, for an exhibition cricket match against the "old boys" of Christ's College of Christchurch, a traditionally fierce competitor on the sports field. A photograph of the event shows the two teams arrayed in a variety of dress, from school uniforms to three-piece suits, with Jolly seated in the front row, looking compact, mustached, neat, and determined but rather worn and older than his thirty-five years.[30]

Perhaps the largest and most moving engagement of this nationwide speaking tour took place in the city of Auckland in May 1939 to commemorate the five New Zealand International Brigaders killed in action. An estimated nine hundred people attended the ceremony, organized by local poet and Communist Party member Ron Mason. The famed brass band of the Auckland Waterside Workers' Union played Handel's "Dead March," and in the course of the evening, a tableau depicted "a Spanish refugee woman with her baby in her arms on the French border."[31]

Local newspapers were eager to interview this articulate and recently returned veteran of a still-not-quite-concluded war. Alongside accounts on its international pages that the former Spanish premier Dr. Juan Negrín had left the country, that Republican general José Miaja had assumed leadership of the government, and that Franco continued to spurn all peace negotiations, the Wellington daily *Evening Post* reported Jolly's views of the Spanish people:

> [They] are filled with an amazing joy of life, and having had very little real liberty as a people, they are bent on achieving it. My own opinion is that government by Franco would be impossible without terrorist methods, as so large a proportion of the people have been governed by themselves for three years. They are not a people to accept lightly the loss of the thing they have fought for. . . .
>
> I met Dr Negrín, and have a very great admiration for him. He is a young man and a statesman. Dr Negrín was in the physiological department of the University of Madrid at the outbreak of the war. I met two famous military leaders, El Campesino [Valentin Gonzales] and Enrique Lister, lieutenant-colonels in the Government Army, commanders of two of the most famous units. They were men of the people, not cultured in the university sense, but innately very fine fellows.[32]

To the Communist Party paper the *Workers' Weekly*, he was a little more forthright:

> I went [to Spain] because I am a convinced anti-fascist, believing that a world victory for Fascism will be an irrevocable step back towards barbarism. . . . The association with the Spanish people in the fight for their liberty and with the Europeans in the International Brigade, many of whom had come from the concentration camps in Fascist countries, and my experience of

> Fascist totalitarian war, fortified my decision to be on the side of democracy against Fascism. . . . The so-called democratic Powers of Western Europe, Britain and France, which countries, by taking the initiative in denying to the Spanish Government the arms necessary to defend itself against its insurgent generals, bear a moral responsibility for the prolongation of the war and the defeat, if it comes, of the only people in Europe to take up arms in the defence of real democracy against the rising tide of Fascism in Europe.[33]

Not all of New Zealand's newspaper readers were prepared to accept such views without challenge, and for some weeks after Jolly's interview by the Christchurch *Press*, its letters page ran a lively correspondence by defenders of Franco who objected to a medical man's engaging in such a torrid political debate. "Surely Dr. Jolly would do better to confine himself to recounting his experiences in Spain, without making propagandist statements about matters of which he is evidently ignorant."[34]

Within a very short time, however, Jolly's outspoken anti-fascist stance would become sharply relevant and almost universally shared by his fellow New Zealanders. His speaking tour took place only four months before Germany invaded Poland, an intervention that made the rising threat of fascism impossible to deny any longer, and with scarcely a dissenting voice, New Zealand joined Britain and France in declaring war on Germany. In a letter to a friend in Auckland, published in New Zealand newspapers in February 1940, Jolly explained his views on his country's decision to enter a world war against Nationalist Spain's recent allies. He said he had no sympathy whatever for the British Communist Party's position, in adherence to Hitler and Joseph Stalin's recently concluded Nonaggression Pact, that the war with Germany was a conflict between capitalist powers and that communists should therefore remain aloof from it. "I'm certain that we see in Germany, in its actions against the European states with virtual enslavement of whole white populations, a new phenomenon in history. I believe that this war is a war of desperate defence by Britain and France against sharing the fate of such countries as Poland and Czechoslovakia."[35]

His family was similarly unhesitating in their support for the war. Two of his brothers, Stanley and Harold, both dental surgeons, enlisted with the New Zealand Army Dental Corps.

While traveling around his homeland, Jolly evidently conceived of supporting the developing anti-fascist war effort by compiling his recent experiences in book form:

> I was convinced that some record of the surgical advances of what had happened in Spain must be recorded to augment, or supersede, the only help the new, young war surgeons would have ie. the evidence of the experiences of those who had worked in ADS [advanced dressing stations], CCS [casualty clearing stations] and Base Hospitals from 1914 to 1918. I was certain that we *had* learnt a lot under fire when bombers and strafing aircraft had become, tactically, an almost unlimited increase of the range of heavy artillery; I had learnt something of the truth of the fact that, if you must operate surgically under this sort of new "artillery," you might as well be dug in nearer to the front line as to do so far from it. You might be obliterated anyway, but if you were lucky enough (or wise and experienced enough) to survive, your wounded had a much greater chance (especially the vascular and abdominal cases) if they could be on the operating table within an average of 5–6 hours "time lag" instead of the 18–24 hours that was accepted in 1914–18.[36]

Recognizing that the book he envisaged was potentially of value to the medical services of all Allied forces, Jolly determined to return to Britain and write and publish it there. He was booked to leave on the liner *Arawa* in October 1939, but Britain's declaration of war against Germany in September forced a change of plan. The New Zealand Army had commandeered the *Arawa* for conversion into an auxiliary cruiser to escort troopships to the Middle East, "so Shaw Saville were good enough to appoint me as ship's surgeon to an old freighter going by the Panama Canal and hugging the American coast to Halifax, Nova Scotia, to join a slow convoy bound for the Thames estuary." This unprepossessing vessel was not required under maritime regulations to include a ship's surgeon in its crew, so Jolly was taken on board as an unpaid crew member. During the voyage, he agreed to serve with the purser as a decoding officer. "This meant hours and hours of work decoding all Admiralty messages appropriate to the sector we were sailing in."[37]

His slow and monotonous but militarily uneventful voyage brought Jolly back to Britain in February 1940 with the primary intention of enlisting in the

Royal Army Medical Corps and reentering the fight against fascism under a new flag. He postponed those plans after several of his medical colleagues urged him instead to proceed urgently with writing the book he had envisaged. "I have been advised by surgeon friends here in London," he told one friend, "that there is a need for someone who has war surgical experience of more recent vintage than 1918 to write a book about 'Surgery in Forward Areas.' Most that has been published on this subject has two faults—it is 20 years old, and all treats of the viewpoint of the base hospital. As my time in Spain was spent in 'Forward Areas,' they think I have something that will be useful to younger, inexperienced surgeons who will be operating, in this war, in the casualty clearing stations."[38]

Although Jolly cannot have known this, the mobile field hospitals staffed by skilled surgeons that proved so effective in Spain were then already being emulated in an utterly different wartime setting. When the tempestuous Canadian doctor Norman Bethune, who had left Spain in unhappy circumstances in early 1937, traveled to China the following year to offer his services to Mao's Red Army, he explained his proposed model of military medical organization to the "Great Helmsman" himself. "Mao rose and began to pace the floor. 'A mobile operating unit,' he mused. 'Functioning close to the front. . . . Yes, that would be good. It would be good for our fighters to know they would receive immediate treatment for their wounds. . . . You will organise the mobile operating unit at once.'"[39] Bethune did so and operated on thousands of Red Army troops over the following two years. A chronic lack of medical supplies, extending even to a lack of surgical gloves, caused him to die of blood poisoning after cutting his finger during an operation and developing a fatal infection.

Jolly spent the next several months writing at an extraordinary pace while supported, as ever, by the devoted Grants. He owed Irene Grant, he acknowledged, "a special debt of gratitude for her invaluable help in the preparation of this work for the press."[40] In long hours at his desk, he presented his experience in Spain and its implications for future wars in precise, clear, and measured language that would have gratified his teachers in distant Dunedin. His only diversion was a modest resumption of his former involvement with the Christian Left. One of its early members was a progressive Anglican cleric named Rev. E. O. Iredell, who, along with John Macmurray and others, had visited Spain in 1937 to investigate religious persecution. At his parish in Barnsbury, North London, Iredell had begun holding ecumenical discussion groups attended by the likes of Labour MP and Left Book Club co-founder John Strachey and future prime minister of India Jawaharlal Nehru, who had also visited International Brigaders in Spain in 1938. On at least one occasion, Jolly left his writing desk and made the journey from Hampstead to Islington to take part in these discussions.

To illustrate the innovative, complex, and often dramatic medical advances he described, Jolly was fortunate to have access to a wealth of photographs taken by a young Englishman named Alec Wainman who had traveled to Spain at the outset of the civil war, hoping to help in whatever way he could. He first drove an ambulance for the British Medical Unit and, as a keen amateur photographer, aimed his Leitz Leica camera at every scene "that caught his eye or touched his sensitivity." He recorded combat on the Aragón front, civilian life in Barcelona, the Lincoln Battalion's arrival from the United States, and the work of doctors and nurses in many of the International Brigade hospitals.[41] These remarkable photos were supplemented by others, perhaps taken by Jolly himself since he was known to have access to a camera in Spain, that show technical details of wound treatment, modified medical equipment, and other subjects of interest primarily to fellow military surgeons.

Like many writers, Jolly flirted with alternative titles—*War Surgery in Forward Areas*, *War Surgery in Besieged Areas*—before settling on the punchier *Field Surgery in Total War*. On the basis of his initial outline, the newly inaugurated medical division of the venturesome London publisher Hamish Hamilton accepted his book proposal. The head of that division was Maurice Newfield, a doctor, editor, and staunch eugenicist for whom the Spanish Civil War was a personally significant crusade. He had raised funds among his colleagues to buy medical supplies to send to Republican units in Catalonia and had offered accommodations and other forms of support for Basque children evacuated to Britain in the wake of Franco's air attacks such as those that destroyed Guernica.[42]

Dr. Newfield had almost single-handedly built up a book list that included *Treatment of War Wounds and Fractures* by the outstanding civilian surgeon Josep Trueta, who had escaped to London shortly before his city of Barcelona fell to the Nationalists. Trueta's book, like Jolly's, was directed at medical professionals preparing to treat war casualties, and some overlap between their contents was to be expected. Trueta, however, had spent the civil war working in a large urban base hospital, and Jolly's unequaled frontline surgical experience promised a very different clinical perspective.

Seeking the imprimatur of a distinguished medical name, the first-time author asked the most prominent military surgeon in Britain to provide a foreword to his book. Sir Gordon Gordon-Taylor, surgeon rear admiral OBE, FRCS, FRACS (Fellow of the Royal Australasian College of Surgeons), had served in World War I and in 1939 became a consulting surgeon to the army with the rank of major general. He described himself as "an incorrigible Tory" but, after reading Jolly's manuscript in proofs, replied that he would be flattered and delighted to oblige its author.[43] His earlier dealings with Antipodean medicine may have influenced this decision. Sir Gordon had served with New Zealand and Australian surgeons in France during World War I, and as a councillor of the Royal College of Surgeons, he had traveled to those countries in 1934 to conduct its entrance exams, a development introduced just too late for Jolly to take advantage of it.[44]

After seven months of phony war, sudden and profoundly unexpected developments across the English Channel brought home to Britons the reality of the Third Reich's grandiose goals and forced their attention to their own self-defense.[45] Germany's highly mechanized army swept across France, demonstrating a seemingly unstoppable integration of the air and ground forces that they had earlier tested on the dry plains of central Spain. British troops who had entered the war in France with confident bravado were forced back toward their landing points in a succession of desperate retreats, and their chaotic and anguished evacuation by sea from the Dunkirk coast revealed to soldiers and civilians alike the inadequacies of Britain's war preparations. Ambulances loaded with wounded men would race to the departure points on the Normandy coast but find no docked ship ready to receive their patients. RAMC surgeons ran a small operating theater from the basement of a nearby chateau, but dressings, rations, and even anesthetics were in critically short supply. "The inevitable delay in operating on the wounded meant that even those lucky enough to escape from France had a much reduced chance of survival."[46]

Through the nightmarish months of May and June 1940, military hospitals in the south of England received floods of desperately wounded men who had survived without treatment for four or five days and perhaps had been immersed in salt water for much of that time. "Coated with grime and sand, unshaven, exhausted by lack of food and sleep, shaken by many hours of continual bombardment, and with fearful wounds, it was amazing to us how they had survived at all."[47] Surgeons were required to explore infected shell, bomb, and bullet wounds riddled with fragments of cloth and equipment, leather, cigarette packets, and cuff links. They treated these wounds much as Jolly and others had done in Spain: "opening up, cleansing, debridement of dead tissues, removal of the accessible projectile fragments, loosely packing with gauze soaked in [the disinfectant] proflavine and immobilisation in plaster of Paris."[48] Crucially, however, the patients evacuated from Dunkirk typically received this treatment several days after experiencing their dangerously infected wounds, and the results were correspondingly discouraging. As the RAMC's official history acknowledged, "There was, inevitably, a tendency of medical planners to think along the lines that they had learned as young officers during the largely static struggle from 1914 onwards. Mobility of the surgeon and his team was not much in the official mind, and one service textbook which was standard reading for promotion stated that 'the finest surgeon is powerless unless the patient . . . can be brought to him.' Clearly some fresh thinking was needed."[49]

12 The System, Not the Surgeon

In 1940 Doug Jolly could assure Irene Grant that "my work goes on merrily—am now in the middle of the fourth chapter, having already written the introduction and the first three (with the exception of some necessary polishing and here and there rewriting before typing)."[1] Working at a pace impelled by the deeply dismaying turn in the course of the war, the surgeon-turned-author completed his manuscript in time for publication in October 1940, as the Battle of Britain scrawled across the skies overhead and the first bombs of the blitz fell on English towns. A U.S. edition appeared simultaneously through the medical book department of the New York publisher Harper & Brothers. Second and third printings were produced in March 1941 and June 1942.

The book's timing was exceptionally fortuitous and met a large and immediate gap in the market. Several other English speakers with experience of the war in Spain had recently turned those experiences into print, but none aimed their works at the many doctors on both sides of the Atlantic who, like Jolly himself, were now preparing for active military service. Two years earlier the scientist J. B. S. Haldane drew upon his firsthand knowledge of bombing raids in Madrid to produce a general guide to surviving such raids in Britain. His book, he wrote, "is intended for the ordinary citizen, the sort of man and woman who is going to be killed if Britain is raided again from the air. . . . I have seen the results of air raids during the present year, and I feel that I should be guilty of innocent blood if I did not make every effort in my power to save the people of Britain from the fate which is now befalling the peoples of Spain and China."[2] A British doctor, Gerald Shirlaw, had served with Jolly in the Thirty-Fifth Division in Spain and distinguished himself at a first aid post during the battle of Brunete. He wrote two books drawing on the advances achieved by the Republican Army's medical services, but both were aimed at Britain's Home Guard and other civil defense organizations. One featured an introduction by Tom Wintringham that specifically singled out Jolly's contribution to the restructuring of wartime medical services to address the consequences of aerial warfare.[3]

Wintringham's endorsement was significant since he had become one of the most influential British voices on the need for more intelligent military preparedness. After his shoulder wound at Quinto in May 1937, he underwent emergency surgery by Jolly and was invalided home to Britain. He then became a prominent writer on military issues who constantly urged the need to prepare for a new and unprecedently mobile form of warfare based on aviation. After the resignation of Nazi-appeasing prime minister Neville Chamberlain in May 1940 and the strategic crisis of the unfolding disaster in France, a rebellious and disenchanted public was ready to urge the adoption of Wintringham's battle-forged tactical prescriptions.[4] By the following month, with the evacuation of Dunkirk and the signing of the German-French armistice, the threat of a German invasion of Britain had become imminent. Winston Churchill, Chamberlain's successor as prime minister, made his "finest hour" speech in the House of Commons, acknowledging in his distinctive gravelly and high-pitched tones that "the Battle of Britain is about to begin" but asserting that the British people would withstand a sustained attack by the Luftwaffe "like the brave men of Barcelona."[5] Finally, Allied as well as Axis leaders were willing to learn the lessons of the Spanish war.

In its promotional material for *Field Surgery in Total War*, the publisher described it as the first book "to deal comprehensively with methods of organisation and techniques adapted to mechanised warfare." Its fundamental element was a historically unprecedented system for speedily recovering the wounded from the battlefield and providing them with prompt and medically appropriate treatment. This procedure, seemingly straightforward but in practice complex, flexible, and requiring rigorous management, departed significantly from the rigid processes of casualty evacuation and management employed in World War I. In that war, first aid treatment, classification, and frontline surgery were all carried out at a single field hospital that was typically large, immobile, and sited both too close to the front for safety and too distant from it for prompt treatment of the most urgent cases. That concept was perpetuated in standard texts such as T. B. Nicholl's 1936 *Organisation, Strategy and Tactics of the Army*

Medical Services in War, and at the outbreak of World War II, many senior figures in military medicine remained firmly wedded to it.

By contrast, Jolly's book described a triage system of casualty evaluation. The wounded, he wrote, were first carried by *camilleros*, or "stretcher-bearers," to a small *puesto de socorro* (battalion aid post) just three hundred to five hundred meters behind the front line. There a medical officer, usually a captain or lieutenant, administered whatever basic lifesaving measures were necessary: dressing wounds, splinting fractures, and perhaps giving an intravenous transfusion and morphine, anti-tetanus, and gas gangrene injections. The seriously wounded, each bearing a card indicating the nature of the wound and any medication given at the first aid post, were then taken by ambulance to a classification post perhaps five kilometers from the front line. The walking wounded made their own way there on foot. This post, like the aid post, was highly mobile and might be based in a tent, a cellar, or part of a bombed-out building. Although its staff might give further basic treatment, such as minor surgery or stitching, its main function was triage. A specially trained triage doctor assessed the wounded as requiring either immediate emergency surgery or less urgent treatment. The former cases were taken to a mobile surgical unit, or No. 1 field hospital, and the latter to more distant and generally larger No. 2 base hospitals via a shuttle system of rapid ambulances.[6]

The No. 1 field hospital, the type in which Jolly himself worked throughout his time in Spain, was typically set up within ten kilometers of the front line in locations such as tents, tunnels, and caves or requisitioned buildings such as stables, mills, schools, and convents. Its size and surgical capacity were flexible depending on its proximity to larger and more established field hospitals. It was typically supported by a truck loaded with beds, marquees, ward furnishings, and kitchen equipment; an ambulance with a triage officer; a clerk; two ward nurses; four stretcher-bearers; and a cook. "This combination of units allowed the chief medical officer of an Army Corps to provide a flexible medical service to support military operations."[7] The No. 1 field hospital usually contained fifty to a hundred beds, although sometimes up to three hundred, and had three surgical teams working in round-the-clock shifts.

Jolly placed great emphasis on reducing the time between wounding and treatment. Critically injured troops, especially those with abdominal and chest wounds, should reach the mobile surgical unit no more than five hours after being wounded and sooner, if possible, to minimize infection and complications from blood loss and dehydration. They must also be retained at the field hospital for at least eight days for postoperative recovery, since any attempts to move them too soon raised the risk of death significantly. "Serious cases stand movement even worse in the few days after operation than in the few hours preceding it," Jolly wrote.[8]

As early as safely possible, they were evacuated back to No. 2 base hospitals staffed by more specialized surgeons, usually sited at least thirty to forty kilometers behind the line and near a railhead. These surgeons performed operations such as cranial and jaw surgery, and treated the less urgent chest cases and those fractures that could not be safely transported the considerable distance to evacuation hospitals for lengthy orthopedic treatment.[9] The main Republican base hospitals were in Huete, Benicàssim, and Murcia. According to Jolly's colleague Moisès Broggi, he and other frontline surgeons made a point of visiting these hospitals whenever possible "to follow the course and recovery of the wounded we had treated and, above all, to check the results of the methods used."[10] If necessary, patients were sent on yet again from these hospitals to more specialist rehabilitation or convalescent facilities.

To distinguish it from the single treatment point of the World War I field hospital, Jolly called this the "three-points-forward" system. It was deceptively straightforward but in practice carefully structured on the basis of travel time rather than physical distance. It could select various alternative routes between each of its points, and differing modes of transport, each with their particular advantages and drawbacks. If the battlefront shifted suddenly either forward or back, the various elements of the system could replace each other—for example, with the aid post becoming the classification post, which in turn became the No. 1 field hospital, and so on. Most importantly, each of the three points could potentially be relocated if the time taken to reach any of them rose above the limits Jolly regarded as acceptable.[11]

From the perspective of traditionally trained military surgeons, the siting of the No. 1 field hospital much nearer the front line than previously considered possible was perhaps the most startling and contentious element of the entire system. According to one study, "The concept of a completely self-contained surgical unit with a holding capacity of 50 beds, capable of undertaking any form of surgery as close to the front as possible while retaining a capability of rapid deployment, was something quite unique to the army medical services of the time."[12]

One of the greatest differences between the military medical services of the Great War era and those developed in Spain was the latter war's large-scale use of aircraft as weapons of attack. Jolly noted that this technological advance posed many new problems for frontline medical organizations, and his book details the need to protect hospitals from aerial bombardment. As Sir Gordon acerbically noted in his foreword, "It is a sad commentary on the word 'Kultur' and on modern civilization that in Spain the use of the Red Cross on hospitals had to be abandoned, since it was found that this emblem no longer gave sanctuary but invited, nay provoked, air-attacks by those brought up in the countries of . . . crafty, ambitious, bloodthirsty dictators of the so-called Axis States."[13]

Extensive use of airpower meant that all military units, including their medical services, became vulnerable to enemy action. "During the earlier part of the war in Spain No. 1 Hospitals could be set up in villages conveniently near to the front and near main evacuation roads. . . . Later, however, this became impossible. With the increase in aviation, and the numerical superiority of the opposing forces, it became certain that, in any active sector, all villages would be rapidly demolished."[14] In addition, towns and cities became targets regardless of their military significance, "negating any protection that might have been afforded to civilians. Thus medical units had to adopt the same principles of dispersion, camouflage and protection employed by combatant units. Large aggregations of transport or wounded men at hospital sites had the potential to become targets for aerial bombardment."[15]

Among the precautions Jolly advocated was the formation of a system of "air-alarm sentries" as soon as a medical unit arrived at the site where it planned to establish a hospital. Thereafter, transport movements in the vicinity of the hospital had to be reduced to a minimum whenever enemy aircraft appeared. "Dust clouds from ambulances approaching a hospital are the surest revelation to aircraft of a hospital's position." In addition, a narrow zig-zag trench, camouflaged from the air, must immediately be dug to shelter hospital staff, and "an absolute rule must be enforced against the false heroism of those who scorn to take shelter." These protections, he insisted, were necessary both for the safety of patients and staff, and for their psychological benefit. "A device that may have little practical bearing on the safety of the hospital in the face of a determined bombing attack may have an unassessable but good effect on the morale of the hospital patients and personnel."[16]

In a further sharp contrast with Great War practice, decisions on the siting of field hospitals seem to have been left largely in the hands of the medical staff themselves rather than with the Republican Army's general staff. This drastic departure from the long-standing hierarchy of military command appears to have arisen not so much from the Spanish Republic's democratic ideology as from the chaos and enforced improvisation of the war's early months. "In building a military medical service to meet the new conditions of warfare," Jolly wrote in the book's preface, "the medical profession in Republican Spain had to begin almost from zero, for the greater part of the Army Medical Service had passed in the first days of the war to the insurgent forces."[17] He and the several hundred other doctors who arrived to replace them, both from Spanish civilian ranks and from overseas, enjoyed exceptional freedom to use their own initiative in developing new systems to address unprecedented conditions. "We witnessed the birth of a new military medical service, and watched it grow from infancy to flourishing maturity under conditions of total war." The process, he acknowledged, was a painful and imperfect one. "It grew by methods of trial and error—sometimes very costly error."[18] Yet by the end of the war, Jolly told a New Zealand paper, the Republican Army's medical corps had changed "from a rudimentary, ill-equipped inadequate organisation to a disciplined, efficient body of which no modern army need be ashamed."[19]

Field Surgery in Total War comprises two distinct parts. The first makes the case for a radical reorganization of frontline surgical services on the three-points-forward model. Its single strongest message is that the most important factor in wartime wound treatment is the system, not the surgeon. Although an exceptionally gifted and skilled surgeon himself, Jolly gave equal importance to the role of every member of his team, from the stretcher-bearers and ambulance drivers to the orderlies, theater nurse, anesthetist, and assistant surgeon. The second and longer section is a manual for treating the main types of wounds encountered in wartime. Here Jolly describes, briefly but with unequivocal precision, the best surgical techniques for dealing with those injuries. He evidently aimed to simplify the work of battlefield surgery by breaking down the steps before and after the surgeon's work on the operating table into specific actions that could be carried out by nurses, orderlies, anesthetists, and junior doctors, as well as trained surgeons.

Most of these procedures, such as those for serious head injuries, limb injuries, and chest wounds, are not significantly different from those practiced during World War I apart from the shorter time lag before an operation that was achieved by placing the surgeon near the front line. The main innovations Jolly describes in this section are the use of blood transfusions in the field and the so-called closed plaster method for treating fracture wounds. He was evidently deeply impressed with the blood bank collection and delivery systems introduced by Frederic Duran i Jordà in Barcelona and Norman Bethune in Madrid in the early months of the war and maintained and further developed by the English doctor Reginald Saxton. "Very few of the more seriously wounded among those treated in No. 1 Hospitals did not receive a transfusion, either before or during the operation. In the few instances in which supplies of the appropriate conserved blood were not available, direct transfusion was carried out from donors among the members of the hospital staff," and a large proportion of his patients, Jolly believed, owed their lives to this intervention.[20] This major medical advance, he saw, was unquestionably of immediate application in other countries, and his personal papers include contemporary articles from the *British Medical Journal* describing the origins of a wartime blood transfusion service for Britain.[21]

The treatment of bone fractures represented another major departure from the World War I–era practice that British military surgeons still followed at the time Jolly's book appeared. Most of those surgeons accepted without question that broken limbs should be splinted but not enclosed in plaster to avoid the risk of a chronic infection leading to amputation. By contrast, the closed plaster method adopted in Republican Spain immobilized the wound, caused far less trauma to the injured soldier during transport, aided healing, and actually reduced the risk of gangrenous infection to near zero. Through the widespread introduction of this form of treatment, wrote Jolly, "countless men wounded in the extremities in the present [1939–45] war will, unlike their fathers who fought in the War of 1914 to 1918, survive to work with their own arms and legs."[22]

The closed plaster technique was greatly developed in the 1920s by the young and innovative Barcelona surgeon Josep Trueta, who worked mainly with the victims of industrial accidents. Before applying a plaster cast, he carefully cleaned and drained the wound and removed all damaged tissue, achieving remarkable results at controlling infection and recovering the use of the healed limb.[23] During the civil war, he remained working as the head of surgery at a large Barcelona public hospital, treating thousands of victims of aerial bombing. As word of his principles of wound treatment spread, frontline doctors from throughout Republican Spain traveled to Barcelona to study them. The English volunteer George Orwell gave an uninformed and unfavorable account of this method after he was wounded on the Aragón front in early 1937. "Men with dreadful shell wounds, smashed bones and so forth, were swathed in a sort of casing made of bandages and plaster of Paris; a description of the wound was written in pencil on the outside, and as a rule the casing was not removed till the man reached Barcelona or Tarragona ten days later. It was almost impossible to get one's wound examined on the way; the few doctors could not cope with the work, and they simply walked hurriedly past your bed saying: 'Yes, yes, they'll attend to you at Barcelona.'"[24]

Orwell's anxieties at this apparently laissez-faire treatment proved wholly unjustified. By 1938 the Trueta method was almost universally employed among Republican forces, and over twenty thousand cases were treated in this way with a death rate of less than 1 percent. According to Jolly, "During the Ebro offensive one surgical team operated on 220 cases in the forward zone without having to perform a single amputation," a record that was unimaginable during World War I.[25]

Abdominal wounds, Jolly's particular area of expertise, are understandably given more attention in his book than any other form of injury. His instructions for dealing with them are detailed and sometimes strikingly direct and dogmatic. "In wounds of the abdomen," he declares bluntly, "the only successful haemostatic [means of stopping bleeding] is the knife of the Surgeon, and the only adequate external splint the flat metal top of the operating table."[26] In other words, an early operation must precede splinting since there was no point in splinting if bleeding was not controlled. More strongly than anywhere else in his book, Jolly stresses that "the recovery rate in abdominal cases depends less on the individual ability of the surgeon than on any other single factor in the forward system. In fact young, comparatively inexperienced surgeons working well within the five-hour period can usually show far better figures than more practised surgeons who are condemned to operate on similar cases farther back."[27]

Certain injuries, he readily acknowledged, had a poor rate of recovery no matter how quickly and skillfully they were treated. They included crush injuries caused by aerial bombing that resulted in organ damage and tangential bullet wounds—that is, those striking the body from the side rather than in the front or back. Patients with severe chest wounds, in particular, very often died before they could undergo surgery, and Jolly refers repeatedly and with great compassion to the situation of the surgeon presented with a case which is likely beyond help:

> When there is a long time lag (from wounding), the judgement of the surgeon is sufficient to determine whether an operation would serve a useful purpose or be merely a "sentimental intervention." . . . Conservative (non-operative treatment) should only be given when a patient arrives at the No. 1 hospital so late that peritonitis is already advanced, or where it is certain no hollow viscus is perforated [that is, where no organs such as the bowel, liver, or kidney are perforated, such that organisms within them could contaminate and infect the abdominal cavity, leading to generalized infection or peritonitis] and that haemorrhage is not sufficient to endanger life. . . .
>
> When a great wound or prolapse [rupture of the abdominal wall, exposing the bowel to the air] is present and . . . repair is impossible, it is a great kindness to take the patient to the theatre and simply return the gut to the abdominal cavity, suture the wound and give repeat large doses of morphine. A man with a large prolapse, who knows that he will die unless operated on, and who lies in the corner of the ward or Reception Room waiting hopelessly for his turn, is the most heartrending object in a field hospital. Five minutes given to him will allow him to die in comparative peace.[28]

All of Jolly's instructions on clinical techniques were underpinned by an extraordinary depth of experience. In less than two years in Spain, he had treated over four thousand wounded and carried out almost one thousand abdominal operations. In his foreword, Gordon Gordon-Taylor stated categorically, "No living British surgeon before the author of this book, and probably no surgeon of any race, has ever personally operated upon almost a thousand gunshot wounds of the abdomen." Jolly's publisher claimed that he had "what is probably an unparalleled experience in the diagnosis and treatment of wounds produced by modern weapons."[29]

As in his 1938 article for the journal *AMI*, Jolly acknowledged in *Field Surgery in Total War* the potential conflict of interest between purely surgical roles and purely military roles. The professional duty of the former is to provide aid to the most severely injured at the earliest opportunity, but the latter's primary goal is to return as many fighting men to the front as possible. Jolly's three-points-forward system, he maintained, provided the most effective way to address both imperatives. An efficient and dedicated field medical service also made a valuable impact on the troops' morale, whether injured or not. "Men fight and stand strain much better when they know that if they are wounded they will be given every chance of survival."[30]

The book's writing style is brisk and military in its precision but with occasional flashes of dry humor and a rigorously practical attitude forged in the fires of battle. The wounded, Jolly warns, should always be carefully searched on arrival at a casualty clearing station, and any ammunition such as hand grenades should be located and removed. "It is disturbing to have the field hospital incinerator blown up when burning old clothes." Also, an initial blood transfusion should be started just before the operation itself. "This also is easier in the theatre than in a room where stretcher-bearers are liable to trip over the outstretched arm."[31]

Reviews of the book were uniformly glowing and indicate that its influence was widespread, immediate, and profound. The book "should be read at once," declared the *Lancet*, "by every young surgeon who may be called upon to treat war casualties, and by every consultant who is still uncertain how far his memories of the last war fit into the actualities of this one."[32] In its journal, the Royal Army Medical Corps, in which Jolly himself had by then been commissioned, foresaw that "his views will not only command attention, but be worthy of close study. . . . It is now generally appreciated that the whole medical organisation in warfare . . . must be built around the surgeon as a nucleus, and that the time factor is of such importance that if the wounded man cannot be brought to the surgeon, the surgeon must go to him."[33] The *British Medical Journal* found that the author "has approached the subject with a mind not unduly trammelled by tradition . . . it describes the gradual development of a system not handicapped by set ideas and a rigid traditionalism. . . . Dr. Jolly's clear directions on the surgery of wounds of the chest and abdomen, based on extensive experience, cannot but be helpful to the Army surgeon."[34]

Several reviewers also saw the book as having value beyond the sphere of military medicine. *Medicine Today and Tomorrow*, the journal of the Socialist Medical Association, believed "it should be placed in the hands of every doctor who is a member of any casualty, hospital or medical service."[35]

Field Surgery in Total War quickly became required reading for young aspiring war surgeons in the United States as well as Britain.[36] Maj. James Mason of the U.S. Army Medical Corps noted:

> The timelag between the sustaining of the wound and the surgical intervention . . . is the crux of the organisation of the Medical Corps of the Army in the field. . . . A lesson that certainly might well be taken by our Army is the location of the echelons of evacuation within the five-hour, ten-hour and 18-hour time periods following the receipt of a wound, rather than by the fixed distance of miles. . . . The chapter on Abdominal Wounds is one of the highlights in war surgery at the present time. His description of the manner of organisation, the simple and yet compelling instructions he has given in the handling of many conditions, are arresting.[37]

The eminent surgeon Edward Churchill, who left his post as chief of general surgical services at Massachusetts General Hospital to enlist with the U.S. Army Medical Corps, later recalled, "One of the few books I had tucked into my luggage to take to North Africa was *Field Surgery in Total War* by Douglas W. Jolly. This described the 'three-points-forward' developed in Spain, and influenced my thinking greatly. Jolly's book was unknown to our AFHQ [Allied Forces Headquarters] group of medical officers. Even the word 'triage' required explanation."[38] Another American surgeon, William Pike, who had worked as second in command to Ed Barsky in the U.S. medical unit in Spain, noted that the concept of triage was also unfamiliar to him and his colleagues until they first encountered it in Spain as an integral part of Jolly's system. "Triage—French for the classification of the wounded to determine priority of operation—[was] initiated by the New Zealander surgeon, Dr. Jolly."[39] That claim is much too sweeping, but it is nevertheless true that "the concept of triage by destination was implicit in Jolly's 'three-point forward' system." By categorizing patients on the basis of the urgency of their treatment, his system "ensured the earliest possible diversion of seriously injured casualties to a surgical facility away from the flow of the majority of casualties in the evacuation chain." Although later adapted to take account of very different geographical conditions and military strategies, the U.S. and UK armed forces employed the same system in the Mediterranean and northern European theaters in World War II and in many later conflicts.[40]

"This principle of triage based on the urgency of the wound," wrote Dr.

Churchill in his memoir, "with separate hospitalization for the two categories of cases, subsequently became the basic principle followed by the US Medical Corps in World War II. To a great extent it resolved the dilemma between the mutually contradictory 'military' view and the 'surgical' view, and established clearly that the function of the Army medical service is to save life irrespective of the future military potential of the individual battle casualty."[41]

In Jolly's country of birth, where in 1940 an imminent Japanese invasion was greatly feared, the medical military establishment proposed setting up mobile surgical units for home defense use.[42] That idea was soon abandoned, but it was put into practice with New Zealand forces serving overseas. In almost every English-speaking sector of the Allied forces, it appears, the small, sturdily bound, and blue-covered work by a first-time medical author with unorthodox but unarguably extensive field experience was read and its advice put into practice. According to one American authority, Jolly's book "undoubtedly contributed more to the saving of lives of patients with abdominal wounds than any other single factor."[43]

Further, and just as remarkably, *Field Surgery in Total War* remained unsurpassed as a standard work of military medicine for decades after World War II. In 1948 during the Korean War, the US Army and its allies established the mobile army surgical hospital (MASH), a sixty-bed unit with its own vehicles and infrastructure based directly on the mobile units that Jolly described. In the first six months of that war, almost all U.S. and allied casualties requiring immediate surgical treatment received it from a MASH.[44] The off-duty antics of their staffs gave rise to a comedic novel that became a hit film and eventually a long-running TV series.[45]

The enormous importance of helicopters for transferring patients rapidly from remote and inaccessible frontline locations to the nearest MASH marked a dramatic advance on earlier systems of wartime transportation and one that was presumably barely imaginable to Jolly. In Korea, army medical helicopters minimized the effect of shock and delay before surgical intervention, while their return journeys solved the problem of refilling depleted supplies of stored blood.[46] In fact, rapid helicopter evacuation and other innovations such as well-trained paramedics and advanced methods of treatment for shock were said to be "not effectively matched in the civilian world for another 15 to 20 years"; then they became "the model for future modern metropolitan trauma centers."[47]

In the 1960s, a young New Zealand surgeon named Michael Shackleton, assigned during the Vietnam War to a civilian hospital in the coastal town of Qui Nhon, carried his well-worn copy of *Field Surgery*, just as his father-in-law, Capt. Stan Wilson, had done more than twenty years earlier in World War II.[48] In Vietnam, military surgeons found the wounded could seldom be evacuated by road since there were few secure road networks in the combat area; therefore, helicopters were used in even greater numbers than in the Korean War. At first helicopters designated for purely medical use evacuated large numbers of patients to central medical facilities. Those hospitals only had to be moved when major new combat operations began elsewhere in the country. At that point, pending the construction of permanent facilities, trucks or helicopters carried MUST (medical unit, self-contained, transportable) hospitals into the new combat areas. Each MUST was based on two large, self-inflating tents: One was used as a surgical ward, and the other provided power, water, and compressed air.[49] Even in the tropical jungle, they could provide far more sophisticated, sanitary, and climate-controlled conditions for emergency surgery than those Jolly had endured in Spain; yet, they were recognizably based on his system.

Thirty years later, still another air-transportable hospital unit was developed by Jolly's own compatriots. More than five thousand New Zealand Defence Force staff served from 1999 with a United Nations (UN) peacekeeping force in East Timor, at that time a violence-wracked province of Indonesia. They took with them a specially developed forward surgical team, and for three years, until East Timor achieved independence, the team provided medical support to its own and other UN troops and to the local population.[50] "One of the important lessons learned," a report on the mobile hospital unit concluded, "was that humanitarian medical care should be included as a tool in strategic military planning," a finding with which Doug Jolly, who delivered more than one baby in Spain, would undoubtedly have agreed.[51]

In his survey of the development of frontline surgery, New Zealand surgeon Michael Shackleton concluded, "The treatment descriptions in Jolly's book retained their relevance for many years. Such principles as adequate resuscitation, early surgery and complete postoperative rest for several days before facing the hazards of evacuation down the line still apply, even in this modern era of helicopter and ambulance transport."[52]

13 The Tobruk Plaster

This author can well imagine the sense of satisfaction when, after several months of concentrated effort, Jolly dispatched the final manuscript of *Field Surgery in Total War* to his publisher in mid-1940. Immediately afterward, he enlisted in Britain's Royal Army Medical Corps, giving Irene Grant as his next of kin and stating his relationship with her as "friend."

The RAMC, he soon found, was a male-only domain. Britain's women doctors were eager to serve in frontline roles but were excluded from doing so for the duration of the war, although they were permitted to work in ancillary units such as the Blood Transfusion Service.[1] With the rank of lieutenant (a considerable demotion from his final rank in Spain), Jolly was initially posted as a surgical specialist to a succession of military hospitals near the coast of southern England. By late 1940, he was working at a dressing station in Folkestone, the narrowest point of the English Channel and therefore a vitally important military port. The town was within range of Nazi Germany's heavy artillery bases in northern France and a popular target for its bombing runs. The ululating wail of air raid sirens sounded frequently, day and night. Working in a role by then grimly familiar to him, Jolly treated troops and civilians injured in the raids who were carried directly to his station by stretcher-bearers and ambulances. He received a promotion to major in February 1941.

The injuries inflicted by aerial warfare in Britain, as it had in Spain, called for large volumes of transfused blood, and the British Army could now claim to be the only one in the world with a transfusion service capable of meeting this need. "Experience in the Spanish Civil War," declared the *British Medical Journal*, "has shown that modern war, waged largely from the air, affects the civil population almost as much as it does the fighting forces. Experience in Spain showed, again, that at least 10 per cent of air raid casualties are seriously wounded and require blood transfusion. It is essential, therefore, to organise an adequate scheme for the supply of blood for the large number of transfusions which might be necessary in wartime."[2]

The Army Blood Supply Depot was accordingly created in late 1938 in a public hospital in the port town of Bristol, a location selected as unlikely to suffer enemy bomb attack (although that prediction was later shown to be optimistic). The maternity ward became a transfusion laboratory, and the depot supplied both fresh blood and liquid and dried plasma.[3] At collection points set up around the country, more than 750,000 civilian donors gave blood during the war. Jolly's personal papers include an account of one of those local depots, "housed in the country at a social centre." It describes the enlistment of volunteer blood donors from the local factories, with "both men and women coming forward with quite extraordinary willingness . . . some of the donors have professed themselves feeling better for what has been done to them, and have even intimated a desire to come back before the stipulated minimum interval (a month) to undergo it again." The stored blood, in glass bottles packed twelve to a wicker crate, was then delivered to hospitals in refrigerated vans.[4] "Of the medical advances that have contributed to surgical progress," wrote an RAMC surgeon near the end of the war, "the most outstanding is undoubtedly resuscitation as practised by the Army Blood Transfusion Service."[5] According to the RAMC's own historian, "Right down the line, from the private soldier acting as a donor to the nursing orderly controlling the transfusion under fire, the huge organization worked superbly. . . . Not many years before, even in good civilian circumstances, transfusion itself involved the patient in serious risks, mainly from faulty matching between the patient's blood and the donor's. This was now an extreme rarity."[6]

The work of treating the mangled victims of bombing raids on southern England was demanding and often literally lifesaving, but it had become routine to Jolly. As the news from overseas battlefields reached his small coastal town, his role must also have seemed peripheral to the direct confrontation, in which many of his former colleagues in Spain were already serving, against the Axis powers that had recently secured a victory for Franco. The anti-fascist battle, although finally lost in Spain, was now being fought throughout Europe and beyond it. In North Africa, directly across the Mediterranean from southern Spain, the front lines zig-zagged back and forth as Mussolini's troops attacked

British defenses in Egypt and, after initial success, were driven back as far as Tunisia and Algeria.

In September 1940, Irene Grant informed Karl Polanyi by mail that Jolly had been issued draft papers for overseas service "and told us not to expect any news of him for six or eight weeks. . . . He was here on his last leave, was well, and glad—since he *must* go abroad—to be with a very fine outfit of men." Jolly had heard, he told Irene with evident satisfaction, that his newly released book was "being used a lot by the high-ups" in the British military hierarchy. She and Donald, she admitted to Karl, hated the prospect of their close friend leaving the country for another foreign conflict zone, but nothing would deter him. His two brothers in the New Zealand Army Dental Corps were already serving in Greece together with their sister Ruth's husband, but the latter had been wounded and invalided to Egypt.[7] For Jolly himself, remaining on Britain's home front was now out of the question.

As the new year began, British and Australian troops took the key port of Tobruk in Libya, and it became their supply base, receiving reinforcements by land and sea. However, in February 1941, Field Marshal Erwin Rommel—whom Churchill described as "very daring and skilful"—arrived with his desert-trained Afrika Korps and large supplies of matériel to regain the lost territory. By the following month, he was besieging Tobruk and soon forced the British back eastward across the Egyptian frontier, leaving a single Australian division to hold the port.

Jolly reached this desert war in June 1941 when he embarked from Britain to join the Western Desert Force, made up of both British and Commonwealth Divisions, including troops from India, Australia, and New Zealand. He found himself part of a much larger and vastly better-equipped military machine than Spain's Republican Army, with well-drilled professional troops and freed of the crippling constraints on resources that had sealed the fate of the Spanish Republic. The Axis forces opposing them, however, were similarly well armed and trained, and the desert environment, desolate and bare apart from patches of camel thorn that inflicted painful scratches, posed daunting medical as well as military challenges. Inland from the Mediterranean coast, decades might pass without rainfall, and the punishing midday heat produced dehydration, heat exhaustion, and burns whenever skin touched metal. Yet in the winter months, temperatures could plunge below freezing overnight, a strange and even dangerous experience for troops from tropical climates. Fresh water, crucial to survival, was constantly inadequate. A gallon (4.5 liters) was the daily ration for each man, and half of it was required for cooking and topping up vehicle radiators.

Jolly was first posted to the British No. 2 General Hospital at El Tahag, a vast, tented transit camp near the Suez Canal that served as the main British military base in Egypt. This railhead for the war on the Libyan frontier to the west sprawled over miles of desert. Seared for days on end by the khamsin desert winds, the camp was subdivided into fifty blocks of tents, with each block measuring five hundred by a thousand yards and identical apart from the numbered signs at their entrances. Everyone carried a fly swatter and, when visiting the latrines, a stick to beat off the swarms of rats.[8]

In a small but telling distinction between the under-resourced and haphazardly improvised army medical services of the Spanish Republic and those of the vast and rigidly hierarchical structure of the Allied forces, the hospitals where Jolly now worked were not named for the nearest local settlement but were simply allocated numbers by the military high command. Consequently, Jolly's succession of hospital postings was no longer known by place-names resonant of the wartime conditions they saw but by bland numerical titles. Forward hospitals in World War II were frequently relocated as the fortunes of war changed, but their titles remained constant as they shifted between countries and even continents.

Although Jolly apparently never learned of this, a mobile surgical unit (MSU) inspired by his experiences in Spain and his book based on them was being assembled at that very moment by New Zealand medical personnel less than a hundred miles west of El Tahag, a trifling distance in the context of this vast battlefront. The proposal to form this pioneering unit arose from the series of talks Jolly gave in Britain in the early months of 1939 with the aim of exhorting the torpid British military and medical establishments into more realistic preparations for the forthcoming world war. At one of these talks, the audience included a wealthy New Zealand businessman named Arthur Sims, who was deeply impressed by Jolly's description of field surgery in wartime and began high-level lobbying to replicate it within his own country's army medical service. Sims, like Jolly, came from New Zealand's South Island. He achieved commercial success in the frozen meat export trade and based himself in London, and by the outbreak of World War II, he was able to leave his business affairs in the hands of others and contemplate philanthropy. He made an offer to the New Zealand government to fully fund a mobile surgical unit to support the Second New Zealand Expeditionary Force (2NZEF) serving in the Western Desert.[9] In August 1940, New Zealand prime minister Peter Fraser learned of the offer, and it was accepted the following month. Duncan Stout, consultant surgeon to the 2NZEF, used Sim's funds to buy theater equipment and instruments and a three-ton truck chassis to convert into a vehicle to carry surgical and anesthetic apparatuses, an electricity generator, and lighting.[10] Fred Bowerbank, director general of medical services to the NZ armed forces, endorsed the project. He also considered Jolly's book "a most important and a very valuable contribution to Military Surgery. There is no doubt that we still do not realise the rapidity of modern war, and if the combatant units are to move at a rapid rate, as they are doing, then it is essential we should do the same. For this reason I consider the Casualty Clearing Station as it is at present situated, is obsolete."[11]

The experimental surgical unit was set up at the Maadi military camp south of Cairo. A fleet of customized vehicles had been equipped with sterilizing and lighting equipment and complete surgical instrument kits. The first staff included a young surgeon named Stanley Wilson who, like Jolly, had studied first at Otago University and then in London. With the rank of captain, Wilson left for the Maadi camp with New Zealand forces in August 1940. Early the following year, he wrote to his wife in Wellington and asked her to send him military medical manuals including *Field Surgery in Total War*. "The war surgery books came yesterday," he informed her in April 1941. "It was grand to get them and they will be very useful; we have no library worth speaking of here. . . . Douglas Jolly's book is first class; in it you could read all about a MSU and you will see the work which we will be doing . . . our unit follows his ideas very closely."[12]

By May 1941, the unit was fully staffed, with Maj. Fred Furkert as its commanding officer and Captain Wilson as second in command. Unlike Jolly's original and minimally equipped unit, these surgeons could rely on medically qualified anesthetists who would also act as triage and resuscitation officers. The role of anesthetist had gained greater recognition and status since Jolly had trained his own, practically overnight, in Spain. During World War II, by contrast, specialist anesthetists held the same field rank as surgeons, and if they had the most seniority of service, they were placed in command of their field surgical units.[13] Theater staff and orderlies, however, were all recruited from the New Zealand troops based at the Maadi camp and given training in their new noncombat roles. The total strength of the all-male unit was forty-two, including five medical officers and nine Army Service Corps drivers. They were required to work in tents since the desert landscape offered no other suitable shelter.[14]

The consultant surgeon to New Zealand's forces in the Middle East who inspected the unit regarded it "as a war surgeon's dream from the surgical point of view. Its advantage lies in its mobility, independence in regard to transport, and the excellent power plant in the surgical lorry."[15] Four months later, the staff saw their first action on the border between Egypt and Libya, moving to a new location every few days as the battle conditions against Rommel's armored troops altered. Their three tents received a steady stream of wounded, many with injuries from Germany's deadly 88mm field guns, which could smash a British tank from a range of a mile. Patients were immediately triaged on the principles Jolly had established in Spain—as abdomen, chest, head, and flesh wounds or as compound fractures.[16]

The New Zealand Mobile Surgical Unit had no equivalent in the Western Desert Force, and it soon proved that field surgery capability could be taken much closer to wounded troops than was previously considered possible. During a critically important phase of the desert war, when Rommel's tank corps routinely outpaced and outmaneuvered the Allies, the unit provided a valuable stimulus not just to the New Zealand Medical Corps but also to their allies within the Western Desert Force, particularly the British.[17] In November 1941, it saw action at Sidi Oman on the Libyan border. After a lightning thrust by Rommel's forces, two German officers armed with Luger pistols appeared in the theater tent where Stanley Wilson was operating on a stream of casualties. In perfect English, they ordered him to carry on with his work but to move the wounded German troops to the head of the triage queue. For the next week, the unit worked steadily on both Allied and German wounded, with help from German medical officers. The German forces then pushed eastward, leaving the unit in the control of Italian troops who soon proved far less collegial, withdrawing several of the New Zealanders as prisoners of war and looting their supplies. Eight of the remaining MSU staff, including Captain Wilson, managed to disguise themselves in German uniforms and escape into Egypt in a stolen truck. Wilson was forced to leave behind his precious copy of *Field Surgery in Total War*, but he recovered it several weeks later, its cover badly stained by the desert conditions, when an armored column of his own troops evacuated the rest of the unit.[18]

Despite the ill-defined battle lines and sweeping movements of troops and armor during the El Alamein campaign, the mobile surgical unit demonstrated a remarkable operative success rate and a capacity to function independently of larger facilities, and it earned the ultimate tribute from the summit of New Zealand's military hierarchy. The commanding officer of the New Zealand Expeditionary Force, Gen. Bernard Freyberg, considered the unit "a rare example of medical ingenuity. . . . Jolly's principles of triage, early resuscitation and surgery sooner rather than later, followed by an appropriate period of complete rest, began for the NZ Medical Corps with the Mobile Surgical Unit."[19]

Nevertheless, Col. Duncan Stout, the expeditionary force's senior medical officer, was concerned that placing surgeons so close to the battlefront exposed them to unacceptable risk. A World War I veteran, Colonel Stout never lost the conviction that emergency battlefield surgery should be carried out at relatively static casualty clearing stations. Even better, he suggested, "was a delayed operation by a better surgeon operating under better conditions with better post-operative nursing, preferably female."[20] Accordingly, in early 1942 the mobile surgical unit was officially disbanded, and most of its personnel transferred to a newly formed casualty clearing station. Wilson wrote, "We all regret the passing of the MSU. . . . The days drag on slowly as we organise a CCS—it is an awfully cumbrous affair compared with the MSU and many of us wish that the change had not been necessary . . . now New Zealand have a CCS with an establishment little different from 1914–18!"[21] A medical historian later wrote, "It was a pity that younger, more flexible minds could not have prevailed and maintained the initiative, perhaps adding another similar unit to the divisional structure."[22]

Jolly was spared the disappointment of seeing the unit he had inspired so abruptly terminated. Although he spent more than a year as a surgical specialist in British general hospitals during the several battles around El Alamein, he apparently never encountered the New Zealand surgeons who worked according to his own guidelines. From mid-1941, he was stationed at the British No.

62 General Hospital at Tobruk on Libya's Mediterranean coast. This acted as a staging section in the line of evacuation from the forward areas of the fast-moving desert war back to the British bases in Egypt. The road and single-track railway following the coast were littered on both sides by burned-out trucks, tanks, and aircraft, while Tobruk harbor was glutted with the sunken vessels of both armies, its beaches putrid with oil and debris. The hospital was based in a school built some years earlier under Mussolini's regime. Its single-storied earth-brick buildings formed a quadrangle with the six classrooms on each side repurposed as wards. Offices at the western end were converted into a large operating theater with eight tables, while the storerooms and cookhouses at the opposite end of the courtyard retained their former functions.[23]

Jolly found that in this setting pests of various kinds proved a constant problem—not simply the swarms of flies that were attracted by food, human waste, and corpses and that settled on everyone's lips whenever they opened their mouths to eat or drink, but also sandflies, mosquitoes, scorpions, and rats. The sand itself permeated everything, aggravating existing skin diseases and causing galling "desert sores" that eventually affected almost everybody, patients and staff. "These painful and demoralizing skin ulcers were difficult to prevent without ample soap and hot water, and many resolute soldiers were laid up for long periods with these intractable and multiple sores."[24]

Although nominally a base hospital in terms of the three-points-forward system, No. 62 General functioned in practice more as a static field hospital, receiving wounded directly from dressing stations along the rapidly shifting front and later evacuating them to rear hospitals. Its patients typically arrived in an exhausted state after long, jolting truck journeys over boulder-strewn desert tracks. "It was found that the patient suffered least if the truck was half-filled with sand till the springs were flat and then the patient himself was partly buried, a peculiar but effective form of splintage."[25] Ambulances began arriving in the courtyard in the late afternoon, and their patients were carried on stretchers into a reception room for triage. Men in immediate need of plasma or blood transfusions were moved to a room used only for that purpose, and the severely shocked were taken to a "resuscitating room," where specially trained staff gave them whole blood, plasma, or glucose saline and monitored their condition until they were capable of withstanding surgery. "The desire to do something in the theatre," wrote one of Jolly's colleagues, "must be curbed till the general condition has been made satisfactory."[26] Less urgent cases were held in a long room behind the main building to await their turn to enter the theater. Here English, Scots, French, Indians, Australians, and New Zealanders mingled indiscriminately with wounded Germans and Italians who, one American ambulance driver noted, "received exactly the same care given to the British troopers."[27] The operating theater worked day and night on eight-hour shifts, apart for an hour or so each afternoon when it was cleaned.

The ready availability of fresh blood was a literally vital component of emergency treatment, new to many hospital staff but not to Jolly and other veterans of Spain. As noted earlier, his colleague Reggie Saxton's expertise at field transfusions and the establishment of donor blood banks influenced the creation of blood banks for both civilian and military use.[28] This early adoption of the practice developed in Spain made Britain the only nation to enter the war with a fully functioning transfusion service, "which meant that [its] transfusion in the field was far better organised than in the armed forces of other combatant nations, especially Germany."[29] To supply blood to overseas forces, blood transfusion units were formed at military bases, and smaller field transfusion units and advanced blood banks carried the precious supplies to casualty clearing stations and field ambulances. Each field transfusion unit consisted of an officer specially trained in the technique of resuscitation, some technical assistants, and a refrigerator van to carry the store of whole blood. These units radically transformed the process practiced as recently as 1940, when a transfusion might require half an hour's work, mainly by the surgeon himself. "It became recognised that the Field Transfusion Officer was the key man of a forward surgical group . . . without him a surgical team was robbed of half its value."[30]

The service eventually delivered the extraordinary total of 430,000 liters of blood to the battlefront, of which 10 percent was whole blood with a "shelf life," even when refrigerated, of only twenty-eight days. By far the bulk of the donated blood was converted into liquid or dried plasma, the portion of blood without red blood cells. This refinement, developed by American scientists at the outbreak of the war, greatly simplified storage and transportation problems, and was highly regarded during the first months of the Battle of Britain.[31] "Plasma is undoubtedly of great value," wrote the commander of one blood transfusion unit, "and plasma alone is sufficient for the resuscitation of large numbers of the less seriously wounded men." Eighth Army surgeons, however, dealing with casualties of desert war with severe blood loss, grew convinced that whole blood was vital to restore the oxygen level in the blood supply.[32] They found it revived patients more quickly and enabled them to stand the added trauma of an operation much better than plasma alone.[33]

The great stretches of treeless, hazardous desert lying between frontline primary medical services and the Tobruk hospital made a mockery of the maximum permitted time delays specified in the three-points-forward system. However, even men who had been wounded days earlier generally arrived with injuries less severely infected than those Jolly had seen in Spain. This was attributed to a combination of the dry and almost sterile desert conditions and the increasing use of sulfanilamide powder as an antiseptic. "In the Middle East campaigns," wrote one of Jolly's RAMC colleagues, "this form of chemotherapy proved a magnificent asset—but never a substitute for sound surgery."[34]

Much of Jolly's own work in the theater consisted of limiting postoperative infection. He and his colleagues developed and refined a two-stage surgical process that allowed them to monitor wounds for sepsis after the initial operation. The first stage involved removing all accessible foreign bodies; debriding, or removing, dead tissue; and then packing the wound with gauze soaked in sterile grease. Fractures, particularly compound fractures where the broken bone had penetrated the skin, posed special difficulties. Early traction toward the ankle was necessary to realign the break and reduce pain by preventing the broken ends of bone from rubbing, but it was not easy to manage in the desert. In Spain, Jolly and other Republican Army field surgeons had widely adopted the Catalan surgeon Josep Trueta's closed plaster technique. This simple yet remarkably effective technique required fewer medical personnel, and leaving the wound undisturbed in its plaster cast, protected from constant reinfection, promoted a natural healing process.[35] It proved equally effective and convenient to the desert war.

The need to avoid moving patients after major operations, even in forward hospitals, was becoming generally recognized, and in besieged Tobruk, No. 62 General provided postoperative wards with wide, airy verandas for these patients. As soon as they were in a condition to travel, they were evacuated 150 kilometers eastward to the town of Bardia. Some were transported "in austere conditions on stretchers under a tarpaulin suspended over goal-post-like frames from the back of a lorry."[36] The more fortunate traveled in ambulances, driving five to a convoy. The outward journey was made slowly to protect the worst stretcher cases, taking up to five hours on the dangerously overcrowded road and often having to detour through the desert. The empty ambulances returned in half the time.[37]

In September–October 1941, six months into Rommel's siege of Tobruk, the port was pounded by a force of a hundred Stuka dive-bombers, while Panzer tanks made repeated ground attacks. To insulate the hospital's shock patients from the horrifying vibration and noise, they were cared for in a special tunnel ward dug into a nearby hillside under forty feet (twelve meters) of sand and rock.[38] The besieged port had become the key to the entire North African campaign, and the tanks of the newly formed Eighth Army (which replaced the Western Desert Force in October 1941) crisscrossed south and southeast of the town as they confronted Rommel's forces during the second Western Desert Campaign. The Eighth Army's goal was to regain the territory lost to Rommel earlier in the year and to relieve the port's beleaguered garrison, which grew desperately short of water after a Stuka destroyed its desalination plant.[39]

Jolly's patients at the Tobruk general hospital were now evacuated by ship to base hospitals in Alexandria, Egypt, as soon as they were considered sufficiently recovered to withstand the two-day voyage. This was a hazardous journey. The hospital ships could moor no closer than half a mile from the shore, since the port was thronged with sunken Italian vessels and bombing had destroyed all its wharves. Stretcher-case patients were transported to the ships in small boats known as lighters, which were towed out and hauled aboard the ships using their hoists.[40]

The many patients with broken legs faced journeys of several days without proper nursing care on the voyage to Alexandria. To reduce the patients' discomfort, the surgical staff at No. 62 General Hospital developed a variant on the closed-plaster technique using the captured enemy supplies available to them, including a large number of Italian metal splints. The staff encased the broken limb in a plaster cast and placed it within one of these splints.[41] They then wrapped the splint itself in more plaster of Paris bandages. Fractures of the arm were encased in a massive plaster shell incorporating both the arm and the trunk. By this unorthodox method, blood circulation for the affected limb was unimpeded, but the fracture was rigidly yet comfortably immobilized. The technique became known as the Tobruk plaster, although Jolly often referred to it, with a nod to its Spanish origins, as the "yeso de Tobruk." Reflecting on its use many years later, he recalled that it "proved so efficient for evacuating men with wounded lower extremities down the long line of communication to the hospitals in the [Nile] Delta."[42] A patient with "a fractured femur could now travel without danger or discomfort for four or five days after the primary surgery had been carried out," wrote another army surgeon. He added, "I was never able to discover who first evolved this magnificent advance in war surgery," although as its name makes clear, this technique was developed and first practiced by Jolly and his colleagues in Tobruk.[43]

The hospital ships were clearly marked with large red crosses to protect them from attack, and enemy aircraft and artillery generally honored the convention that they should not be treated as military targets. On at least one occasion, however, patients were evacuated by vessels not displaying these internationally recognized markings and suffered tragic consequences that must have had specially painful resonance for Jolly. In December 1941, during the height of the battle for Tobruk, the *SS Chakdina* prepared to leave the port for Alexandria with a number of prisoners and 380 wounded, including ninety-seven New Zealand stretcher cases, placed in the aft holds. Just as the moon rose, spreading its greatly feared "good bombing light" across the harbor, a torpedo-carrying German aircraft at little more than fifteen meters above the sea approached the ship. It released a torpedo that exploded in one of the aft holds and sank the *Chakdina* in less than five minutes. Few of those belowdecks managed to survive, "but there were several remarkable escapes when the exploding boilers caused an upward surge of water that thrust some to the surface. These and others were picked up by ships of the convoy which carried out rescue work for two hours despite continued air attacks . . . the decision to use the *Chakdina* as a hospital ship, without markings, appears unjustifiable."[44]

Five days after this tragic incident, and after further heavy losses on both sides, New Zealand infantrymen with fixed bayonets linked up with British tank units and relieved the siege on the port, forcing Rommel's Afrika Korps westward. Over the following five months, he would build up his forces for yet another offensive to retake Tobruk.

Logistics of all kinds, both purely military and medical, were a key factor in this desert war, where the grueling terrain and constant sand abrasion on engines caused vehicles to break down with monotonous regularity. The location of each point in Jolly's three-points-forward system required constant reevaluation under the punishing conditions of motorized desert war, where a rapid advance could suddenly become an equally hasty retreat. The senior American surgeon in the North African and Mediterranean theater of the war, although a firm admirer of Jolly's system, found that the distance between the field hospital and the casualty clearing station needed to be eliminated in desert conditions. "This provides for the immediate transfer of wounded from the clearing station to the first-priority surgical hospital by hand litter. No pause is required for resuscitation or interference with splinting or dressings. . . . Surgeons assigned the responsibility of caring for the wounded in a first-priority surgical hospital must be highly trained and experienced, as their tasks are the most exacting of military surgery."[45] Greater importance was now placed on the time lag between initial emergency surgery, the kind in which Jolly excelled, and subsequent reparative surgery aimed at restoring the full use of limbs and reducing disfigurement. "To fail to take cognisance of the potentialities of early reparative surgery . . . will be as unthinkable as a failure to plan for the removal of the wounded from the field of battle."[46]

Taking advantage of the temporary lull that followed the relief of Tobruk, a conference of senior RAMC officers in Cairo in February 1942 addressed these and related medical issues. Its deliberations resulted eight months later in a smaller and more mobile medical formation, the field surgical unit (FSU), suggesting that the impact of *Field Surgery in Total War* was filtering up the chain of command.[47] Surgeons attached to an FSU could work at the front with field ambulances, using nothing but a small lean-to tent attached to a truck to perform lifesaving surgery.[48] In this period, wrote eminent U.S. Army surgeon Edward Churchill, "the Royal Army Medical Corps attained mobility for their forward surgical teams which made the relatively cumbersome and static British CCS [of the World War I era] appear obsolete."[49] It is a peculiar irony of the Western Desert Campaign that just as British surgeons at the Cairo conference were reinventing mobile field hospitals developed during the battle of Madrid five years earlier, their New Zealand colleagues were dismantling well-proven mobile surgical units derived from the same harsh experience.

14 Merry Hell

By May 1942, Rommel was prepared to launch a massive, renewed offensive on Tobruk. Its British, Indian, and South African defenders were outgunned and outnumbered, and after two weeks of heavy fighting, the order came to evacuate the town. Patients capable of withstanding overland travel were either driven to a South African hospital about two hundred miles away or taken another eighty miles to the British military base of Mersa Matruh. Three hospital ships arrived from Alexandria to evacuate the remaining wounded, all stretcher cases and many extremely ill.[1] In this critical period, according to one contemporary account, "conditions for careful surgical work in the No. 62 General Hospital became increasingly difficult owing to the large number of casualties, inadequate water supply and other adversities. Four enamel bowls of water served eight operating tables and were [refilled] once an hour. The surgeon broke the crust of blood, sand, dirt and soap suds on the top and washed as best he could beneath this."[2]

Jolly was then head of the surgical division of the hospital. "This was at a time when Tobruk was under close siege . . . and no part of this enclave was not under direct German shell fire." Over two days, he organized the evacuation of the remaining 750 wounded by British hospital ships such as the HMHS *Somersetshire*. The ships were unable to dock alongside the wharf since Tobruk harbor was clogged with sunken vessels, so these patients, mainly casualties of Rommel's tanks in the Libyan desert, were evacuated on stretchers laid across lifeboats. The boats were towed out to the hospital ships through choppy seas and under constant shelling. To prepare his patients for their nightmarish journey through the harbor, followed by a four-day voyage to Alexandria, Jolly relied greatly on the Tobruk plaster technique, "convinced that it was preferable for treating all soft tissue injuries as well as compound fractures."[3]

One of the *Somersetshire*'s British nurses, Mary Evans, recalled being dive-bombed and machine-gunned three times and finally torpedoed. "Luckily it happened as we were on our way back into Tobruk, so no patients were on board. Six of the nursing orderlies and one Indian seaman lost their lives . . . and the rest of us were in the [lifeboats] within five minutes of the ship being hit."[4]

In late June 1942, Tobruk finally fell to Rommel. Its thirty-three thousand defenders, including their commander, the hapless South African general H. B. Klopper, became his prisoners, and Rommel's forces acquired a giant stockpile of Allied munitions, fuel, and other supplies. The Eighth Army, wrote Winston Churchill later, "was reduced to bits and pieces and oppressed by a sense of bafflement and uncertainty."[5] Jolly did not witness this surrender, the most humiliating British defeat of the war apart from the fall of Singapore four months earlier, as he had left Tobruk on the last outward voyage of one of the hospital ships. He spent the next several months at the British No. 42 General Hospital in Alexandria, Egypt, one of the very few periods of his wartime service when he was not based at a forward area.

The Alexandria hospital received evacuated patients from the confused series of engagements in July 1942 around El Alamein, at that time an insignificant railway halt near Egypt's western frontier. Under their new and buccaneering commander, Bernard "Monty" Montgomery, the Eighth Army's desperate defense succeeded in halting Rommel's advance into Egypt, and he again retired westward into Libya. Over the following months, a reinvigorated Eighth Army, now larger and better equipped than ever, prepared for a final campaign to drive the German Army permanently out of North Africa. By September, Jolly could report to Irene Grant that "there is nothing but confidence here—well founded, I trust. . . . I'm as brown as brown, with swimming two or three days a week in the salt water. . . . And very fit, Irene—haven't had a day off-colour since I came out. Nearly everyone else has had malaria or dysentery or some such specific malady but they all just pass me by."[6]

As part of the medical services' preparations for the next epic confrontation with Rommel, in October 1942 Jolly was transferred to No. 2 General Hospital at Quassasin military camp east of the Suez Canal. With the rank of lieutenant colonel and again as head of its surgical division, he found the camp sited in a bleak stretch of desert, parched by day and bitter by night, and with no shelter from gritty sandstorms and whirling dust. No. 2 General was nominally a base hospital situated well east of the battlefront; however, during the final months of 1942, Jolly once again found himself responsible for the early surgical management of large numbers of battle casualties, this time with few of the usual facilities of a base hospital.

Montgomery's Allied forces now greatly outnumbered Rommel's tired and undernourished troops, who also faced critical shortages of fuel and ammunition. In anticipation of the assault to expel them, the Axis troops reinforced their defenses by laying half a million mines (the "Devil's Garden"), most of them acquired from the Allied stockpile captured at Tobruk five months earlier. The decisive battle of the campaign began under a full moon on the night of 23 October 1942, with an Allied artillery barrage followed by an infantry advance to clear a path through the minefields for their tanks. This signaled the start of three weeks of hellish and often close-quarter attacks and counterattacks. Monty had planned the battle as a First World War–type exercise of attrition, with corresponding numbers of casualties. To prepare for them, the British Army's medical services put into practice the principles agreed to at the Cairo conference in February 1942 and formally deployed both field surgical teams and field dressing stations, siting them well forward to receive the bulk of casualties.[7]

The fighting was characterized by long and dangerous lines of communication and by highly mobile light equipment; therefore, the forward surgical units constantly had to move. Treating injuries on the battlefield with sulphonamide drugs neither sterilized contaminated wounds nor prevented infection in those who had not received surgical treatment, but surgical units on the battlefield "were able to keep a local infection local and to prolong from a few hours to many days the period during which the excision of dead and contaminated tissues was safe and profitable."[8] Once the wounded arrived at the Quassasin hospital, even those who had received initial treatment at the battlefront more than twelve hours earlier were found to have reasonably clean and manageable injuries that Jolly and his staff could treat with a high rate of success.

By early November 1942, the German and Italian forces were shattered and retreated westward in disarray. The second battle of El Alamein was the first clear-cut and irreversible victory for the Allied powers, and it proved to be a major turning point of the entire war. Yet Rommel refused to admit defeat and conducted a fighting withdrawal toward the port of Tripoli on the Libyan coast. Along almost two thousand kilometers of coastline, his exhausted troops conducted a textbook retreat, peppering the ground behind them with mines and booby traps to delay their pursuers. The Allied forces, however, were both more numerous and more mobile, and Rommel abandoned Tripoli and instead withdrew even farther westward to make a final stand at Tunis, capital of Tunisia.

Once again based on the coast at Alexandria and now in the blessedly cooler conditions of the desert winter, Jolly's letters to Irene exuded confidence and exhilaration:

> This country is at its most glorious. The days are like wine—bright, clear sunshine with just a zip in the air to set the sense of beauty soaring. I'm up with the sun each morning just after six, indeed . . . sometimes I'm up before it. Not even any need really to be up so early except for the joy of being human, conscious and abroad in the beauty of sunrise in the desert. Then on to an early breakfast and off round the surgical division to see the most serious cases before becoming involved in the routine business of the day. . . . The food is excellent throughout the Army in this country—far better than it must be with you in England. I never sit down to breakfast without knowing that after grapefruit or porridge there will be fried bread with two eggs and bacon or sausages. . . .
>
> Here the Christmas festivities intervened, one day of which I've spent in the city with a name a bit like Karli's [i.e., Cairo]. . . . And on three occasions I've sung at various functions "Frankie and Johnny" and "Abdul the Bulbul Amir"—and the news continues to be good.[9]

The very next letter, however, dated January 1943, sounded a strikingly downbeat note, indicating the fast-moving pace of the battlefront and the huge distances and varying landscapes to be negotiated.

> Since I last wrote to you at the beginning of November I've travelled a long way and was separated from my unit—had no fixed address so did not get any mail until I rejoined my unit. . . . I don't seem to be able to remember when I wasn't in a war. . . .
>
> This place is horribly cold and wet, frost every night. We are in tents again and I pine for the comfort of a fire. Fortunately, our patients are in

buildings. We are very busy and the work is more onerous as we haven't settled down again yet after our move. It always takes time to get equipment sorted out and functioning again.[10]

By March 1943, the Eighth Army had taken Tripoli and crossed westward into Tunisia. Jolly and his staff followed behind the advancing Allied forces and relocated their hospital at Tripoli, nearer the new battlefront. Italy had seized this ancient trading port before World War I and made it the capital of its colony of Libya, which was occupied by 150,000 Italian settlers. The staff of No. 2 British General Hospital arrived to find that most of its colonizers had prudently abandoned it, leaving broad main streets lined by date palms and elegant Italianate buildings. The staff reestablished their hospital in a collection of modern, flat-roofed concrete buildings that offered protection against the glare and ferocity of the desert sun.

With its large and well-equipped port and imposing public facilities, Tripoli was designated by the Allied military command as a crucial element in its future operations, including the planned invasion of southern Europe. For the present, however, Rommel remained an active and immediate threat. His formidable defenses were based on the Mareth Line, a fifty-kilometer-long string of desert fortifications that the French had built a decade earlier to protect Tunisia against an anticipated invasion from Libya by Mussolini's forces and that German military engineers had reinforced and extended. The Eighth Army launched a full-scale attack on the Mareth Line in March 1943, and a flanking maneuver by New Zealand troops decisively encircled it. The Afrika Korps was driven from Tunis by the end of March. By then the Eighth Army had been joined by a newly formed First Army made up of British, U.S., and French divisions, and this combined force pressed its advantage by driving north-westward toward Algiers and Morocco. Two months later, the last German and Italian troops in North Africa surrendered, and the Eighth and First Armies prepared to cross the Mediterranean into Sicily.

At this point, the Allied health services acquired the very first sample doses of a new chemical antibiotic that would eventually transform the entire practice of medicine, both military and civilian. Some of its first tests on military patients were carried out in Jolly's Tripoli hospital, and this opportunity to witness medical history in the making was a privilege he valued all his life.

The discovery of more effective treatments for controlling infection had directed surgical practice for generations, and even in the two decades after Jolly entered medical school, significant innovations appeared. Nineteenth-century disinfectants such as Listerine were augmented in the 1930s by the introduction of sulfa drugs, developed first by German chemists working for the textile dyeing industry. By World War II, sulfa drugs were being produced in large quantities by both sides and were heavily used in the Western Desert, where troops were issued with packets of sulfa powder before battle and instructed to pour them into their own wounds at the first opportunity. Eighth Army surgeons, Jolly included, were delighted with the relatively mild infection rates among wounds incurred in the desert environment, and they initially attributed this to the protection that the new drugs supplied.[11] Yet when these surgeons met with their First Army equivalents, with recent experience of treating wounds incurred in the cooler, damper, and more fertile regions around Algeria, they learned that sulfa drugs had been far less effective there at controlling wound infection and that widespread debridement and even amputation at World War I rates were still regarded as essential.[12] It was primarily the harsh, arid, and almost sterile desert environment, Jolly and his colleagues discovered, and not sulfa powder alone that produced the good results they had witnessed. As they now prepared to leave the desert for the much cooler and intensively cultivated terrain on the opposite side of the Mediterranean, they could expect the effectiveness of sulfa drugs to decline precipitously.[13] Furthermore, some conditions, such as the devastatingly widespread gonorrhea, already seemed to show increased resistance to sulfa powder, perhaps from overuse.

The war was evidently entering a final phase, with the Allies preparing to retake Axis-occupied territories in Europe. As they calculated the extent and nature of the casualties this giant military operation might entail, the Allied armies' medical services exchanged rumors of a new and miraculous antibiotic. Penicillin had been discovered and named in the 1920s when the Scottish microbiologist Alexander Fleming stumbled upon the antibiotic properties of mold spores, but the difficulty of isolating and propagating its active ingredient had prevented its use for medical purposes. In 1938, with global conflict looming, research into the drug intensified at Oxford University under an Australian pharmacologist named Howard Florey and Ernst Chain, a German-born Jewish refugee. By 1940, as bombs rained down on British cities and their civilian hospitals' staffs watched casualties die from massive and untreatable infections, the Oxford trials finally delivered promising results. Penicillin's only apparent limiting factor was the time required to produce the necessary quantities. Unlike the artificially created sulfa drugs, penicillin was cultivated from live organisms, and treating even a single patient with severe sepsis might require two thousand liters of culture medium.[14]

The United States entered the war the following year after Japan's attack on Pearl Harbor and therefore had its own urgent reasons for developing large supplies of the drug. It was soon being produced at a frantic pace in both the United States and Britain. As a military-scientific project, only the efforts toward developing the nuclear bomb exceeded those of mass-producing penicillin. By May 1943, enough of the precious substance had been cultured and refined to carry out trials on military subjects, and RAMC surgeon Lt. Col. Ian Fraser, along with a pathologist and a technician, left for North Africa with 10 million units, the entire stock then available worldwide. The men were joined in Tripoli three weeks later by Professor Florey himself, a pale and donnish figure under a trilby hat who made a most unmilitary appearance among the bronzed warriors of the Western Desert. At three military hospitals in the town, including No. 2 General, Florey supervised some of the earliest tests of penicillin on war wounds. "We had only enough material for 20 patients by systemic injection but enough for about 200 or more casualties if the powder was used diluted with sulphonamide," he later wrote.[15] He quickly established that the new drug was less toxic than sulfa drugs used alone and more effective against certain microorganisms.[16]

An instructional film of this unquestionably historic development in medical science shows Florey injecting the drug into a soldier's severe leg wound. A few days later, the patient is seen walking with no more than a slight limp.[17] Although dosages and treatment protocols were still barely understood, it was apparent to the delighted witnesses to these trials that penicillin was significantly more effective at preventing infection than sulfa drugs or any existing surgical techniques including the "delayed suture." It also proved miraculous at curing that eternal soldier's complaint, gonorrhea, a condition that was disabling thousands of troops who would soon be needed to take part in the invasion of Sicily. Its use for this purpose, however, was delayed on moral grounds. Professor Florey found it unacceptable that his life- and limb-saving panacea, developed to treat the heroic victims of battle casualties, might be used in much greater quantities by those suffering a condition he regarded as the self-inflicted consequence of their sinful behavior. This impasse was referred to Winston Churchill himself, who sent a carefully worded response to the effect that "this valuable drug . . . must be used to best military advantage." This was interpreted in Tripoli as license to treat the venereal disease sufferers with penicillin and restore them to their units.[18] "Without a doubt," states one recent authority, "penicillin gave the allies an advantage over the German forces."[19]

In the month after this world-changing medical breakthrough, Jolly's commanding officer, Col. L. M. Rowlette, recommended his head surgeon for the OBE, an award established during World War I to honor those serving in noncombatant roles. It was awarded in both civil and military divisions, with the latter reserved for those in the nursing services and commissioned but noncombatant officers. Rowlette wrote that Jolly

> has probably the widest experience of war surgery of any surgeon of the present day, both in forward area and base. . . . During the period covered by this citation he has used his experience to the fullest advantage in organising his division to cope with an abnormal rush of casualties at a critical time when the hospital had moved to a new site [in Tripoli] and was not properly established and lacked the normal facilities of a base hospital. Despite this, his cases received every care and attention and the remarkably good results obtained must, in a large measure, be attributed to Lt. Col. Jolly's professional and administrative ability and sound judgement. . . . Lt. Col. Jolly's untiring zeal and quiet but thorough methods have been an inspiration and stimulant to all the staff.

Jolly's military OBE was accordingly awarded in July 1943.[20] Writing to Irene Grant to tell her the news, he sounded typically offhand about this honor but noted that "Mother will be happy."[21]

Early July marked the beginning of the next phase of the Mediterranean theater of war. The wedge-shaped island of Sicily off the toe of Italy's boot was the chosen invasion site for the Allied reconquest of Europe. Before sunrise on 10 July, almost 200,000 troops from the U.S. Seventh and British Eighth Armies launched an amphibious invasion of its southwest shores. Medical units were attached to each of the combat forces and equipped with blood plasma, morphine, and sterile dressings. Jolly and his team at Tripoli were not among them since No. 2 General Hospital was designated as a base hospital to receive patients evacuated, either by sea or by air, at the earliest opportunity.

During the landings on the precipitous and rocky Sicilian coast, navy as well as army first aid stations were set up on the beaches to treat and evacuate the wounded until the first field hospitals could be brought ashore. Within two days of the initial assault, the ground forces had secured a third of the island. They then advanced rapidly across dangerously steep terrain threaded only by narrow mountain trails. The swift Allied advance demanded maximum mobility from the field medical units, but the first air evacuations began four days after the initial attack. "The backbone and single indispensable element in the evacuation system was the litter bearer. It took strength, stamina, gentleness, and a high order of courage to collect the wounded on the field while the fighting, often enough, was still in progress, and by relays of four-man teams to carry the casualties sometimes as much as ten or twelve miles over mountain trails impassable to any vehicle, too steep even for mules."[22]

These casualties reached Tripoli after a blessedly short, two-hour flight, and Jolly and his surgical colleagues were delighted with the condition of those whose injuries had been treated in the field with the precious new supplies of penicillin. Rather than attempting complex and risky operations at the battlefront, field surgeons now simply cleaned up wounds to remove infection and foreign materials, sprinkled them with penicillin powder, and stitched them closed. Patients received further regular penicillin injections en route to Tripoli, where they could be operated on in near-ideal conditions. "The results were magnificent, with clean wounds ready for definitive surgery on arrival at the forward base hospitals."[23] The Sicilian casualties included many civilians, and some of them, most distressingly for Jolly, were children who had stepped on mines. Allied troops also learned by punishing experience that in that perilous midsummer, the vineyards clinging to the hillsides and displaying luscious purple grapes had been heavily mined.[24]

By late August 1943, the crucial eastern port of Messina fell to the Allies. The fascist dictator Mussolini had been deposed, his successor was suing for peace, and the last German and Italian troops had withdrawn across the Straits of Messina into Italy. The Sicilian campaign had delivered its principal objectives of diverting pressure from the German advance on the eastern front, opening up the Mediterranean seaways to the Allied fleet, and providing a strategic stepping stone for the much larger and more protracted liberation of mainland Italy. That campaign began, with barely a pause, on 3 September, a fortuitous date for the Allies since it also marked a formal armistice with the Italian government. German forces now braced to hold Italy without the support of its national army, but they had prepared a strong line of defenses along the Apennines, the country's mountainous spine. Just before the new invasion began, a medical conference in Algiers agreed that Eighth Army casualties would be evacuated by air to North Africa and the Middle East rather than to Sicily and that base hospitals would be established in Naples as soon as possible after its capture.[25] As in the Sicilian campaign, air evacuation was used for almost all surgical cases capable of withstanding transportation, including the most severe abdominal wounds. Jolly's surgical team received the first planeloads of wounded men within days of the initial landings in southern Italy, and in the face of stubborn resistance, as the Allied troops pushed the Germans slowly northward, the evacuation runs did not cease for the next two months.

The injuries that the infantry incurred in the cultivated soil and under increasingly cold and damp autumnal conditions included blast wounds from German minefields and booby traps that produced devastating tissue damage, typically strewn with dirt and other debris. Treating and evacuating troops with these grievous wounds were hampered by the daunting terrain, which was well suited for the German defenses but not for the motorized desert warfare familiar to the Eighth Army. In these conditions, Allied surgeons evolved a variant of the delayed suture technique to take account of both the use of penicillin, when available, and the long, airborne evacuation route to a base hospital. At the earliest opportunity, wounds were treated in the field by "a wide and drastic excision of all dead or damaged tissue, especially muscle. The whole wound is exposed . . . it is left open *without sutures* and is then dusted with calcium penicillin powder and evacuated." Three to five days later, at a base hospital such as Jolly's, the wounds were sutured for the first time. "This procedure led to the direct healing of wounds without sepsis in 80% to 90% of cases, a remarkable result," and without precedent in medical history.[26]

By the end of September 1943, after fighting through rain and mud, and crossing trackless marshlands and valleys raked by enemy fire, the Allied forces reached the key southern port of Naples. They found the city virtually destroyed after months of aerial bombing but especially from demolition by its former

German occupiers. Within a month, however, supplies were moving steadily into the city by air and sea in preparation for an assault on Rome and northern Italy. Among the hundreds of tons of equipment and thousands of military personnel assembled for this phase of the war was Jolly's general hospital, now ordered to transfer from Tripoli to the newly conquered Italian mainland. Colonel Rowlette commended all his staff on their past year's activity:

> This hospital has just completed another chapter in its history, a history full of hard and conscientious work during its stay in Tripoli. Our previous records have been far exceeded and a very large number of patients have passed through our hands and I have never in my long experience encountered happier or more contented patients. You have set up a standard of hard and efficient work which I have good reason to believe is widely recognized throughout the Middle East, and at home, and of which I am very proud. This very gratifying result has only been achieved by each and every individual pulling his or her full weight for the good of all.
>
> On behalf of innumerable patients who have thanked me for the care and attention they have received at your hands, and on my own behalf as your Commanding Officer, I ask you one and all—Officers, Nursing Officers and Other Ranks, to accept very grateful thanks for your zealous work. You have accomplished a big task and added much honour to the record of the Medical Service.[27]

The historic town of Caserta, forty kilometers north of Naples, was chosen as the new location for No. 2 General Hospital largely because the Allied headquarters in the Mediterranean was also based there in a vast four-hundred-room royal palace. Jolly's hospital, however, was housed in the more spartan premises of a nearby Italian Army barracks, a series of unlovely three-storied stone buildings surrounding a rectangular parade ground. Over the next two months, the six-hundred-bed hospital was transported there through winter blizzards and across a blasted landscape of crashed planes, burned-out tanks, and shattered buildings. Jolly would spend the rest of his war at this site, serving both as the head of surgery for the No. 2 British General Hospital and as the senior medical officer of the No. 2 New Zealand General Hospital, which shared the same site. He was thus able to work and socialize alongside compatriots a decade after leaving his homeland.

For the next six months, as the Allied forces advanced toward Rome, these two hospitals were nearer the front line than any others of the Italian campaign. Jolly and his colleagues no longer received casualties by air evacuation, as at Tripoli, but directly from the field of battle—from ambulances, field dressing stations, and casualty clearing stations. "This demanded that the hospital be primarily surgical," wrote Jolly's medical colleague George Komrower, "and a large number of available beds were earmarked for this purpose."[28] In both hospitals, most patients were held in large wards, holding 120 beds or more, and tended to prefer the social interaction this system provided. Entertainment was organized for them in the form of occasional concerts and dances provided by the more musical members of the British hospital staff, who created a small orchestra.[29]

Several parallel lines of defenses spanning the width of Italy rigorously defended the route to Rome. In January 1944, the Allies began a series of costly attacks across freezing rivers and mountain passes, finding that the German defenders had made skilled use of every feature of the landscape to obstruct their advance. In this flinty ground, a shell or mortar bomb or even a single bullet sent shards of rock flying in all directions, and facial wounds were frequent.[30] Evacuating these casualties under enemy fire, and through terrain ambulances often found impassable, required great effort and ingenuity. New Zealand troops winched their wounded across the swollen Sangro River by dangling stretchers from a "flying fox" (zip line) along a 120-meter cable. Elsewhere stretchers were lashed together and covered with a tarpaulin to make an eight-man raft. Sleds, mule litters, and ski-towed stretchers—all were employed to make the agonizing journey that ended at the Caserta hospital.[31]

Each day Jolly made a round of the surgical wards, and to prepare for this ritual, the nursing staff first washed and shaved the patients and tidied their beds. One young English patient at the New Zealand General Hospital later recalled, "Orders were given to all patients, 'Do not speak unless the O. C. [officer commanding the surgical division] speaks to you first.' A few moments later, a large party consisting of doctors, nurses, the Matron and others came into the ward." The bedbound Englishman heard the most senior figure present addressed as Colonel Jolly, "and my ears immediately pricked up." During the battle of Ebro six years earlier, Johnny Longstaff had been treated by Jolly for facial injuries at the railway tunnel hospital in Flix, Catalonia. With his eyes heavily bandaged, he never saw his surgeon, but he remembered his distinctive name and, in defiance of the nursing staff's strict instructions, now addressed the doctor in Spanish. "The Ward Sister's face was not pleasant to behold but he stopped." Ignoring the matron's outraged glare, Longstaff persisted in reminding Jolly of their earlier meeting in the gloomy surroundings of the Flix hospital.

> "I was there and I believe that you helped to save my eyesight," I said. It was him. What a coincidence! He gave me a few kind words and said he would return after his inspection. Sometime during that afternoon he returned and told the Ward Sister not to worry about his presence. For over an hour we talked. He told me that the hospital had operated on me and had left two pieces of foreign body in the wound. I would have no trouble as the penicillin had saved my leg from being amputated. Almost every day Dr. Jolly came to see me, bringing books and cigarettes.[32]

Under this kindly treatment, and with four daily doses of the miraculous new penicillin, Longstaff soon improved sufficiently to have his bed moved to the hospital's outside veranda, where he felt cooler and less bored. Jolly then offered him a job as the hospital's librarian, assuming he had seen enough of combat duties. However, Longstaff and two other members of his company who were also receiving hospital treatment heard that "our boys were now fighting near Perugia . . . and the battalion had suffered very bad casualties. And we decided we would get back."[33] From his convenient outdoor convalescing station, Longstaff managed to escape the hospital and rejoin his company with his injury barely healed. Two days later, he was returned to a different ward with two bullets in his left forearm and another "that had ploughed through the top of my back. . . . This time Dr. Colonel Jolly played merry hell with me. I had to give him a promise that I would not desert his hospital again until I was really fit and well."[34]

The amphibious assault on the port of Anzio, sixty kilometers south of Rome, during the late winter of 1944 was one of the toughest battles in the Italian campaign. The beachhead, heavily shelled by German artillery, became known as "Hell's Half-Acre." British casualty clearing stations used tents that, according to one of their surgeons,

> let in water very freely at the junctions and during the heavy rains it just poured in. . . . On either side of the ward were placed the stretchers of the men awaiting operative treatment for their wounds. . . . Some were unconscious,

> these chiefly head wounds, whose loud snoring breathing distinguished them. Some were carried in dying with gross combinations of shattered limbs, protrusions of intestines and brain. Some carried in, gasping and coughing, shot through the lungs. Others, less badly wounded, looking around with curious eyes, clutching mounds of equipment and agitating about pieces of their kit which had gone astray. All were exhausted after being under continuous fire and lying in the mud.[35]

Even these critically injured men, given emergency treatment under such unsanitary and distressing conditions, were usually found to be progressing well when they reached evacuation hospitals to the south. A vital factor in this success rate was the provision of fresh blood from a blood bank set up in Naples in early 1944. By June that year, as the Allies were approaching Rome, a Dakota plane known as the "Blood Wagon" carried blood and plasma daily to the front. No injured soldier on either side was denied it, and "many a Yugoslav, Pole or German prisoner of war . . . owes his life" to blood donated by British troops.[36]

In June 1944, Rome fell to the Allies, and two days later, far to the north, the invasion of Normandy began. As the front line moved farther away from them, Jolly's Caserta general hospitals assumed the duties of base units, with many patients delivered to them by air ambulance, a journey of only forty minutes.[37] Increasingly, their surgical patients also arrived in satisfactory condition due largely to the growing use of sulfanamide and penicillin.[38] The frantic British-U.S. project to produce penicillin in industrial quantities was gathering pace, and the drug was at last becoming available in tablets rather than the less convenient liquid form. Its effectiveness at preventing sepsis in wounds, even with a long delay between a first treatment and definitive surgery, was steadily transforming Jolly's profession.[39]

The combination of penicillin and large-scale blood transfusion, together with improved means of transporting severely wounded patients and increasingly sophisticated surgical treatments of abdominal wounds, made the successive campaigns in North Africa, Sicily, and mainland Italy "a veritable crucible of military medicine."[40] By the end of the Italian campaign, the rate for complete healing for limb wounds reached 90 percent, a previously unheard-of figure.[41] These and related innovations were analyzed at length during another congress of Central Mediterranean Forces army surgeons in Rome in February 1945.

On one day of the congress, the pope granted an audience to the delegates, who included Jolly.[42] (The pope's predecessor, Pope Pius XI, had offered a benediction to Franco's forces eight years earlier.)

Several months later, Jolly carried with him a small quantity of the precious penicillin, then still in short supply, to Egypt, where he used it to save the life of a fellow Spanish Civil War veteran and compatriot. While visiting the general hospital in Alexandria, he learned that a female patient with an intractable high fever had been "put into a corner of the hospital to die." He scoured the wards until he found the critically ill forty-one-year-old nurse Dorothy Morris and immediately injected her with the drug. When she recovered sufficiently to speak to him, he learned that the slender, dark-haired woman he had found clinging to life had served in Spain as the administrator of children's hospitals and, furthermore, that she was a New Zealander from the same small town of Cromwell as himself. She recovered sufficiently to be invalided back to London for VE Day in May 1945.[43]

In August, just before the Caserta hospitals were decommissioned, Jolly made the journey to the United Kingdom, bringing to an end his seven years of combined service as a military surgeon, most of it near the front line. In preparing to return to civilian practice, he bore a glowing testimonial from his senior officer, Brig. Harold Edwards, consulting surgeon to the Central Mediterranean Forces. Brigadier Edwards summarized the work of his senior staff in the previous eighteen months and its significance for the future:

> In the Italian campaign, you have:
>
> (1) Brought the specialism of forward surgery to a remarkably high standard
> (2) Developed the Two-Stage concept of wound treatment to a truly astonishing level of success
> (3) Reduced chronic sepsis to negligible proportions
> (4) Perfected the use of penicillin, and established its role in the treatment of war wounds
> (5) Reduced mortality and morbidity for most types of war wounds to a level rarely equalled and never surpassed in any campaign in history
> (6) Advanced the technique of early skin grafting and early and late wound closure by plastic methods

(7) Appreciated the importance of maintaining the normality of the blood throughout convalescence, and acted accordingly
(8) Contributed scientific data at the Rome Conference, and in medical publications, which will be of historic medical value
(9) Unselfishly allowed devotion to the welfare of the patient to triumph over professional rivalries so that segregation of cases to a new degree of intensity became possible. . . .

It will of course be for the historian to assess the worth of your contribution in relation to advances in all theatres of war, present and past, but I am confident . . . that the record of your fine work will find a prominent and permanent place in the archives of war surgery.[44]

15 Phantom Pain

Unlike many of his friends and companions from the years of war, Doug Jolly returned to civilian life physically unscathed. He was a decorated veteran, deeply admired by his colleagues, and seemingly well placed to build a peacetime career. Yet his first and most pressing requirement, in early 1946, was rest and recovery from disabling emotional strain. As often in the past, Irene and Donald Grant found room for him at their latest address in North London. In this familiar and comforting setting, Irene took care of Jolly with great devotion for some months.[1]

As soon as he recovered sufficiently, he began to write to old friends and former members of his various surgical units. Some of their replies were heartbreaking. "Cher ami," wrote his former nurse Anna-Mária Basch, "I was very happy to learn in your letter that you are in good health and that this terrible war—that I call global hellfire—is well over for you. [Son] Jean and I spoke of you often, asking each other: in which corner of the world are you busy opening and sewing bellies?"[2]

She revealed that she had spent much of the war working with the anti-Nazi Resistance in Brussels.

> For two years I worked as a night nurse in a *German* military hospital and afternoons at Dr. Lavaud's place—a man you know. So I was only able to sleep 3–4 hours a day, but at the doctor's it was very easy to organise meetings with friends in my little room. One day however I became exhausted and my situation in the hospital was already dangerous. I left my two jobs, and devoted myself entirely to the Resistance. Moreover Dr. L. also worked for the Resistance, we were already compromising each other. He was wanted by the Gestapo in 1943, he left and became an illegal.

She and János were often hungry in this period, she told Jolly, "without money, without anywhere to stay, but we had a smile on our lips and joy in our hearts. We worked with the partisans. . . . It was very, very dangerous but very beautiful. You lived day and night in anguish, if not for yourself then for the others."[3]

In March 1944, both were arrested. János, who despite his youth had risen to the rank of sergeant in Spain, was sent to the Buchenwald concentration camp in central Germany. She herself, Anna-Mária wrote, was sent to the all-female concentration camp of Ravensbrück, north of Berlin, as a *politisch* (political) prisoner with a red triangle on her striped uniform. Her Jewish origins might have condemned her to also wear a yellow one, further reducing her chances of survival. Soon afterward she was moved to the nearby subcamp of Neubrandenburg, where more than 130,000 women and children were eventually incarcerated, and at least 50,000 of them died from starvation, execution, or illness. Almost half the inmates were Hungarians like herself. Most were put to hard physical labor: roadbuilding, shifting earth and stones, unloading trains and boats. As a fluent German speaker, Anna-Mária was more fortunate and was sent to a sewing workshop:

> When I looked from time to time through the windows, I saw a wood of fir trees not far away behind which the sun had just risen. It was very beautiful, and often I thought of you in those moments. It was our only pleasure in this accursed camp, and absolutely indispensable that we focus on pleasant memories and think of good things. Otherwise, one would become completely stupid, idiotic. Because there we had to be strong on our feet, and have an iron will to morally resist! I do not wish to write of life in the camps in detail. . . . A normal mind would not believe what the Nazis thought to invent to make us suffer, physically and morally. To work very hard like slaves, to be cold and hungry, without clothes, without shoes, to take blows, insults, fortunes, to be thrown out when one is ill, without care, to live in filth and vermin.

After a year in this camp, with Russian troops just thirty kilometers away, the guards ordered the prisoners to leave:

> The Boche commandant told me that if I stayed behind I would be shot. In the evening I escaped from the column and hid with a lot of wanderers

until the arrival of the Russians. These people were very, very trustworthy and kind to us. When the Russians arrived we were full of joy, and cried like kids. Obviously I do not know how to speak about this in detail. As we say, you can't fit a house in a box of matches. It is better that I do not continue telling stories about the camp, I have to be cured of this nightmare atmosphere. In the depth of my heart I sense the horrors and see again before my eyes the terrible scenes that took place there.

She was reunited with János, who had managed to escape from Buchenwald a month before the Russians liberated his camp, and they returned together to Belgium in May 1945. "I came back from Germany exhausted and very sick. Already I'm feeling better, but I'm not the same. Firstly because we have no news of my husband, who was arrested in 1943 in France and deported to Germany."[4]

Endre Basch, she later learned, had commanded an artillery until at the end of the civil war, with the rank of lieutenant colonel. He was then held in the Gurs internment camp in southwest France and deported in February 1943 in a "reprisal" convoy after the Resistance killed two Luftwaffe officers in Paris. The convoy, comprising two thousand foreign Jews, was sent to the extermination camp of Sobibor in Poland. Only nine of its members were later identified as survivors. Endre Basch was not among them.[5]

"I congratulate you on the success of your book," wrote Jolly's former lover, "and your decoration. I understand you well, it will not be easy for you either to adapt to normal life. Have you started your studies at the hospital? Do you have news of your family? . . . Of my family not much was left. One cousin and my husband's brother in Budapest—that's all. Those at the front and the few Jews are all dead."[6]

Her son added a brief note to his mother's letter. "Deep down I was certain that you must have taken part in the [Second World] war somewhere in the world, because those who fought in Spain obviously could not sit idly by. . . . Come see us soon because we all have important things to share that can only be expressed in words, face-to-face. Hoping to see you soon, receive dear Jolly, this expression of my cordial wishes."[7]

It appears that no such reunion between Jolly and the surviving members of the Basch family ever took place.

Other friends from Spain, he learned, did not survive their second war.

The mechanic John Kozar had returned to his former occupation of merchant seaman. The courage and resourcefulness he showed in Spain could not save him from freezing to death when his ship, with a cargo of tanks and other machinery, was torpedoed off the coast of Newfoundland in January 1942.[8] The Czech doctor František Kriegel, whom Jolly greatly admired, was a fortunate survivor. He was held for a time, like Endre Basch, in the Gurs internment camp but then succeeded in traveling to China to work with Mao's Red Army and later with U.S. forces in Burma and India. On his return to his own country, he chose political activity over medicine and was clearly delighted to hear from his old friend:

> Your words revive innumerable old pictures of hard and yet so beautiful days! In all those years of war I've met some fine people, many of them became my good friends, but hardly ever did that band of friendship grow as close as it used to in Spain. There was another air we breathed and lived with.... I had a chance to observe the friends in China and India; nothing of the new world around us was able to erase the feelings we held for Spain....
>
> I'm sharing your disappointment with the foreign policy of Great Britain. At a time when modern progress of science should allow to satisfy the most urgent needs of mankind, there is more sabre-rattling, atom-policing and Churchillian forgive-the-German and save-Christian civilisation and save-Greece democracy than in 1938. It shows that many a demagogue believes in a very short memory of the human species.[9]

The fortitude and undiminished spirit shown by his old friends may have contributed to Jolly's recovery from his disabling despondency. By mid-1946, he began to look for work within the great network of London hospitals that was soon to form part of the country's new National Health Service (NHS). The Socialist Medical Association had largely shaped the health policy of Britain's Labour Party, and the party's landslide victory in the 1945 general election (jubilantly celebrated by the Grants and their friends at Pyecombe Corner) ensured that the policy would soon be implemented.[10] The National Health Service Act was introduced four months after the election and passed during the new parliament's first session. There can be no question that Jolly, in common with other doctors with recent military experience, welcomed this development. They had worked for military health services that frequently achieved a higher standard of care than most civilians had received before the war; therefore, they had few concerns about imposing a socialized command structure on an ad hoc, market-driven health system.[11]

Jolly's first postwar employment was with the Royal Cancer Hospital in Fulham Road in central London, the first hospital in the world devoted entirely to the study and treatment of cancer. Its 1951 centenary history proudly declared that "the primary object of the hospital has always been . . . the treatment of the sick poor. Nothing is withheld or refused so long as it is calculated to benefit the patients."[12] After the formation of the NHS in 1948, it became a postgraduate teaching hospital; later renamed the Royal Marsden Hospital, it remains a leading research and treatment institute today. Jolly spent five years at this prestigious public institution, and in that time, despite his unmatched record of recent clinical experience, he practiced no surgery. This would remain the pattern of his later career. The physically robust, politically committed, and compassionate figure who—amid the blood and bombs of Spain, North Africa, and Italy—had shown "a willingness and capacity to do most exacting work beyond what seemed to be the limits of endurance" in peacetime appeared withdrawn, hesitant, and often unwell. According to a longtime friend, he "never regained his enthusiasm and confidence for surgery."[13]

The clearest evidence of this transformation, and both a cause and a symptom of it, was Jolly's failure to gain formal qualifications in surgery. This crushing blow for an outstandingly gifted practicing surgeon was due in part to a succession of unfortunate timings. He had left New Zealand for London in 1932 with the sole aim of gaining his fellowship of the Royal College of Surgeons. For some years earlier, medical graduates throughout the British Commonwealth had been pressing for changes to the royal college's examination procedure that would enable them to qualify without having to spend a lengthy period of study in Britain.[14] Those efforts bore fruit in 1934 when two British surgeons conducted primary examinations for admission to the college in both Australia and New Zealand. The best results were obtained by graduates of Otago Medical School, Jolly's own alma mater, where thirteen out of twenty-three candidates were successful.[15] Since Jolly's final marks in surgery were among the highest in his year, it is most likely that had he remained in New Zealand, he would have been among those successful candidates. Instead, he had left London to go to war just months before taking his second and final FRCS examination.

On his return from Spain, both his speaking tours in Britain and New Zealand and his book writing left Jolly with no opportunity to prepare for the FRCS examination before he enlisted in the British Army. His situation was far from unique among Britain's military medical staff, and their superiors recognized this toward the end of World War II. They sought to ensure that young doctors who chose to enlist before qualifying in surgery would not later be disadvantaged relative to their colleagues who had managed to acquire the precious FRCS qualification during the war. In a report dated May 1943, as Jolly was observing pioneering trials of penicillin in Tripoli, the consulting surgeon for Middle East Forces advised his general headquarters that "the situation of those young surgeons, often the most brilliant men of their year, who took the Primary [examination] shortly before the war and joined up at the beginning, is one of genuine hardship. They have the humiliation of seeing their less gifted but more astute contemporaries and their juniors come out with recent fellowship and specialist status, while they remain CDOs." Jolly's name appears on a list of seventeen medical officers in this category. "It is suggested that these men be recalled to the UK in order that they may renew their contacts with civil surgery and have the opportunity to sit for their final examination."[16] That considerate recommendation was apparently not acted upon, and Jolly was not given the opportunity to sit for his surgical fellowship before his demobilization from the RAMC.

On their return to civilian life, some of his medical colleagues in similar circumstances managed to acquire their fellowship in the years soon after the war. Unlike its U.S. counterpart, the Royal College of Surgeons assessed candidates for membership purely by its examination of a "high and uniform standard" and not by a record of the surgical operations they had performed.[17] This method of assessment greatly disadvantaged Jolly, who had gained a vast and perhaps internationally unique practical experience, especially in abdominal surgery, but had probably barely touched a textbook in the previous decade. The final FRCS examination typically consisted of a written paper or papers, a clinical examination, and two oral examinations—one clinical and one in pathology. While employed at the Royal Cancer Hospital, Jolly spent long evening hours preparing for this daunting, daylong ordeal, and in early 1947, he arranged to sit for it. When he reached the examination venue, he found himself unable to go through with the process.[18] This outstandingly gifted surgeon thus never gained his final qualification and was never afterward permitted to practice surgery in Britain. This strange anomaly was an ongoing mystery to colleagues such as Archie Cochrane, who later wrote that he "could not understand why [Jolly] never got his FRCS."[19]

After fifteen years away from his homeland, Jolly looked and sounded archetypically English, and he was to spend the rest of his life in England. Yet his New Zealand origins remained important to him, and when a law change prevented him from holding dual citizenship, he took out a second, New Zealand, passport.[20] He maintained close contact with his family members and in late 1947 made a four-month trip to visit them, especially his mother, Elizabeth, who was by then ailing and almost blind. She died not long after his visit. He found that the Cromwell general store owned and run by three generations of Jollys had passed out of the family's hands during the war, presumably because none of his siblings wished to manage it.[21] The eldest, William, was a high school teacher. Two other brothers were dental surgeons, the fourth was an agricultural scientist, and his lone sister, Ruth, had married a farmer in the fertile province of Blenheim. He visited most of these relatives on this trip and for the first time met nephews and nieces such as seven-year-old Barbara, whose father, Harold, was a dentist in the small North Island town of Otorohanga. Her celebrated uncle "seemed larger than life," she recalled. "I asked him to be my pen pal and we wrote to each other occasionally for years. I collected foreign stamps and he sent some from Morocco."[22]

As a prominent and temporarily returned expatriate, Jolly was interviewed during his visit by the provincial newspaper, the *Otago Daily Times*. He chose to talk about atomic energy, a subject of absorbing worldwide interest and anxiety in the wake of the destruction at Hiroshima and Nagasaki two years earlier. His London hospital, Jolly told the paper, was researching the use of atomic energy as a potentially valuable asset in the fight against cancer. "If nations will refrain from blowing one another to bits and we have a period of peace, there is no doubt that we can learn a great deal from radioactive elements. This is a period of hope for advances in the realm of physiology and, in consequence, pathology."[23]

This observation, borne out by later developments in nuclear medicine, showed that Jolly felt proud of the world-leading research in radiotherapy then carried out at the Royal Cancer Hospital. Nevertheless, after returning to Britain, he clearly felt discontented at his ineligibility to practice surgery, and he attempted to build a new career in writing and editing. A proposed *Biographical Dictionary of Men of Science*, for which he wrote a number of draft entries, was rejected by several publishers including Penguin.[24] He applied for mid-level positions with the World Health Organization, the Nuffield Foundation (which had supported other Spanish Civil War doctors including Josep Trueta), the Medical Research Council, and the *British Medical Journal*.[25] He even offered to serve part time on the Ministry of Pensions medical boards, assessing the fitness of those applying for state support. None of these applications was successful.

One consolation in this dismal period was the steady support of friends from his early years in London. Writing in a hasty, prescription-pad scrawl, he maintained a regular correspondence in particular with Karl Polanyi, who in 1937 had tutored on social and economic history and international affairs for the Workers Educational Association, the extramural adult education program of the University of London and Oxford University. Polanyi then spent three years as a resident scholar at Bennington College in Vermont, where his notes from the association lectures formed the basis for his magisterial 1944 work, *The Great Transformation*, a sweeping survey of the development of the modern state as a product of the market economy.[26] It resulted in an offer three years later to lecture at New York's Columbia University. Jolly sent his congratulations on this appointment by post, adding, "but the knowledge that you will not be living in England is very hard to bear."[27]

Polanyi's wife, Ilona, however, was still living in London at this time. Her political stance was well to the left of her husband's, and the U.S. immigration authorities advised the couple that given her radical persuasion, she would not be permitted to join him in New York. This situation placed enormous stress on the couple's relationship, and as with other crises in their lives, the Polanyis turned to their old friend of Christian Left days for emotional support and advice. "The bare fact of the refusal of the visa must be to you, as it is to Ilona, such a devastating blow," wrote Jolly in September 1947.[28] In a subsequent letter, phrased with the directness that only an intimate friend could risk, he took Karl to task for apparently urging his wife to repudiate her Marxist convictions to gain a U.S. visa. "You must not, for *your* soul's sake and the sake of *your* work ask [Ilona] to do something that she *cannot* do with any hope of becoming the person she could be."[29] That stern injunction was evidently heeded, and Ilona migrated instead, with her political principles intact, to the more socially tolerant nation of Canada. The couple bought a tiny house on the outskirts of Toronto, where Ilona lived, and her husband joined her on weekends after his week's teaching duties at Columbia. A few years later, Karl Polanyi was able to tell Irene Grant that "Ilona is working on a social history of Hungary in our Canadian shack, where we love to be together."[30]

Jolly spelled out his own individual and non-ideological brand of socialism in a long letter to his brother Stanley in New Zealand. He freely acknowledged that since the heady days of the Christian Left, he had become

> disillusioned about Russia. . . . But perhaps my "illusions" were never so bright as those of many people who were Russia-worshippers. Also, never having been under the discipline of the party line, I've always been free to take an un-idealised view of that great and important country. Certainly my basis in Socialism has never depended on the success or failure of the Russian experiment. That Russia is of great importance and that the achievements, along certain Socialist lines there, have been tremendous and exciting, I do not doubt. But whether, under the continuous and increasing pressure of the external and over-riding situation, Russia can come through to that freedom which for me, is the sine qua non of Socialism, I wonder. Whether, on the other hand, Labour Britain, or any other Social Democratic country, in attempting to preserve *all* the freedoms, can be ruthless enough to make the Social equation irreversible is also, I believe, open to doubt. I can never forget Spain in 1936. . . .
>
> I am sufficient of a Marxist and a Socialist to believe that, having transformed the economic basis of society and established at least the institutions of a Socialist society, the Russians must have the basis of a free society—however overlaid it may now be by the super-structure and excrescences of the power-political struggle now raging between Russia and the Western world.[31]

Jolly's emphatic intervention on the question of Ilona Polanyi's U.S. immigration status seemed only to reinforce his friendship with the couple, and in late 1950, he sent a vivid account of his latest overseas travels to their Toronto address. After a further bout of serious illness, and perhaps to distract himself from the unexpected loss of his surgical career, he spent several months touring southern Europe. George Komrower, a physician who had served with Jolly in the Caserta hospital (and would eventually write his friend's obituary for the *British Medical Journal*), was due to attend a pediatric conference in Zurich, and Jolly accompanied him and his wife on a long and rambling journey there via France and Italy. They spent several days in a villa with a "glorious view, by day and by night, over Florence and the valley of the Arno," as guests of a young American poet, William Jay Smith, and his wife, Barbara Howes, a short story writer. The trio then pressed north through the Passo della Mendola, high in the Tyrol near the Italian-Swiss border, where Jolly exulted in seeing "the Austrian-speaking peasants who had come up between the grain and grape harvests to cut the hay on the high alps, the exhilarating walks at 5am in the high beech and pine forests, the wonderful variety and bloom of the wild-flowers that grew everywhere there was room to grow."[32]

On the return journey, he met Irene Grant in France, and they spent a week in "an old walled town set at a height of about five hundred feet above the headwaters of the Marne and the Rhone." The final stage of this long and restorative holiday was a side trip to the town of Armentières, near Lille on the Franco-Belgian border. On the edge of the town lies the Cité Bonjean Military Cemetery, containing the graves of more than two thousand war dead, including Jolly's father. Practicing his intended new profession of writer, Jolly described this experience in a feature article for the *Otago Daily Times*, which had earlier published his reflections on peaceful uses of atomic energy. "The cemetery is extremely beautiful and lovingly cared for by a Scot from Inverness" who "in 1916 was fighting in this sector himself with the 51st Highland Division." Jolly then listed each of the New Zealand officers and troops buried in the cemetery, many of them killed on the same night as his father. He recognized that in the economically constrained postwar period, few of the relatives of these men could travel to the other side of the world to visit their grave sites, and he generously supplied photographs of each of their headstones to the newspaper, whose editor promised to forward them to their next of kin.[33]

With no sign that he might find work outside the field of medicine, yet still prevented from practicing surgery, in 1951 Jolly joined the staff of the limb-fitting center at Queen Mary's Hospital in Roehampton, southwest London. Like the Royal Cancer Hospital, it was an internationally regarded institution specializing in fitting prosthetic limbs for amputees. Standing in twenty-eight acres (eleven hectares) of landscaped grounds dominated by the gracious Queen Anne–period mansion of Roehampton House, it was founded to treat the forty-thousand-plus troops who had lost limbs in the First World War and became Britain's main hospital for this purpose. Its workshops turned out custom-fitted artificial limbs, and its newly limbless patients were trained to use them, given physiotherapy and other forms of rehabilitation, and received vocational training in those trades still open to them.[34] The hospital acquired a unique level of expertise in treating amputation cases and took on a further teaching and research role. In the 1930s, one notable patient was a Royal Air Force pilot, Douglas Bader, who lost both legs when his Spitfire crashed. The metal replacements supplied by Queen Mary's enabled him to return to flying, and he became a celebrated and highly decorated air ace during the Battle of Britain.

In the years after World War II, numbers of civilian patients arrived to replace the war casualties. From 1948 the hospital's limb center took responsibility for about twelve thousand patients with amputations resulting from accident or illness. Many were aged fifty and older, and suffered arteriosclerotic conditions and diabetic gangrene. Others required artificial limbs as a result of industrial or vehicle accidents, poliomyelitis, or congenital deformities. By the 1950s, Queen Mary's had become a general hospital, although it retained a primary responsibility toward disabled ex-servicemen.[35] Jolly would spend the rest of his career in this sprawling, ever-evolving institution, eventually becoming its chief medical officer. He commuted in his Jaguar or by train from a one-bedroom flat beside St. James's Park in central London, although from time to time Donald and Irene Grant would again take in their accomplished but erratic friend as a lodger. Their children had all left home, and two of them chose to study medicine, perhaps influenced by the friend they had first met in childhood in Dunedin.[36]

At Queen Mary's, Jolly held a series of increasingly senior but invariably non-surgical roles and this reserved, mustached, and upright figure was regarded fondly by staff and patients who had little, if any, idea of his former achievements. His duties included checking the stumps of recent amputees, recording their progress ("phantom pain: present but not severe"), and advising on a limb-fitting regimen.[37] Douglas Bader, now Sir Douglas, continued to arrive at the hospital for limb refittings and adjustments, and formed a friendship with his fellow military veteran despite the ex-RAF man's loudly proclaimed arch-conservative views.

Those who worked with Jolly described his years at Queen Mary's as a somewhat unhappy period of his life. His successor as the chief medical officer felt that he was "regarded rather as a 'caretaker', extremely quiet, and shied away from decision-making. He was in no sense innovative."[38] Other colleagues had valued Jolly's cheerful and helpful attitude, but the formerly energetic and gregarious iconoclast was now seen as introverted and vaguely aloof. He was a mild and smiling presence at the garden parties and other social events held in the hospital grounds each summer throughout the 1960s.[39]

In his personal life, Jolly was known for his generosity and loyalty to friends. In 1953 his publisher's son, Gabriel Newfield, appealed to him for help with "the cumbersome procedure for recognition as a C.O. (conscientious objector)." Gabriel had decided to abandon the study of medicine for sociology and was therefore required to carry out compulsory military service, an obligation he felt unable, on principle, to fulfill.[40] Jolly provided an impressive letter of endorsement. "It is my firm belief, from having known Mr Newfield in his formative years, and from a close friendship with his family, that there can be no question at all of the sincerity, nor of the mature feeling and thinking behind his inability to continue his military service. Although I do not agree with his point of view, and do not hold his conviction about military service, I respect him highly for the stand he has taken."[41] This ringing imprimatur from a distinguished and decorated veteran proved decisive, and a military tribunal gave the young Mr. Newfield a light sentence that enabled him to enter the London School of Economics by the following term.[42]

Tess Simpson, an animating spirit of the Society for the Protection of Science and Learning, was a friend of even older standing than the publisher Maurice Newfield. In 1956 Jolly wrote to congratulate her on receiving an OBE. "I think you are the very sort of good and valuable person who should be so honoured."[43] Her decades-long campaign to repatriate and find academic postings for endangered scholars did not abate after the war, as such admirable figures as the doctor František Kriegel, by then a prominent political figure in his native Czechoslovakia, came under threat of a state purge. He had become one of his country's strongest proponents of democratic reform and was forced out of his post as undersecretary of health in an attempt to limit his influence. In August 1968, when Russian tanks rumbled into Prague to crush the budding reforms, Kriegel was the only member of the Czechoslovak leadership who refused to sign the humiliating document drawn up by Moscow to validate the invasion.

The Austrian philosopher Karl Popper, who had been assisted to find a teaching post in the unlikely setting of Christchurch, New Zealand, returned after the war to the London School of Economics. He and Jolly became acquainted and presumably exchanged impressions of the distant South Pacific country they had both chosen to leave.[44] Popper was eventually knighted and became a Companion of Honour and a Fellow of both the Royal Society and the British Academy, yet he was just one of scores of distinguished academic refugees who owed their later careers, and perhaps their lives, to Tess Simpson and her society. Others included seventy-four Fellows of the Royal Society, thirty-four of the British Academy, and sixteen Nobel Prize winners. She told a friend that since 1968, "there have been waves from Czechoslovakia, Greece, Poland, Brazil, some South Africans, the occasional Hungarian, Rumanian, ex-Biafran, Bangladeshi—there is no end." Later refugee scholars came from Argentina, Chile, Uganda, Zimbabwe, and, after the 1989 Tiananmen Square massacre, China. Simpson continued supporting them almost until her death in 1996.[45]

16 Light in the Darkness

> Manic-depressive illness is, by any measure, gravely serious—complex in its origins, diverse in its expression, unpredictable in its course, severe in its recurrences.
>
> —FREDERICK K. GOODWIN AND KAY REDFIELD JAMISON

Jolly's romantic life in this postwar personal limbo was as intriguing as ever. He formed a short-lived but intense relationship with the widow of his old friend Tom Wintringham who, after returning from Spain with a shoulder wound, formed a guerrilla training school to resist an anticipated invasion of Britain. In 1942 Wintringham founded the libertarian socialist Common Wealth Party with, among others, the philosopher John Macmurray of the Christian Left.[1] Tom died suddenly of a heart attack in 1949, leaving children by three women including his second wife, Kitty, an American journalist he had met in Spain. Whether Jolly also met her in that period is unknown, but the two evidently had a brief, volcanic affair in the 1950s that Kitty recalled later with "gratitude for all the times you have lightened my darkness."[2] They may have met through overlapping professional interests, as after her husband's death, Kitty Wintringham worked as a medical social worker. She later formed a climbing and camping supplies company in partnership with Elizabeth Neale, Tom Wintringham's sister.

Jolly had by then embarked on a new and less fraught relationship with the widow of another close friend, Alan Kain, a New Zealand–born civil engineer who had married an Englishwoman named Jessica. In the 1930s, the Kains moved to London, and Jolly met them after his second war. Rather surprisingly for someone reared as far as geographically possible from the coast, Jolly became a weekend sailor in this period. He and Kain jointly owned a yacht, the *Grey Heron*, and spent days at a time sailing around the coast of southern England, often accompanied by Irene Grant. Alan Kain died in 1962, and Jessica, known as "Jay," formed a new attachment with her late husband's shipmate.[3] They would remain devoted to each other for the rest of their lives.

The relationship included the complicating but rewarding factor of an adult stepchild. Jay Kain had a daughter, Joanna, who was recently married and held a PhD in marine biology, an unusual career choice for a woman in that period. She worked at the Port Erin Marine Laboratory attached to the University of Liverpool, and as she carried out dives in the clear, cold waters off the Isle of Man, her mother sat in the dive boat and wrote fond letters to "dear beloved Doug."[4] Jolly had always shown great affection toward his various nephews and nieces in New Zealand, and after Joanna's two children were born in the mid-1960s, he welcomed the duties of grandfatherhood.

Old flames continued to flicker periodically. Anna-Mária Basch wrote from her hometown of Budapest, Hungary, in 1960 and chided her former lover for his failure to maintain contact with her. "During the past years I have often thought about you, and have not understood your great silence . . . you did not put in much effort to find me, even though the world is small, 'like my pocket.'" She felt unable, she wrote, to provide a full account of the previous ten or twelve years:

> All I will tell you I will do in broad strokes, in telegram style, . . . From 1952 till 1955 I worked for a doctor at the College of the Party as a nurse. After that I received my retirement and from then on I did voluntary work for the Party. My pension does not allow me to live without daily worries. . . . We live together with Jean [her son] and his family. André [her grandson, named for her late husband] is already 13 years old, intelligent, very playful, pretty good student, speaks French. . . . The old ones from Spain have remained brave. There is a great solidarity between us. Unfortunately we have lost many.[5]

Always the committed left-wing activist, Anna-Mária Basch received a decoration in 1968 at a ceremony in Warsaw to honor the volunteers of the Thirteenth International Brigade.[6] Some years later she attended a reunion of former inmates of the Ravensbrück concentration camp.[7]

As another ex-lover, Irene Grant must have followed the news of Jolly's relationship with Jay Kain from a distance and with very mixed emotions. She undoubtedly loved him deeply and continued to do so as they both aged and while she remained married to Donald. In the early 1970s, a nephew asked her to approach Jolly for some information about the Spanish Civil War, and she felt obliged to refuse, telling him, "It's very difficult for me now."[8] She had evidently resolved not to threaten the stability of Jolly's relationship by remaining close to him, although at the cost of her own heartbreak.

Now with the support of a devoted partner, Jolly carried on his daily duties at the great limb-fitting hospital whose function and facilities changed repeatedly in response to new social conditions and demands. From the 1960s, many patients were "thalidomide babies," congenitally deformed after their mothers were prescribed the drug during pregnancy.[9] In 1963 Jolly gave a talk to a London medical symposium on the provision of wheelchairs, pointing out that the national demand for them had risen sevenfold in the past decade. "We are living in the age of rehabilitation. Doctors are less and less content to accept that large numbers of their patients are beyond the point where they can be given independence, at least within their own homes. . . . This consciousness of the need for rehabilitation is not confined to the medical world. It is more and more understood and expected by disabled people, by their relatives and by interested associations concerned with the welfare of their members."[10]

He was an active member of the British Orthopaedic Association and encountered fellow Spanish Civil War veteran Josep Trueta at its conferences. In 1964 Jolly told the association's annual meeting that Queen Mary's Hospital and its many outposts in other towns and cities were treating the needs of eighty-five thousand amputees, most of them the result of vascular disease.[11] The social stigma facing these visibly disabled people was a constant concern to him. "Society as a whole," he wrote, "must learn to accept not only amputees but all handicapped and disabled persons on the basis of their inherent dignity, ability and worth as human beings, not on the superficial basis of individual differences in physical condition due to crippling diseases, congenital defects or debilitating injuries. In the past amputees, like members of minority groups, have encountered unreasoning psychological prejudices unworthy of the brotherhood of man."[12]

This farsighted advocacy on behalf of the disabled may have hastened his retirement from Queen Mary's Hospital. As its chief medical officer, Jolly advised Health Minister Sir Kenneth Robinson on "the question of cars for the haemophiliacs." However, he also tendered advice on aids for the disabled to a parliamentary interdepartmental committee without first taking independent advice from specialist consultants. His action on this occasion, he admitted, was "questionable." It appears to have led to his enforced retirement in 1968, at age sixty-four and after seventeen years at Queen Mary's, under circumstances that left him feeling "very sad."[13] His friend Sir George Godber, chief medical officer of the National Health Service, wrote to express his sorrow at losing such a valuable colleague. "How very well aware I am of the service you have given to the limbless in this country. You were one of the very few in the service who came over to the Ministry of Health able to bring a wide surgical knowledge to bear on the problems of limb fitting."[14]

Earlier that year, Jolly and Jessica Kain were married in a simple registry office ceremony in Hampstead. The groom listed his profession as "surgeon," an indication of how strongly he continued to uphold that professional identity despite having been denied the opportunity of practicing it for almost twenty years.[15] That summer the couple bought a comfortable 1930s brick bungalow, the first and only house Jolly ever owned, in the semirural Surrey village of West Horsley, thirty-five kilometers southwest of London.[16] He and Jay spent the rest of their lives in this quiet village, which had stood since Saxon times, appeared in the *Domesday Book* of 1086 AD, and was once home to the celebrated children's author Beatrix Potter, who set several of her books among its thatched cottages.

The marriage prompted the forthright Anna-Mária Basch to write again from Budapest, not only offering Jolly her congratulations and her hope that she might meet his new wife, but also making clear her view that he had allowed others, especially Irene Grant, to divert the course of his life from his own best interests. "In my opinion you were wrong not to get married a long time ago, have a family home and have children. I remember well how you adored children. You know my opinion on your friendship with Irene. You gave her your best years, and this was also a bit of selfishness on her part. I dare to hope that with your marriage, this matter is over."[17] As Jolly's closest colleague and intimate companion in Spain, and as a loyal friend who had persisted in maintaining contact with him intermittently over the following thirty years, Basch knew Jolly better than most. She was undoubtedly aware of the shadowed corner of his life that he had succeeded in concealing from most other acquaintances as his surgical career rose and fell.

Ever since his early years as a boarding school pupil in Dunedin, he had periodically experienced extreme mood swings, oscillating between euphoric high spirits and crippling depression, a condition that also affected other members of his wider family. Typically, the initiating trigger for such a psychiatric state is a stressful event, and in Jolly's case, the death of his father in 1916, coupled with his family medical history, seems the most likely causative factor. Anna-Mária Basch would have realized that this medical condition, then labeled "manic-depressive illness" and later "bipolar disorder," more than any selfish designs on the part of Irene Grant, lay behind Jolly's several short-term engagements and his unusually late marriage, which precluded the prospect of having children of his own.

For much of Jolly's life, the only medical treatments available for his condition were bromides, or crude and ineffective sedatives. Later, electroconvulsive therapy (ECT) was administered in hospitals, although Jolly, presumably well aware that this treatment was poorly understood even by its practitioners, succeeded in avoiding it. By the mid-1950s, an effective drug appeared in the form of lithium, a naturally occurring mineral that was found to be remarkably fast-acting in reducing and preventing the symptoms of manic depression. Although it also produced unpleasant side effects, such as nausea and trembling, the availability of lithium will have greatly relieved Jolly's periodic manic-depressive episodes and may have enabled him to form the only long and stable relationship of his life.

As he aged, however, Jolly's dark secret became ever harder to conceal, and in a letter to his friend Sir George Godber, he revealed that at the time of his retirement from Queen Mary's Hospital, "I was very depressed. Thank heaven, my consultant has quickly snapped me out of this with large doses of Nardil [an antidepressant]. I am very glad to be alive again," he confided feelingly to his friend, "but am suffering from the multiple side effects of these mono-amine inhibitors."[18]

The medical consultant he referred to was Dr. Nina Coltart, one of the preeminent British psychiatrists and psychoanalysts of her time, whose practice included peers of the realm and famous artists and musicians. A tall, elegant woman, she worked from a consulting room beneath her apartment in a terraced house in Hampstead. Her patients took a flight of stairs to "a small, beautifully furnished waiting room . . . always bedecked with flowers and plants."[19]

Dr. Coltart began treating Jolly in February 1967, and aspects of his past are likely to have especially interested this polymathic and unconventional physician. She had studied English and Spanish literature at Oxford before taking her medical degree at the great London teaching hospital of St. Bartholomew's. She chose to specialize in psychiatry and was working at a psychiatric hospital in Essex when she met another woman doctor, Evelyn "Polly" Lind, a New Zealander who was training in psychoanalysis and encouraged Coltart to enter that field herself.[20] The two became lifelong friends, and in later years, Coltart often visited New Zealand, where Dr. Lind had become that country's first qualified psychoanalyst.[21]

In late 1968, Dr. Coltart wrote a report on Jolly's mental condition. "He has a long history of classical manic-depressive illness, dating from late adolescence. There has been no sustained manic phase, but on emergence from depression he has usually had a period of euphoria. Onset of the depressive phase is insidious but emergence is sudden, and the phase itself may last up to a year or more. It is characteristic symptomatically of severe endogenous illness, but is also marked by extreme resistance to pharmaceutical therapeutic agents."[22] At various times, wrote Dr. Coltart, she had prescribed Jolly large doses of various antidepressants without success. "Finally, in two separate bouts of depression, I used Actomol (mebanazine) . . . and was of the opinion that there was some response to this." (This drug, used as an antidepressant in the 1960s, was later withdrawn due to its toxic effects on the liver.) "Dr Jolly has never had ECT and wishes to avoid it if possible. In spite of the severity of his depression at its worst, he has never missed work, and has never expressed suicidal intentions."[23]

By the time she wrote this report, Dr. Coltart had added psychotherapy to the range of treatments she was qualified to dispense. She was also a longtime practitioner of Theravada Buddhism, finding many correspondences between this tradition's practice of meditation for mindfulness and the calm and open state of mind she aimed to induce in her patients.[24] In cases such as Jolly's, however, the benefits of psychotherapy could generally be enjoyed only if accompanied by a combination of mood-stabilizing drugs. A handwritten schedule among his personal papers records the startling number of powerful psychoactive and other drugs he ingested four times daily in this period, including lithium and the painkiller codeine, which was probably for treating his colitis, or inflammation of the large intestine, a condition that may well have resulted from his long-term use of the other pharmaceuticals.[25]

Given the evident severity and intractability of his psychiatric condition, it seems at first sight extraordinary that for much of Jolly's life he succeeded in functioning at a very high level of professional competence and that few of his colleagues were apparently aware of the mental strain this must have cost him. The times when he practiced advanced frontline surgery with a physical endurance surpassing that of any of his colleagues are likely to have coincided with periods of elevated mood swings, and he evidently controlled this exalted state of mind remarkably effectively. The spells of numbing depression in between may have been obliquely referred to in those letters from Spain when he confessed to feeling "a bit nerveux."

The world's most comprehensive and authoritative publication on his condition has found that highly accomplished people show a higher than normal incidence of bipolar disorder and that it "may, in some individuals, enhance productivity, creativity and sociability."[26] This may help to explain how, in 1940, he wrote *Field Surgery in Total War* in a matter of months. Even episodes of his somewhat bizarre behavior, such as performing the Māori haka for the exhausted members of his equipo, can be interpreted as a deliberate channeling of his disrupted mental impulses to positive effect.

At other times, however, the violent and uncontrollable mood swings Jolly experienced generated behaviors that were potentially damaging professionally and harmful to his personal relationships. Manic depression can produce feelings of euphoria, exultation, and "an inordinate production of written declarations."[27] In the times when he wrote frenetically for long periods, such as in 1935 when he produced an entire novel, Jolly evidently considered abandoning medicine for literature and, as noted, was only dissuaded by the kind and careful intervention of Professor Aitken. A bout of depression is also the most likely explanation for his failure, after returning from World War II, to gain the prized surgical qualification he had sought for so long and for which his breadth of practical experience would otherwise have made the examination process largely a formality.

Those who suffer from mood swing disorders typically find their manic periods exhilarating and creative, but afterward, when the exaltation subsides and is replaced by a debilitating depression, they seek to reproduce their former heightened state with alcohol or other drugs. Opportunities for illicit self-medication were freely available to Jolly, but he consistently abstained from them, perhaps as a valuable vestige of his Presbyterian upbringing. As a result, he frequently succumbed to prolonged periods of severe depression, especially after World War II when he no longer experienced the challenges and rewards of surgery. The many oblique references in letters from Irene Grant and others to his periods of bedridden illness from the late 1940s can be read as evidence of his decreasing ability to function normally, let alone exceptionally, once the stimulus of wartime was denied to him. Hence, Dr. Coltart's 1968 report noting that Jolly "never missed work" as a consequence of his severe and intractable mental illness is surprising.

That observation has been clarified by one authority uniquely placed to understand it from both a professional and personal perspective. Professor Kay Jamison is a renowned clinical psychologist at the Johns Hopkins University School of Medicine and co-author of the standard textbook *Manic-Depressive Illness*. She herself has a manic-depressive disorder and revealed this to her medical colleagues while already holding a challenging clinical and teaching position. "When I went public with my own illness, almost all of my colleagues said they had no idea. It's not unusual for people to be tolerant of deviant behavior, and when people are manic they leave the situation so people don't necessarily see them [behaving unusually]. They give you a pass."[28] Jolly's own periods of depression-induced illness and his postwar introversion were typically ascribed at the time to some other cause. His colleagues at Queen Mary's Hospital seem to have been unaware that a clinical reason may have been behind his lack of professional ambition. According to his successor as chief medical officer, "Most people attributed this to his harrowing time spent in the Spanish Civil War, and this may well have been the explanation."[29]

This justification, coupled with Jolly's attractive personality and his well-recognized clinical skills, must suffice to account for his success at concealing his illness from colleagues and friends for much of his career. His intimate friendship with Irene and Donald Grant, who repeatedly took him into their household and provided unquestioning support when he was unable to function alone, must also have helped him to avoid the worst consequences of his condition. In the 1970s, Irene revealed to him that at times in the past when he had behaved abnormally, "I was often overcome with inadequacy and at least once very frightened. I have often wondered whether or not you actually remember things that happened when you were 'over the top' with exultation?"[30]

Jolly's mental condition became not only more pronounced and apparent as he aged but also more manageable through pharmacological intervention. The family he acquired through his marriage and his own relatives were certainly well aware of his illness but continued to hold him in warm and high regard. In the 1960s and '70s, several of his younger relatives made the long journey from New Zealand to London as part of an Antipodean rite of passage known as "the big O. E." (overseas experience) and were welcomed to his house at West Horsley whenever he was well enough to receive visitors. "He was always most gracious and hospitable to his Antipodean family relatives," recalls one of them, Jacqui O'Donnell, "and would always insist we young and adventurous world travellers join him and his wife Jay for a traditional home-away-from-home Sunday dinner in their charming home and garden."[31] After first training as a nurse in New Zealand, his niece Barbara arrived in 1967 to further her experience in operating theaters. She wrote to her uncle Doug beforehand to tell him to expect her, but by the time she arrived, "he happened to be in one of his downward spirals." It was several days before she received an apologetic and effusively welcoming phone call from him. In the five years she spent in London, Barbara often made the trip by rail to Jolly's home outside London, sometimes finding him in the garden enjoying a reunion with some old comrade from Spain who was now an icon of the medical profession. She remembers her uncle as full of joie de vivre, even though "he had quite a number of episodes in hospital with colitis, probably a side-effect of all the drugs he was given."[32]

In 1969 the recently retired Jolly took his new wife on a voyage back to New Zealand, where he made such a profound impact on the latest crop of nephews and nieces that they remembered it clearly fifty years later. Allan Jolly, later a dental surgeon, recalled his uncle teaching him the vital surgical skill of tying knots one-handed and employing this dexterity to make kites for the family.[33] Allan and other family members were fully aware of the bipolar mood condition that often affected their beloved uncle's behavior and, to their great credit, have never attempted to deny or conceal it from others, including this author.

With advancing age, the cumulative side effects of a heavy and long-term regimen of psychoactive drugs began to produce their own health problems, requiring additional specific medication until it became almost impossible to distinguish cause from effect. Yet even in this bleak stage of diminishing physical as well as mental ease, Jolly retained much of his earlier good humor, vigor, and enjoyment of life. Letters from his family and friends portray him as charming and generous, prone to anonymously paying for presents such as concert tickets and even a car for those who could not afford them, and delighting in playing ring-around-the-rosy with small children. Throughout the remorseless decline of his later years, the still resolutely cheerful surgeon (as he invariably identified himself) spent much of his time puttering in the large garden behind his house, which incorporated several greenhouses. He adapted his redundant surgical skills by teaching himself woodcarving in a garden shed equipped with a lathe and in time developed an impressive ability at this quiet hobby.[34]

It may have been in this calm and reflective period of his life that Jolly also wrote another book drawing on his wartime experiences. His handwritten manuscript for "Surgical Curiosities in Two Wars" runs to some two hundred pages and is illustrated with his own photographs. It is a peculiar but frequently compelling medical memoir, combining bizarre anecdotes with the careful detailing of clinical procedures that characterized *Field Surgery in Total War*. Although clearly intended for publication, "Surgical Curiosities" was evidently not as salable in peacetime as that earlier work, and it remained unpublished at Jolly's death. An edited extract appears as an appendix to this book and is apparently its first appearance in print.

His wife, Jay, practiced her own retirement hobby of pottery and became acquainted with a young Australian potter named Julian Davies, who eventually came to stay with the couple. Julian wrote,

> I was in my mid-twenties when I met Doug and read his *Field Surgery in Total War* on summer evenings while staying in a caravan in his garden in Surrey, in 1978. The intelligence and deeply committed service revealed to me in that book impressed and moved me enormously, as did Doug himself. . . . I saw he was troubled by the stark reality of much of what he had experienced in war and life. But, however that had damaged him, he showed an unusually consistent humanity in his values and actions. I can't think of any much greater commendation.[35]

He recalls Jolly as "obviously a troubled person but with a fundamental positivity. I remember him coming down the garden path whistling the *Internationale*. Even when he began to show the first signs of dementia, he still seemed so chipper."[36]

Julian eventually formed a lasting relationship with Bidda Jones, who was eighteen months old when her grandmother Jay married this unconventional New Zealand doctor. Her own mother, Joanna, recalled long afterward that "Jolly was a special step-grandfather for Bidda—an alert and spry old man with a ready story or joke. His warmth of personality was a wonderful part of her childhood. She remembers him with unqualified fondness. . . . The memory of Doug Jolly's sense of the ridiculous, the shared conspiratorial twinkle in his eye, the way he came around a corner with a jaunty whistle, and his humane companionableness, keeps him vividly alive for Bidda and me."[37]

Marriage to a manic depressive is notoriously challenging, and as a young woman, Joanna Kain often had reason to worry about her mother's late-in-life choice of partner. "He was most difficult when he was in full creative flight. Dealing with his euphoria was as difficult as with his depression." Jolly eventually spent hours on end writing, apparently passages of fiction that proved barely readable once his mood stabilized.[38]

Although he remained a staunch socialist into old age, Jolly, unlike many other veterans of Spain, does not seem to have maintained links with organizations such as Britain's International Brigade Association. Civil war veterans, however, occasionally reached out to him to record his experiences. In 1970 the redoubtable former nurse Fredericka "Freddie" Martin, who was researching a history of international medical services in Spain, wrote to ask him for his memories of that time. "I am now very much out of touch with friends of the Spanish Civil War days," he replied, "but would wish to be of any help to you if any recollections of mine would serve." He referred her to *Field Surgery in Total War*, noting that although it was by then out of print, "there must be copies in a good many medical libraries in USA."[39] Some months later, he sent Martin a ten-page letter, apologizing for the delay in doing so since "my wife and I have been taking every opportunity, in this glorious weather, to be on the sea in our yacht *Grey Heron*." The letter included several pages of detailed information, later drawn upon for this book.[40] A warm correspondence between the two continued over the next two years, each letter signed off by Jolly with the Republican slogan, *Salud y victoria* (health and victory). In early 1972, he wrote to "Dear Freddie" from Queen Mary's Hospital, although now as a patient rather than a senior staff member. "I am hors de combat and have been for some time with a serious illness. I have an intractable colitis.

My only comfort is that it is not carcinoma of the colon which was for some time suspected."[41]

In the late 1970s, Bill Alexander, a former commander of the British Battalion in the civil war and later the vice president of the International Brigade Association, advised Jolly by mail that he had begun tape-recording the memories of those who once worked for Spanish medical aid, including Len Crome, Archie Cochrane, Alex Tudor-Hart, "and many more doctors, nurses and drivers."[42] He hoped to do the same with Jolly, but nothing immediately came of this approach. When Alexander renewed the request several years later, he learned that the opportunity had been irrevocably lost. In 1982, after Jolly experienced a prolonged period of serious illness, Jay moved with her husband into a private nursing home.[43] Soon afterward he was registered as legally blind.[44] In a letter of condolence to Joanna Jones, Bill Alexander wrote, "Many of us who benefited from his skill in Spain—and indeed in the Second World War—think of him with warmth and gratitude. We hope he will make a quick and full recovery to good health. . . . If visits from some of his medical associates in Spain—Len Crome, Archie Cochrane and others—would be welcome and appropriate, I am sure that such visits can be arranged."[45]

"Unfortunately," Jay's daughter, Joanna, replied, "it is clear you would get no reminiscences from him now. He has his lucid moments but is unable to express himself, rarely ever finishing a sentence. . . . One cannot be sure what his reaction would be if old friends from the Association were to visit him—on some days he is quite responsive and on others very withdrawn."[46]

Jolly declined further after his wife's sudden death in March 1983. Fredericka Martin wrote to him from Mexico in September that year, expressing optimism that her long-awaited history of the International Brigades' medical services would soon be completed.[47] "I am sorry to have to tell you," Joanna Jones replied, "that he is now quite unable to read or answer letters. . . . Since my mother's death in March he has hardly recognised anyone."[48] A few days later, on 19 December 1983, Jolly died of ulcerative colitis, complicated by senile dementia.[49]

A small death notice appeared in the Communist Party daily the *Morning Star*: "The International Brigades Association regrets the death of Dr. Douglas Jolly, sincere anti-fascist, whose unique skills saved the lives of many fighters in Spain."[50] Medical journals in Britain and New Zealand ran lengthy obituaries noting Jolly's early eminence as a battlefield surgeon and the subsequent, and seemingly unaccountable, decline in his professional status. The most meaningful tributes, however, came from former colleagues such as Jolly's first anesthetist in Spain, Peter de Sarigny:

> Doug was one of my oldest and dearest friends . . . there was a special bond, inevitably, forged by shared experiences in the Spanish Civil War in circumstances of the greatest stress. All the marks of his absolute selflessness were there manifested, amongst other things by his willingness and capacity to do his most exacting and exhausting work, far beyond what seemed to be the limits of endurance and certainly beyond the capacity of his colleagues.
>
> The rest of his life, to my knowledge, was conducted in the same elevated spirit. His generosity of mind and spirit were unquenchable, and I believe him to be one of the few truly "good" men of my experience. Never the less, there was nothing of the prig in him: he had an easy tolerance of human weakness and a gaiety and wit and an infectious capacity for enjoyment which communicated itself to all around him and I consider myself very fortunate to have been numbered amongst his friends.[51]

17 Saving from Submersion

> As a doctor I regard war as a terrible thing; but I believe there are things worth fighting for.
>
> —DOUG JOLLY

For seven decades, the Jolly family's pungent-smelling, dimly lit, and serendipitously stocked general store stood at the literal and figurative heart of the old Cromwell township. After its founding proprietors relinquished ownership during World War II, the centrally located building was bought by a succession of new occupants, reflecting the local economy's gradual transition from resource extraction to pastoral farming, then horticulture, and finally to tourism and other services. During the 1950s, it was a grain and feed store, and by 1969, when Doug Jolly returned to Cromwell for the last time together with his new bride, he found the building in which he had spent much of his childhood was serving as the local doctor's surgery.[1] By the time of his death, it stood vacant, awaiting its most dramatic repurposing to date.

A massive and gracefully curving hydroelectricity dam was constructed thirty-four kilometers (twenty miles) downstream from Cromwell through much of the 1980s, rising eventually to a height of a hundred meters and requiring a million cubic meters of concrete. As the project neared completion, the level of the surging, snow-fed Clutha River crept up behind the dam until it drowned the original coach road, the railway line, the apricot orchards surrounding Cromwell township, the magnificent junction with the Kawarau River, and finally the township itself.[2] Cromwell residents were moved to higher ground nearby; there they could watch their former houses and workplaces become slowly submerged under sixty meters of clear, cold mountain water. A few of the most historic and substantial of the old buildings were dismantled and reassembled two hundred meters uphill on the shore of the large and limpid artificial lake thus formed, and the Jollys' one-time general store was among those fortunate transplants. The family home surrounded by a sunny garden also survived since it was built high above the river junction and is now sited almost on the banks of the new lake.

In the thirty years since that systematic flooding, Cromwell has grown larger and more prosperous than the hardy gold-mining settlement that now rests on the bed of the artificially created Lake Dunstan, since the town lies within a region that has experienced a similarly dramatic recent transformation. Central Otago's remoteness from large population centers and its sharply oscillating subalpine climate once deterred all but the most desperate gold seekers. Now those same characteristics attract skiers, wine drinkers, and other aficionados from many countries. They water ski on the sparkling and sheltered new lake, cycle around it, and sample intensely flavored pinot from the high-priced vineyards cloaking otherwise barren hills. It is a remarkable economic and social metamorphosis from the cold-bath days of Doug Jolly's upbringing a century ago, and few indications of that more spartan era remain.

Relatives who share Jolly's surname still live in and around Cromwell, and his descendants take pride in their family connection with the rather mysterious young doctor who went overseas and achieved a measure of renown there. Yet among the general New Zealand population, Jolly's name is practically unknown, even within medical and military circles. The confident prediction made by his final commanding officer, that his senior staff's achievements in Italy would find "a prominent and permanent place in the archives of war surgery," proved true for many of them but entirely unfounded in Jolly's case. That the man described elsewhere as "one of the most notable war surgeons of the 20th century" is unmentioned in the official war histories of both New Zealand and Britain is surely a matter of some curiosity.[3]

There can be no doubt that Jolly's companions on the Spanish battlefront regarded him as one of the great figures of that war. Archibald Cochrane later described him as "the most important volunteer to come from the British Commonwealth," and their colleague Alexander Tudor-Hart felt that Jolly "was the best surgeon we had."[4] After his return to civilian life, Jolly appears to have watched without evident bitterness as many of his former colleagues from the Spanish Civil War ascended to the uppermost heights of their professions while he toiled in relative obscurity. Cochrane was knighted in 1968 and is today regarded as a father of evidence-based medicine. The Catalan surgeon Josep Trueta became a professor of orthopedic surgery at Oxford and later the director of the Nuffield Orthopaedic Centre. Meanwhile, Jolly remained a well-regarded yet undistinguished practitioner in a quiet backwater of his profession. His sole published work instructed and influenced military surgeons in every Allied theater of war, yet its author was largely forgotten.

The several compounding reasons for this strange lacuna in the historical record include Jolly's own unassuming personality. He was a modest man who made no effort to seek public recognition in his lifetime. It is also possible, although not provable, that his nationality and frankly left-wing views rendered him less employable than his peers within the conservatively run British medical establishment during the professionally formative years that followed his discharge from the RAMC. The common link among these factors, and perhaps more significant than any one of them, is Jolly's intermittent yet increasingly debilitating mental ill health. Poorly understood, ineffectively treated, and often not even correctly diagnosed until the 1960s, his bipolar condition is likely to have repeatedly sabotaged his attempts to build a civilian medical career. During the exhilarating chaos of wartime, his episodes of peculiar behavior could be readily accounted for as understandable, and even at times helpful, reactions to extreme stress. Once those tumultuous days were over, he likely experienced fewer periods of elevated spirits and more of deeply disabling depression, which caused him to withdraw at the last moment from his final FRCS examination, condemned him to lengthy and reputation-damaging spells of housebound inertia, and led him to accept and remain within relatively undemanding nonclinical posts. In recent years, improved treatment protocols and greater social acceptance have enabled some bipolar sufferers to manage their condition with considerable success and to achieve professional standing commensurate with their abilities. Those opportunities were largely denied to Jolly, who contributed to major advances in medical science but lived to experience only very preliminary progress in addressing his own pernicious medical condition. The central theme of this book is that Jolly's wartime reputation deserves to be restored, albeit posthumously, to the historical record.

Some of his closest friends and acquaintances provide instances of such belated professional recognition. By the time the philosopher John Macmurray died, as a Quaker, in 1976, his influence had greatly diminished from his days as a radio don in the 1930s. Even in that period, he was more popular among listeners and readers than with his academic colleagues, who disliked his emphasis on the importance of emotion as well as reason, while mainstream Christian thinkers distrusted his questioning of church hierarchies and doctrinal orthodoxy. He fell further into disfavor in the technocratic 1950s, when British social democracy had little patience with his persistent advocacy of the ethical individual. The key tenet of Macmurray's philosophy—that the self-sufficiency of the individual is an illusion, since to be a person is to be in relation with others—placed him at odds with the individualist thinking of his peers and with the main economic and political currents of his later years.

Only some decades after his death, in a political climate less dominated by neoliberalism, was Macmurray's focus on human relationships and community seen as freshly relevant, including in fields of inquiry barely explored in his own day. According to a recent biography, "Macmurray's ideas are proving to have contemporary relevance in the fields of philosophy, psychology, mental health, education, sociology, politics, theology and feminist theology."[5] His rejection of the traditional distinction between reason and emotion, for example, anticipates recent ideas on emotional intelligence, while his departure from orthodox Christianity leads to a belief system that values the spiritual over the strictly religious in accord with the demographic trend in most Western countries. For both Macmurray and Jolly, an ethical foundation was vital to social and economic life, and that precept, passé for much of their later lifetimes, has outlasted them.

The later career and intellectual influence of Jolly's close friend Karl Polanyi followed a similar trajectory—from the unfashionable to the posthumously acclaimed. His 1944 work *The Great Transformation* drew on his experience of Red Vienna in the late 1920s, a social-democratic middle way between unfettered private enterprise and full state control that he considered "one of the most spectacular triumphs of Western history." Only through such a "great transformation," he believed, could markets provide a stable and satisfying future for all their citizens, while an unrestrained free market would lead, as it had done in Vienna in the late 1930s, to democratic breakdown.

In the later decades of the twentieth century, Polanyi's historically driven economic theory lost ground to the ebullient deregulation of neoliberalism.

His peers also found suspect his lack of formal qualifications in economics and his readiness to transgress traditional disciplinary boundaries with his theories. By the twenty-first century, however, rampant economic inequality and popular disillusionment with the dubious versions of freedom permitted under free market capitalism largely vindicated Polanyi's historical analysis and gave fresh impetus to his ideas. "The great prophet of how market forces taken to an extreme destroy both democracy and a functioning economy was not Karl Marx," declared a recent article, "but Karl Polanyi."[6] In a foreword to a new edition of *The Great Transformation*, Nobel Prize–winning economist Joseph Stiglitz says, "It often seems as if Polanyi is speaking directly to present-day issues. His arguments and his concerns are consonant with the issues raised by the rioters and marchers who took to the streets in Seattle and Prague in 1999 and 2000 to oppose the international financial institutions."[7]

Just as the works of Polanyi and Macmurray have been found to hold enduring value in an age very different from their own, so Jolly's contributions to trauma surgery may eventually restore and extend the reputation he earned during the wars of the mid-twentieth century. There are grounds for confidence in this prospective reassessment. The events of the Spanish Civil War in particular refuse to fade into the historical shadows. More than eighty years after the war ended, its key incidents and figures are repeatedly revived through the rediscovery and reexamination of significant historical records. The work of Gerda Taro, the young photographer who died under Jolly's care in the summer of 1937 in the final days of the battle of Brunete, was dramatically brought to international attention with the discovery in 1995 of three shabby cardboard boxes filled with rolls of 35mm negative film. They had been shot by Taro, Robert Capa, and their friend David Seymour (known in Spain as Chim), and spirited to Mexico after the civil war for safekeeping. In 2007 the boxes and their irreplaceable contents were gifted to New York's International Center for Photography, which Cornell Capa founded after the death of his brother Robert. After developing the more than 120 rolls of negative film, 32 were identified as unequivocally shot by Taro, and they have prompted a comprehensive rethinking of her professional reputation—from Capa's acolyte to a photographer-documentarian of genius in her own right. Since that extraordinary discovery, Taro and Capa have each had streets renamed after them in Madrid. The Calle de Gerda Taro, however, is by far the smaller of the two. A tiny byway just eighty meters long in a residential area on the northwestern outskirts of the city, it perpetuates Taro's unjustly subordinate status as a photographer.

As Spanish society persists with the prolonged and uncomfortable reexamination of its recent history, a growing number of sites of importance to the civil war have been restored as public monuments. One of the most physically striking is the massive Cova de Santa Llúcia in rural Catalonia, Jolly's former field hospital during late 1938. After the local council bought and restored the cave for public access, information panels have been erected to explain its historical significance, and several times a year Spanish and foreign visitors attend commemorative events there and at the nearby municipal cemetery.

The process of uncovering the concealed or forgotten past of the civil war is ongoing and frequently traumatic. The Catalan government's General Directorate of Democratic Memory researches the fate of those who disappeared during the Spanish Civil War and the long Franco dictatorship that followed it by investigating the mass graves and conducting genetic identification of the remains. During early 2021, an archaeological team excavated a site in a mountainous region 150 kilometers southwest of Barcelona. An abandoned and derelict farmhouse lies near the site, although the hermitage of Santa Magdalena that once stood alongside it no longer exists. The general directorate's research team believed that both buildings were used as a Republican Army field hospital during the battle of the Ebro, a belief based partly on Jolly's description in *Field Surgery in Total War*. The archaeologists discovered more than sixty graves in the vicinity with the remains of 177 bodies and an additional nine amputated limbs, most likely of Republican fighters and patients of the hospital who did not survive. Medical instruments and other remnants of surgical operations were also found. After the graves were exhumed, the general directorate's archaeologists and anthropologists studied their remains. Genetic testing compared the human remains with DNA samples supplied by potential relatives in the hope of identifying at least some of the bodies.[8] In May 2022, the general directorate handed the remains of Josep Aubeso Rovira to his daughter and grandson for reburial in a civic cemetery in Barcelona. Aubeso Rovira's grandson said this ceremony made possible "a farewell that has had to be postponed for 84 years."[9]

On the opposite side of the globe, the first modest efforts to honor Doug Jolly's achievements began around 2010, after the publication of a book on New Zealanders in the Spanish Civil War.[10] This prompted Patrick Medlicott, a retired orthopedic surgeon then living near Cromwell, to begin advocating for a memorial to Jolly in the town. Another New Zealand doctor, intensive care specialist David Lowe, was independently inspired to learn more about this intriguing colleague and compatriot whom he had never met. While holding a senior position at a Sydney public hospital, Dr. Lowe conducted research worldwide, including trips to the UK National Archives and to New York University's Tamiment Library, which holds many records by American volunteers in the Spanish Civil War. In the course of long evenings combing the internet, Lowe also discovered an extraordinary cache of Jolly's personal papers in the possession of his step-granddaughter, Bidda Jones, in Australia, and they have formed the core of this book.

Gradually yet ineluctably, like the waters of the Clutha slowly banking up behind the Clyde hydro dam, public pressure grew for a Douglas Jolly commemorative memorial in his hometown. It took the form of a plaque to be placed on the stone wall of the store built by his grandfather 150 years earlier that is now relocated, minus its original deep veranda, to Cromwell's "historic precinct," a spectacularly scenic location just above lake level. The building now houses a tourist café.

On a crystalline autumn morning in March 2018, when the subalpine peaks on the far side of the lake glistened with an early season snowfall, a quietly poignant ceremony took place in front of the store to mark the plaque's unveiling. Local mayor Tim Cadogan attended along with Spain's ambassador to New Zealand and half a dozen of Jolly's relatives who had assembled from around the country. His niece Barbara recalled the warm-hearted, hospitable, and unassuming man she had often visited in London, and she credited her uncle's example for her decision to become an operating theater nurse, a profession she followed for fifty-three years. Other speakers noted unsettling similarities between geopolitical conditions in the present day and those that had led to Spain's civil war, and they commended Jolly's example of dedicated yet even-handed and noncombatant engagement in the conflict. His memorial plaque describes Jolly as "one of the greatest war surgeons of the 20th century," an assessment endorsed by medical historians such as the American surgeon David Adams. His journal article on this "forgotten pioneer of trauma surgery," published in the decade after its subject's death, marked a key stage in resurrecting Jolly's professional reputation and historical status.

With the placing of this plaque, the first public acknowledgment in his own country of his achievements, Jolly has in some sense returned permanently to the home that he left in the 1930s. Work continues to ensure that his contributions to military medicine and civilian trauma care are appropriately recorded and recognized, and Bidda Jones has donated his extensive personal papers to the Hocken Library at Otago University, where he began his medical studies.

Most unusually for a biographer, it has proved difficult in the course of researching this book to find a single hostile or even critical opinion of its subject. Doug Jolly's personal character, as well as his professional attainments, seem to have prompted only affection, gratitude, and admiration from patients, colleagues, family, ex-lovers, and friends alike. The former nurse Penny (née Phelps) Fyvel, although in her late eighties by the turn of the millennium, still remembered Jolly quite clearly and "obviously worshipped him," according to Irene Grant's nephew Desmond Painter, who met both these civil war veterans.[11] Throughout the lethally partisan ideological campaigns within Spain's Republican Army, Jolly retained the trust and goodwill of all parties.

Even those who encountered him while his behavior was governed by either pole of his psychiatric condition appear far more inclined toward sympathy and consideration than alarm. The devastating loss of his father in battle may have triggered the lifelong mental illness to which his family was prone, but his mother's subsequent insistence on higher education aided him to adjust to this insidious disability and even to triumph over it. In a period when his mental illness was poorly understood and treated, Jolly appears to have addressed it with courage and creativity. His moral compass and leftward convictions then led him to engage directly and with exemplary commitment in the most urgent and decisive political issues of his time.

ACKNOWLEDGMENTS

Doug Jolly spent most of his working life in Europe, including two intensely formative years in Spain, a country lying precisely on the opposite side of the world from his and the author's birthplace. Nevertheless, a global pandemic required this book to be written, in its entirety, without leaving Aotearoa, New Zealand. That dislocation included the daunting task of remotely accessing archives in Europe, the United States, Russia, and elsewhere at a time when even their own staffs were prevented from using their workplaces. In this perverse situation, I have been greatly privileged to work with a worldwide network of specialist researchers who gave their services willingly, unstintingly, and without regard to remuneration.

In particular, I am indebted to my co-researcher, Dr. David Lowe, who is a practicing intensive care specialist in the Sydney public health system, in a department placed under exceptional strain during the Covid pandemic. Nevertheless, David remained a tireless and skilled historical researcher and faithful friend, and in many ways a living embodiment of Doug Jolly himself.

I have no medical knowledge and have therefore relied very heavily on the advice and guidance of expert advisers, especially David Lowe but also retired orthopedic surgeon Patrick Medlicott, psychiatrist Sarah Romans, and psychologist Kay Jamison.

The polyglot character of the International Brigades is reflected in their archival records, which required translation from at least a dozen European languages. I am therefore very grateful for the expert services of Éva Cserháti, Denise Grobben, John Jamieson, Alicia Garcia Lopéz, Mary Mowbray, Reuben Kura Sanderson, and Peter Verbrugh. The multilingual professional translator Éva Cserháti also read and corrected the entire manuscript more than once—a contribution beyond price.

Thanks go to historian Jim McAloon for sharing his insights on the ideology of the Christian Left and on John Macmurray's lasting significance, and to economists Dennis Rose and Geoff Bertram for advice in tracing and understanding Karl Polanyi's influence in the present day.

I have received photographs and other images, often rare and previously unpublished, from many countries. I am especially grateful for those supplied by Éva Cserháti and Gabor Basch. Dr. Luis Enrique Sanmiguel Castillo generously traveled to and sent images of both the Calle Gerda Taro and Calle Robert Capa in Madrid.

Thanks also to David B. Adams, Serge Alternês, Peter Barton, Gabor Basch, Richard Baxell, Tim Cadogan, Peter Carroll, John Carvell, Alfonso del Barrio, the Diamond Deli café in Lyall Bay, Ron Easthope (Wellington Medical History Association), Gavin Edwards, Ian Fletcher, Tony Fox, Adam Hochschild, Ray Hoff, Hans Houterman, Anthony Hubbard, Meirian Jump, Knox College in Dunedin, Julian Kuzma, Robert Llópis i Sendra, Duncan Longstaff, Sylvia Martin, Marshall Mateer (Imperial War Museum), Sophie McKinnon, Anne McMurray (Cromwell Museum), Dr. Clair Mills, Doug Munro, David Nordström (Svenska Spanienfrivilligas Vänner), Otago Medical School Museum, Jennifer Phillips-Bacher (Wellcome Library), Desmond Painter, Linda Palfreeman, Amy Proctor (London Metropolitan Archives), Annabel Shackleton, Graye Shattky, Brendan Shirley (National Army Museum, NZ), Marlene Sidaway, Marta Simó, Ricard Simo, Gillian Skilton (Otago Boys' High School), Phyll Smith, Alan Warren, and Kip Wilson. Long as it is, this list is undoubtedly incomplete, and I extend my apologies and gratitude to those I've failed to name.

Thanks to Diane Lowther for generous support with indexing, to Vicki Chamlee for her relentless copyedit, and to Bridget Barry and her colleagues at the University of Nebraska Press.

My greatest debt of gratitude goes to the support and goodwill of Doug Jolly's relatives, especially Jessica Kain, Joanna Jones and Julian Davies, Ro (née Jolly) Lange, Barbara Jolly, and Jacqui O'Donnell. Special thanks also to Núala Grant, daughter-in-law of the late Reverend Donald and Irene Grant, for her generosity, trust, and friendship.

I am grateful to the NZ History Research Trust Fund (Ministry for Culture and Heritage) for a grant toward the research costs for this project.

Finally, and as ever, deepest thanks to my family.

APPENDIX

"Surgical Curiosities in Two Wars"

This is an extract from a longer unpublished manuscript by Jolly, apparently from the mid-1950s, now held in the Núala Grant papers, Hocken Collections Uare Taoka o Hākena, University of Otago Library, Dunedin. Explanations for medical terms in this extract, kindly supplied by Dr. David Lowe, are given in square brackets.

FUENCARRAL—SIEGE OF MADRID, 1937

There are exceptions to the admirable rule that wounds involving joints should hold a priority in surgical treatment next below that of wounds with gross destruction and haemorrhage.

To a school-house in the Madrid suburb of Fuencarral during the fierce battles of the university city in January 1937 was brought, among an ambulance load of seriously wounded men, a Frenchman of the International Brigade. This was in the days when soldiers going into battle in the Ciudad Universitaria could go by tramcar to within a few hundred yards of the front line trenches.

He was a man of middle age, an "ancien combatant" of the 1914–18 war, who had been living in Barcelona prior to the outbreak of the civil war. When the Brigadas Internacionales were formed in November 1936, he made his way to Albacete, the depot of the Brigades, and was embodied as a machine-gun instructor in the 14th Brigade together with some three thousand other Frenchmen.

When Jean Pierre Marchaud was received in the "triage," or classification and preliminary treatment room, of the Field Surgical Unit [F.S.U.] in the school house at Fuencarral, his field card bore the diagnosis: "Heridas por bala de fusil a través del muslo izquierdo y el geniculo derecho" (Through and through bullet wounds of the left thigh and right knee joints). As there were no more serious wounds to be dealt with at that moment the triage medical officer put Jean's name at the head of the priority list and rightly did not inspect the wounds, leaving this to be done in the operating theatre. Jean was carried in and placed on the screened, second table of the "Sala de operaciones" where the surgeon was just closing the abdominal incision of a laparotomy case [stitching up an operation on a belly wound].

Leaving his assistants to complete the dressing of the abdominal case, the surgeon moved behind the screen to inspect Jean's wounds before ordering the anaesthetic to be given. A few minutes later those in the theatre were astounded to hear him say, "No need to operate on the clean entry and exit wounds in this man's thigh. I won't operate on the right knee joint. It's a job for Oliver—will an orderly fetch him please?" Oliver was the chief motor mechanic of the unit, and in civil life a metal worker in Paris. When he came into the theatre, the surgeon passed to him across the screen an aluminium artificial leg with bullet holes neatly punched through the knee joint. The unit M.O.'s [medical officer's] joke had worked.

PRIVATE ARMY—SPAIN, 1937

Any surgeon who has been operating for a long time on patients with wounds of "first priority," sooner or later asks himself, "who among all my patients, was the most-wounded and yet survived both wounds and surgery to fight again?" It is not easy to answer such a question, but in the experience of each surgeon will stand out a few men who are candidates for this "honour."

In the Spanish Republican attack from Híjar towards Saragossa in the autumn of 1937, the towns of Quinto and Belchite were quickly taken and occupied by the advancing Republican troops. (It was in the final clearing of a nest of Italian snipers from the Quinto church tower that the late Tom Wintringham, then a Staff Major of the 45th Division, received his second and most severe wound of the campaign. While trying to direct the fire of a tank to bear on the church tower he was shot through the shoulder by a sniper in the belfry. Here too died, by a bullet from the same rifle, the famous commandante médico Dubois, senior medical officer of the 14th Brigade.)

As soon as the town had been cleared, even before it was out of artillery range of the enemy retreating up the Zaragoza road, a Field Surgical Unit was moved into Quinto to take up its quarters and operate in the basement of a shell-ruined flour-mill. It was not the enemy gun-fire, but the presence of seven very dead mules in an adjacent stable that made the site at first almost untenable. When the mules had been dragged away by a Pioneer detachment, life was much sweeter.

On the fifth day of occupation of the mill a breathing bundle of shred and tatters was brought to the resuscitation room, or "hot box," of the unit. This turned out to be Major Miguel Moreno. He, like the famous "Popski" of Eighth Army and Italian fame, had built up his own small, private army to work at harassing the enemy's lines of communication, working with the Partisanos in occupied territory and doing as much damage especially to the Germans and Italians as the fertile brain of Miguel could imagine. His small band of heroes were drawn both from the Spanish Republican army and the International Brigades—handpicked men with previous knowledge of the use of explosives; miners from Oviedo, German antifascists with experience of sabotage against Hitler, Jews whose brothers were proving their nuisance value even then against the Arabs and the British Army in the "troubles" in Palestine.

Like Lawrence of Arabia before him and Popski after him, the main targets of Miguel's depredations were railway bridges and viaducts, aerodromes and large concentrations of enemy transport vehicles wherever they could be found. In preparation for the attack on Zaragoza, Miguel, with a small party of four or five men, had penetrated the enemy lines in the Lérida sector. They were disguised as Spanish peasants leading three small donkeys in whose panniers, hidden below pea sticks and maze cobs, were slabs of gun cotton and "plastic" explosives.

Having successfully broken their way well behind the enemy lines one dark moonless night, they worked their way at leisure to the eastwards to the Barcelona–Zaragoza railway. Here Miguel left two men and one donkey-load of explosives while he and the other three men worked their way round to the west of the Zaragoza to cut the main Zaragoza–Madrid line. The plan was to blow up viaducts to the east and the west of the city simultaneously, early in the morning of D-day of the Republican offensive, and so cut the main railway communication at that vital moment.

But one night before they could carry out their plan Miguel and his party were surprised by a railway guard while they were investigating the pylons of a viaduct. By extremely bad luck the sentry's first shot hit one of the panniers of explosives on the leading donkey. The donkey and the young Spanish miner leading it disappeared in the volcano-like explosion. Miguel, who was walking behind the first donkey and ahead of the second was mown down by the explosion, while the remaining two men received only minor splinter wounds of face and hands—the second donkey was quite unscathed.

When the two unhurt members of the party found Miguel in the dark, it did not seem possible that he could still be alive. There was no part of his body that did not seem to be riddled through and through with missiles. But he still breathed. Lying in the dark until the sentry had gone further up the line for help, they picked up Miguel, tied him across the donkey and made off into the mountains.

Four days later, having again penetrated the enemy lines in the dark, they made contact with the forward elements of the 45th Division and Miguel was brought by ambulance to the F.S.U. in the flour mill at Quinto.

He was barely recognisable as anything human except in vague outline. His body was everywhere covered by suppurating wounds in which were buried pieces of wire, pea sticks, maize, donkey harness and boxwood from the explosive containers. He had a compound fracture [broken bone that had pierced the skin, therefore increasing potential for infection] of the left ulna [one of two bones of the forearm] and another compound fracture of the middle of the shaft of the left femur [thigh bone]. In addition to all these wounds about one third of his body was burned (first and second degree) by the flash of the explosion.

After receiving a blood transfusion, anti-gas gangrene and anti-tetanus serum in large quantities, he was taken to the operating theatre, the worst of his wounds cleaned up and the left arm and leg set and immobilised in plaster. Three days later his condition was improving after further blood transfusion, when the O.C. [Officer Commanding] Unit received an order from General Pozas, general officer commanding the armies of Alto Aragón [probably Sebastián Pozas Perea] to evacuate all wounded from Quinto—immediately. (Our attack on Zaragoza had failed and our troops were about to withdraw to their original jumping-off line between Híjar and Quinto.) Miguel had to be evacuated with the rest of the wounded to the railhead and sector evacuation hospital at Híjar. So he passed out of the control and the knowledge of the F.S.U.

In October 1938, after the attack across the Ebro, the same F.S.U. was working in the Hospital of La Sabinosa, near Tortosa on the Mediterranean coast of Spain, when a rather good-looking, upstanding but rather pockmarked comandante came enquiring at La Sabinosa for the surgeon commanding the Quinto F.S.U.

It was Major Miguel Moreno. He was quite fit except for his pockmarks and an ulnar palsy of the left hand [paralysis resulting in weakened ability to press thumb to ring finger]. He was apparently still very much in command of his private army.

CIVIL SURGERY IN WAR—MARÇA, CATALONIA, JUNE '38

Pneumaturia [air in the urine] must be one of the strangest symptoms in surgery—an intermittent bubbling, whistling stream like a leaking soda-water syphon.

In the days of tranquillity after the Spanish Republican Army had been forced back across the Ebro river in May until the counter-offensive back across the river into Baja Aragón in August, there was only intermittent shelling and small-scale raiding on the Ebro front. The small farming village of Marça was ringed with battalions being re-equipped and training for the coming offensive; but the life of the village went on its busy but drowsy way in the early harvesting days of sweltering June.

At the end of a long day on the threshing floor, driving a mule team over the parching grain, Esteban Gómez, one of the old men of Marça, went behind the ox wagon to pass water. His stream was muddy and came in spurts [indicating infection, dehydration, and obstruction.] This effervescence went on all the week; his own village doctor sent him to see the English surgeon commanding the small holding hospital in the large farmhouse on the hillside above Marça.

Old Esteban didn't much like the passage of the cystoscope [instrument passed up the penis to allow visual inspection of inside of the bladder], and the surgeon was puzzled to see in the posterior wall of the bladder a black circular outline like the neck of a diverticulum [outpouching], from which protruded a shining, white, ragged cylinder about half a centimetre in diameter. In the lateral view of an X-ray plate taken with a small portable machine, an opaque shadow was disclosed in the pelvis at the level of the third piece of the sacrum—it appeared to be about three inches long and impinged on the dark gas-shadow of the ampulla [cavity at lower end] of the rectum. A sigmoidoscope [instrument inserted via anus and rectum for viewing sigmoid, or S-shaped part of large intestine] was passed. In the anterior [front] wall of the rectal ampulla, the upper end of a rabbit's femur was found to be embedded in the rectal wall, and urine could, with light pressure, be made to issue from the fistulous opening around the femoral foreign body [meaning the patient had swallowed a rabbit's femur or thigh bone, which pierced the rectum, making an abnormal connection with adjacent bladder].

A few days later, after renal efficiency tests [blood tests for kidney function], the abdomen was opened by a lower mid-line incision. Coils of small-gut were stuck to the fistulous track between the peritoneal [external] surface of the rectum and the posterior-superior [upper-rear] aspect of the bladder. When these had been separated the shaft of the rabbit's femur could be seen bridging the gap between the two organs. The fistulous openings in the rectum and bladder were excised and the foreign body removed. Both organs were now repaired with layered sutures, and an in-dwelling catheter passed per urethram and a rectal tube per anum [a tube was passed via penis to bladder and another via anus to rectum]. It was decided that, as only the peritoneal surface of the rectum was involved, a temporary sigmoid colostomy, to short-circuit the affected segment of gut, was unnecessary. [The purpose of an external colostomy is to divert feces to allow a lower portion of the bowel to heal without the presence of fecal bacteria.] This proved to be so. Both tubes were removed at the end of seven days, and an olive oil enema given. Convalescence was uneventful, but the E. coli cystitis [bladder infection] persisted for several weeks.

But before the end of the harvesting season, Esteban Gómez was able to return to his mule-team on the threshing floor.

PENICILLIN—TRIPOLI, 1943

If Sir Howard Florey and Sir Hugh Cairns had not come to Tripoli in the summer of 1943 with the first grammes of penicillin to be used on the recently wounded, a young Canadian named Butters (wounded in Sicily and transferred by hospital ship to Italy two days later) would have needed a colostomy and a very long and painful convalescence.

The officer in charge of a surgical division in Tripoli, having been given sufficient of the precious, golden powder to effect the local treatment of six cases of delayed primary closure of wounds, decided that the six he chose in this first experimental stage would be of such a nature as to exclude, beyond all reasonable doubt, any possibility of delayed primary closure without the aid of this new wonder-drug.

Butters had been lying on his face behind low cover at the time of his wounding. A traversing enemy machine gun had found a target in his right buttock. He was operated on by an F.S.U. in Italy and the wound in his buttock was treated as though it had been tangential. The buttock was laid widely open and left open, but the depths of the wound through the ischio-rectal fat [fat between ischium bone—i.e., "sit bone"—and rectum] were apparently not exposed.

When he arrived in Tripoli two days later, the wound was pouring pus (E. coli, Streptococcus Haemolyticus and Staphylococcus Aureus [common infection-causing bacteria found on skin] were cultured from the wound) and there was oedema [tissue swelling] and inflammatory swelling of the tissues of the buttock. Here was a wound, even presuming that it was only a deep, furrowed, tangential wound of the buttock which no-one with the aid of penicillin would dream of closing by delayed primary suture.

But examination under anaesthetic on the operation table showed the condition of affairs to be far, far worse. On separating the ischio-rectal fat forming the walls of the apparently tangential track, a deep prolongation of the wound was revealed. In this track the left, lateral [outside] aspect of the ampulla of the rectum presented with a tear one cm [centimeter] square though all its coats. The track continued antero-laterally [from front to outer side] to the right from the left, passing between the perforated rectum and the bladder, and with the tip of the examining finger thrust into the wound, a partial fracture of the right inferior pubic ramus [lower interior pubic bone] could be felt. This then was not a tangential wound but a penetrating wound without wound of exit. There must therefore be a retained foreign body. None could be palpated with the examining finger extended to the depths of the wound. (See plate 2.)

A quick decision had to be made whether to treat this man by accepted methods—colostomy, wide opening of the wound, suture of the rectum and open packing of the wound—or whether to test the powers of penicillin by suturing the rectum without colostomy and closing the wound of the buttock with penicillin—installation, capillary rubber tubes introduced into the farthest depths of the wound. This latter method was chosen—perhaps a foolhardy choice when the powers of penicillin were still under test. All accessible dead tissue in the wound track was excised; a two-layer closure of the rent in the rectum was made with catgut, working from the wound track; the wound was closed after the introduction of four penicillin tubes by stab punctures with a trochar and cannula [trochar—i.e., sharp-ended tube containing a cannula, or softer tube, left in wound after trochar is withdrawn] left one inch from the ultimate suture line.

For the next few days penicillin solution was instilled twice daily into these four tubes, having first drawn off through them the serous [watery] fluid lying in the depths of the wound. The patient's bowels were kept confined [intentionally constipated] for four days (non-residue [low roughage to promote constipation] diet and morphine), and on the fifth day he was given an olive oil enema through the flatus tube, introduced into the rectum to beyond the site of perforation at the time of operation and left in situ. His bowels were then further confined until the tenth day. On that day the condition was as shown in plate 3.

The buttock wound had healed except for the extremities. There was no discharge from the wound. The bowels were open normally and from then on enemata [plural of enema] were given as required. Butters' general condition was excellent and his temperature and pulse normal.

On the sixth day, X-rays (A.P. [anterior-posterior—i.e., front and back] and lateral) had been done to discover any retained F.B. [foreign body]. He was found to have four machine-gun bullets in the upper part of the right thigh in the region of the obturator externus and the adductors [muscle groups making up thigh]. (The positions of three of these are shown by the X-ray screening crosses in Plate 3.)

There were no complications in his convalescence and, before being evacuated to Egypt of hospital ship, twenty days after operation, he was already ambulant and the wounds were quite healed and dry. Sigmoidoscopy on the fifteenth day showed the wound in the rectal ampulla soundly healed. He still retained the four bullets in his right upper thigh, but they were causing no symptoms. There was therefore no primary indication for their removal.

Culture of the serous exudate withdrawn through the penicillin tubes before each instillation always continued to show a pure culture of Coliform bacilli, but Staphylococcus Aureus and Streptococci disappeared after the first twenty-four hours of treatment. The discharge, although at times copious, never had the appearance or the smell of "E. Coli pus." It was thought at the time (on the evidence of this one case!) that E. Coli in such a wound, when not growing in symbiosis with pyogenic cocci [pus-forming bacteria], were probably non-pathogenic. Events proved that those in Butters' wound were innocuous.

NOTES

1. THE CENTER OF GRAVITY

1. Vaill, *Hotel Florida*, 36.
2. Capa, *Death in the Making*, unpaged.
3. Quoted in Vaill, *Hotel Florida*, 231.
4. Rogoyska, *Gerda Taro*, 199.
5. Allan, *Ted Allan*, chap. 3.
6. Antón, "¡Te has cargado a la francesa!," *El País*, 12 July 2009.
7. Quoted in Spiegel, *Gegen den Faschismus kämpfen*, 15.
8. Zuehlke, *Gallant Cause*, 150–52.
9. Quoted in Ziff, *Mexican Suitcase*.
10. Sir Gordon Gordon-Taylor, foreword to Jolly, *Field Surgery in Total War*, v.
11. Coni, "Medicine and the Spanish Civil War," 147.
12. To name only English-language texts, see, for example, Browne, *Medicine and Conflict*; Coni, *Medicine and Warfare*; and Palfreeman, *¡Salud!*
13. N. Bethune to B. Spence, 11 January 1937, quoted in Hannant, *Politics of Passion*, 147.

2. THE STOREKEEPER'S SON

1. George Rennie quoted in Dougherty, *Dunedin*, 10.
2. Dougherty, *Dunedin*, 120.
3. Clarke, *Living Tradition*, 120, 178.
4. Clarke, *Living Tradition*, 163.
5. Clarke, *Living Tradition*, 122.
6. Pyke, *Early Gold Discoveries*, 15.
7. "Obituary—Mr. D. A. Jolly," *Otago Witness*, 30 August 1916, 44.
8. "Pioneer" [David Jolly], "Early Goldfield History," *Cromwell Argus*, 20 July 1908, 5.
9. Parcell, *Heart of the Desert*, 56.
10. "Obituary," *Cromwell Argus*, 4 September 1916, 5.
11. Walter Keay, "Cromwell Fifty Years Ago," *Otago Daily Times*, 14 July 1930, 13.
12. Betts, *Celebrating a Century*, 8–10.
13. Don, *Memories of the Golden Road*, 330.

14. See, for example, advertisement, "David A. Jolly and Co.," *Cromwell Argus*, 26 March 1872, 1.
15. Laytham and Laytham, *Cromwell Gorge*, unpaged.
16. Cromwell Schools Jubilee Committee, *Celebrating 125 Years*, 9–10.
17. Cromwell Schools Jubilee Committee, *Celebrating 125 Years*, 16–17.
18. William David Jolly, Army Personnel File, Archives NZ, Wellington (hereafter Archives NZ).
19. First Otago Infantry Battalion War Diary, Archives NZ.
20. See the report of Otago Settlers Association, "Otago's First Catastrophe," particularly "The Raid: 13 July 1916."
21. First Otago Infantry Battalion War Diary, Archives NZ.
22. *London Gazette*, 4 January 1917, record no. 398, 261.
23. First Otago Infantry Battalion War Diary, Archives NZ; and Aitken, *Gallipoli to the Somme*, 101–2.
24. D. Jolly, unpublished memoir, Bidda Jones Collection, Hocken Library Uare Taoka o Hākena, Otago University, Dunedin, NZ (hereafter BJC).
25. Barbara Jolly, in-person communication with author, 11 June 2018.
26. D. Jolly, unpublished memoir, BJC.
27. Betts, *Celebrating a Century*, 11.
28. Sweetman, *Above the City*, 173.
29. See the report of Otago Settlers Association, "Otago's First Catastrophe," particularly "The Raid: 13 July 1916."
30. Arnold et al., *Centennial Publication*, 21, 25.
31. Arnold et al., *Centennial Publication*, 116, 133.
32. Sweetman, *Above the City*, 204.
33. Arnold et al., *Centennial Publication*, 82–83.
34. Arnold et al., *Centennial Publication* 73, 86; and *Otago Boys' High School Magazine* 40, no. 1 (April 1924): 24.
35. Austin, *Official History*.
36. Susan Madden-Grey, email to author, 7 August 2019.
37. Mrs. Fulton to D. W. Jolly, 17 April 1924, BJC.
38. Reverend Cumming to acting master, Knox College, 27 November 1923, BJC; and McEldowney, *Presbyterians in Aotearoa*, 89–90.
39. Arnold et al., *Centennial Publication*, 157.

3. ATTRIBUTES

1. Clarke, *Living Tradition*, 67.
2. Hercus, "Eightieth Anniversary," 48.
3. Page, *Anatomy of a Medical School*, 104.
4. Parry, *Otago Medical School*, 36.

5. Dr. Pat Medlicott, email to author, 10 July 2020.
6. Page, *Anatomy of a Medical School*, 71.
7. Chisholm, "Otago Medical School," 208.
8. Robinson, "Otago Medical School," 380.
9. Chisholm, "Otago Medical School," 89.
10. Chisholm, "Otago Medical School," 88.
11. Hercus, "Eightieth Anniversary," 67.
12. Page, *Anatomy of a Medical School*, 71.
13. Bell, *Surgeon's Saga*, 114, 116.
14. Chisholm, "Otago Medical School," 92.
15. Page, *Anatomy of a Medical School*, 72.
16. Jones, *Annals*, 840.
17. Dow, "Hercus, Charles Ernest."
18. Brunton, *Medicine of the Future*, 71, 74.
19. Le Couteur, "Dentist, Doctor, Dean," 61.
20. Page, *Anatomy of a Medical School*, 71.
21. Page, *Anatomy of a Medical School*, 72–73.
22. Hercus, "The OUMC," 15–17.
23. Berry, *New Zealand Student Christian Movement*, 61.
24. "Rebuilding Europe," *Otago Daily Times*, 23 March 1926, 6.
25. Costello, *John Macmurray*, 93.
26. *Open Windows* (magazine of the NZ Student Christian Movement) 2, no. 15 (July 1928): 2.
27. Sutton, "NZ Student Christian Movement," 19.
28. NZ Student Christian Movement Papers, Student Christian Movement Aotearoa (New Zealand): Records, 1896–2014 (Collection), MS-Papers 1171-005, General Correspondence—folder C, 2, 3, Alexander Turnbull Library, Wellington.
29. *Open Windows* 3, no. 2 (May 1929): 3–4.
30. Chisholm, "Otago Medical School," 87.
31. Bell, *Surgeon's Saga*, 156.
32. Chisholm, "Otago Medical School," 96.
33. Page, *Anatomy of a Medical School*, 87.
34. Chisholm, "Otago Medical School," 98.
35. Sutton, "NZ Student Christian Movement," 20.
36. Macdonald Wilson, *Hundred Years of Healing*, 49–50.
37. Barber and Towers, *Wellington Hospital*, 65.
38. Barber and Towers, *Wellington Hospital*, 63.
39. Barber and Towers, *Wellington Hospital*, 66–67.
40. Wellington Hospital Board minutes 1929–1942, 27 February 1930, 34–35, box 6, part 6, code R41827, Archives NZ Te Rua Mahara o te Kāwanatanga, Wellington.

41. Wellington Hospital Board minutes 1929–1942, 27 November 1930, 70, box 6, part 6, code R41827, Archives NZ Te Rua Mahara o te Kāwanatanga, Wellington.
42. Medical Superintendent, Wellington Hospital, 17 April 1931, BJC.
43. "Operation Register, Main Theatre, 1930–1945," in Operation Books, Theatres 1 and 2, 1930–1980, Series 68824, Wellington Hospital Archives, Archives NZ Te Rua Mahara o te Kāwanatanga, Wellington.
44. Louis Cohen FRCS, Wellington Hospital, 9 April 1931, BJC.
45. Pathologist to Wellington Hospital, 9 September 1931, BJC.
46. Kellaway and Maryan, *Century of Care*, 27.
47. Middleton to D. Jolly, 17 June 1931, BJC.
48. King to D. Jolly, 1931, BJC.
49. "Kitty" to D. Jolly, 10 June 1931, BJC.
50. King to D. Jolly, London, 15 September 1934, BJC.
51. Wylie, 6 January 1932, BJC.
52. Downie Stewart to Hon. Sir Thomas Wilford, 11 December 1931, BJC.

4. CHRISTIAN LEFT

1. General Medical Council, *UK Medical Registers*.
2. Stewart, "'For a Healthy London,'" 417.
3. Rivett, *Development of the London Hospital System*, 196–97.
4. Gosling, *Payment and Philanthropy*, 196–99.
5. Burns, "Post-Graduate Study," 34.
6. Newman, "History of Postgraduate Medical Education," 351.
7. Rivett, "Health Care before the NHS."
8. Harding Rains, "Hand Physician," 257.
9. Addison, 29 May 1933, BJC.
10. Stewart, "'Finest Municipal Hospital Service,'" 330.
11. Stewart, *"The Battle for Health,"* 3, 89.
12. Webster, *National Health Service*, 4.
13. D. Jolly, unpublished memoir, BJC.
14. William Edmarsh, 3 April 1935, BJC.
15. Dr. Louis [illegible], 3 April 1935, BJC.
16. Dr. Peter [illegible], 2 April 1935, BJC.
17. W. Perrin, 1 July 1935, BJC.
18. Brittain, *Rebel Passion*, 191.
19. Cooper, *Refugee Scholars*, 25.
20. Polanyi, *Great Transformation*, 299.
21. Ricolas UK, "Irene Grant and Brecht's Daughter."
22. Quoted in Brittain, *Rebel Passion*, 50.

23. Quoted in Albert Einstein, "The 1932 Disarmament Conference," *The Nation*, 23 August 2001, https://www.thenation.com/article/archive/1932-disarmament-conference-0/.
24. Donald Grant Jr., undated but early 1980s, container (con.) 56, folio (fol.) 15, 39, Karl Polanyi Digital Archive, Concordia University, Quebec (hereafter KPDA).
25. Cooper, *Refugee Scholars*, 27.
26. Ricolas UK, "Irene Grant and Brecht's Daughter."
27. Costello, *John Macmurray*, 202–3.
28. Karl Polanyi to Irene Grant, 13 October 1933; and Karl Polanyi to Irene Grant, Donald Grant, John Macmurray, and Betty Macmurray, Christmas 1933—both in Michael Polanyi Papers, box 17, folder 4, University of Chicago.
29. Costello, *John Macmurray*, 200–201.
30. Cooper, *Refugee Scholars*, 25.
31. Rivett, *Development of the London Hospital System*, 104–5.
32. Cooper, *Refugee Scholars*, 37.
33. Costello, *John Macmurray*, 93.
34. Costello, *John Macmurray*, 179, 182.
35. Costello, *John Macmurray*, 237.
36. Ricolas UK, "Irene Grant and Brecht's Daughter."
37. Costello, *John Macmurray*, 222–35.
38. Costello, *John Macmurray*, 256.
39. Dale, *Karl Polanyi*, 148–49.
40. Lewis, Polanyi, and Kitchen, *Christianity and the Social Revolution*, 359.
41. Lewis, Polanyi, and Kitchen, *Christianity and the Social Revolution*, 11.
42. Lewis, Polanyi, and Kitchen, *Christianity and the Social Revolution*, 507.
43. Ricolas UK, "Irene Grant and Brecht's Daughter."
44. Ted Edwards, unpublished memoir, quoted by his son Gavin Edwards, email to author, 9 May 2022.
45. "Towards a Christian Left," 1 July 1936, con. 20, fol. 10, KPDA.
46. "Towards a Christian Left," 1 July 1936, con. 20, fol. 10, KPDA. Emphasis in original.
47. Ricolas UK, "Irene Grant and Brecht's Daughter."
48. Dale, *Karl Polanyi*, 148–49.
49. Ricolas UK, "Irene Grant and Brecht's Daughter."
50. Costello, *John Macmurray*, 256.

5. BREAD, PEACE, AND LIBERTY

1. D. Jolly, *Sand* (unpublished manuscript), 4, BJC.
2. Aitken to D. Jolly, 5 April 1935, BJC.
3. Costello, *John Macmurray*, 256.

4. Licence, *Living in Squares*.
5. Costello, *John Macmurray*, 210–11; and Dale, *Karl Polanyi*, 148–49, fn 244.
6. Dale, *Karl Polanyi*, 244.
7. Costello, *John Macmurray*, 261.
8. Gavin Edwards, email to author, 22 May 2022.
9. Barnes et al., *Towards a Quaker View*, 24–25. I am grateful to Gavin Edwards for drawing this resource to my attention.
10. Townshend-Stephens, "John Melly," 223–30.
11. "Obituary, John Melly," *British Medical Journal*, 16 May 1936, 1024.
12. "Medical Aid for Spain," *Lancet*, 15 August 1936, 390.
13. Fyrth, *Signal Was Spain*, 28.
14. Wintringham, *Coming World War*, 41.
15. Thomas, *Spanish Civil War*, 62.
16. *Daily Sketch*, 28 November 1936, 3.
17. "Christianity and the Spanish Left," *News Sheet of the Auxiliary Christian Left*, no. 3 (5 October 1936): 2, con. 20, fol. 10, KPDA.
18. Sinclair-Loutit, "Very Little Luggage" (unpublished manuscript), 4, SC/IND/JFY/2/1/7, SC Collection, Marx Memorial Library, London.
19. Sinclair-Loutit, "Very Little Luggage," 4.
20. Fyrth, *Signal Was Spain*, 48.
21. Sinclair-Loutit, "Very Little Luggage," 4.
22. Sinclair-Loutit, "Very Little Luggage," 4.
23. Sinclair-Loutit, "Very Little Luggage," 10.
24. Sinclair-Loutit, "Very Little Luggage," 6–7.
25. Sinclair-Loutit, "Very Little Luggage," 9.
26. Sinclair-Loutit, "Very Little Luggage," 10.
27. Sinclair-Loutit, "Very Little Luggage," 10.
28. Tremlett, *International Brigades*, 49–50.
29. Kenneth Sinclair-Loutit, "An Ambulance in Spain," *Lancet*, 28 November 1936, 1295.
30. Sinclair-Loutit, "Very Little Luggage," 18.
31. Fyrth, *Signal Was Spain*, 52.
32. Cochrane and Blythe, *One Man's Medicine*, 25.
33. Sinclair-Loutit, "Very Little Luggage," 53.
34. Fyrth, *Signal Was Spain*, 52–53.
35. Fyrth, *Signal Was Spain*, 61.
36. Broggi, *Memorias de un cirujano*, 191.
37. Sinclair-Loutit, "Very Little Luggage," 17.
38. Rubin, *Spain's Cause Was Mine*, 111.
39. Paul Preston, "Obituary: Reginald Saxton," *The Guardian* (UK), 8 April 2004, https://www.theguardian.com/news/2004/apr/08/guardianobituaries.

40. Derby and Jorge, "Moisès Broggi i Vallès," 23–29.
41. Sinclair-Loutit, "Very Little Luggage," 19–20.
42. Tremlett, *International Brigades*, 57.
43. Sinclair-Loutit, "Very Little Luggage," 21.
44. Cochrane and Blythe, *One Man's Medicine*, 26.
45. Sinclair-Loutit, "Very Little Luggage." 17.
46. *Medicine Today and Tomorrow*, quoted in Rivett, *Development of the London Hospital System*, 103.
47. D. Jolly, unpublished memoir, BJC.
48. "Help Spain!," *News Sheet of the Auxiliary Christian Left*, no. 5 (4 January 1937): 7, con. 20, fol. 10, KPDA.

6. NINE MONTHS OF WINTER

Epigraph: Ramírez de Lucas quoted in Fuster Ruiz, *El servicio de sanidad*, 23.

1. Tremlett, *International Brigades*, xi–xii.
2. Wintringham, *English Captain*, facing 52.
3. Albrighton quoted in Baxell, "British Battalion," 122.
4. Tremlett, *International Brigades*, 149–50.
5. Cox, *Defence of Madrid*, 49–50.
6. Beevor, *Battle for Spain*, 203.
7. Mikhail Koltsov quoted in Beevor, *Battle for Spain*, 189.
8. Beevor, *Battle for Spain*, 198.
9. Sinclair-Loutit, "Very Little Luggage," 36.
10. Hannant, *Politics of Passion*, 136–38.
11. Mangan, *Never More Alive*, 121.
12. Colodny, *Struggle for Madrid*, 86–87.
13. Coni, *Medicine and Warfare*, 153–54.
14. Wintringham, *English Captain*, 52.
15. Wintringham, *English Captain*, 55.
16. Hannant, *Politics of Passion*, 131.
17. D. Jolly, unpublished autobiographical notes, BJC.
18. Spanish ambassador, London, 1 December 1936, BJC.
19. H. Pollitt to HQ, International Legion, 2 December 1936, BJC.
20. Fuster Ruiz, *El servicio de sanidad*, 50; and "The War in Spain," *British Medical Journal*, 28 January 1939, 168.
21. Cochrane and Blythe, *One Man's Medicine*, 30.
22. R. Neumann quoted in Palfreeman, *Spain Bleeds*, 55.
23. Fuster Ruiz, *El servicio de sanidad*, 59.
24. Fuster Ruiz, *El servicio de sanidad*, 47.

25. Letter, D. Jolly to I. and D. Grant, 9 December 1936, Collection SC/VOL (Spanish/Volunteers), Marx Memorial Library, London (hereafter Marx Memorial Library).
26. D. Jolly, "A Talk by Douglas Jolly: Republican Spain, 1936–1939," undated, unpaged, Marx Memorial Library.
27. Jolly, "Talk by Douglas Jolly," Marx Memorial Library.
28. "Permisio de viaje," BJC.
29. N. Bethune quoted in Hannant, *Politics of Passion*, 154–55.
30. Anna-Mária Basch, unpublished memoir, Éva Cserháti collection, Budapest.
31. Lavinia de Sarigny, letter to author, 8 June 2018.
32. *Daily Sketch*, 28 November 1936, 3.
33. D. Jolly, to Fredericka Martin, 29 January 1972, Fredericka Martin Papers, ALBA 001, Tamiment Library, New York University (hereafter Tamiment Library).
34. Jolly, "Talk by Douglas Jolly," Marx Memorial Library. The following doggerel composed and sung by International Brigaders illustrates the communication challenges they faced: "Ich kam nach Spain in Januar / Yo hablar seulemente English / But jetzt I say Comment Savar / Wie gehts, Que tal, tovarisch / Ich fahren mit mein ambulance / In woikin shoit and panties / No tengo tiempo por romance / Y arbeit más duro que antes." Quoted in Raeburn, "Hammering the World," 225.
35. "Ordre de Mission," 16 December 1936, 545/2/44, 221, RGASPI (Russian State Archive of Socio-Political History), Moscow (hereafter cited as RGASPI).
36. Baxell, "British Battalion," 63.
37. Fernández Suárez, *Fuencarral durante la 2ª República*.
38. "Report of the Head of the Base of the International Brigades," 545/2/32,265, 277–78, RGASPI.
39. "Report of the Head."
40. W. F. Hawkins, "Spain as I Saw It," *Daily Worker*, 22 January 1937, 4.
41. D. Jolly, letter, 14 December 1936, Marx Memorial Library.
42. Jolly, "Talk by Douglas Jolly," Marx Memorial Library.
43. D. Jolly, letter, 14 December 1936, Marx Memorial Library.
44. D. Jolly, letter, 14 December 1936, Marx Memorial Library.

7. A RIVER OF BLOOD

1. Quoted in Bennett, "Abdominal Surgery in War," 556.
2. Dr. Norman Bethune quoted in Lethbridge, *Norman Bethune in Spain*, 113.
3. Palfreeman, *Spain Bleeds*, 60–63.
4. Palfreeman, *Spain Bleeds*, 13–17.
5. Palfreeman, *Spain Bleeds*, 35.
6. Palfreeman, *Spain Bleeds*, 36–37.
7. Palfreeman, *Spain Bleeds*, 49–50.
8. Palfreeman, *Spain Bleeds*, 62–64.

9. Hazen Size quoted in Pinkerton, "Norman Bethune," 255–64.
10. Hannant, *Politics of Passion*, 150.
11. D. Jolly, unpublished memoir, BJC.
12. Jolly, D. unpublished memoir, BJC.
13. Lethbridge, *Norman Bethune in Spain*, 112.
14. N. Bethune, 11 January 1937, in Hannant, *Politics of Passion*, 145–46.
15. Hazen Size quoted in Lethbridge, *Norman Bethune in Spain*, 113.
16. Lethbridge, *Norman Bethune in Spain*, 106.
17. Mangan, *Never More Alive*, 226.
18. Quoted in Hannant, *Politics of Passion*, 126; and Rothman, "Christmas and New Year," 4.
19. D. Jolly, letter, 14 December 1936, Marx Memorial Library. Emphasis in original. *Note*: Parts of this letter were evidently written some weeks after the date it gives.
20. D. Jolly, letter, 14 December 1936, Marx Memorial Library. Emphasis in original.
21. D. Jolly, letter, 14 December 1936, Marx Memorial Library.
22. Desmond Painter, email to author, 20 November 2022.
23. D. Jolly, letter, 8 February 1937, Marx Memorial Library.
24. D. Jolly, letter, 24 December 1936, Marx Memorial Library.
25. Rothman, "Christmas and New Year," 4.
26. D. Jolly, letter, 28 December 1936, Marx Memorial Library.
27. Martin, *Ink in Her Veins*, 164.
28. Beevor, *Battle for Spain*, 231.
29. D. Jolly, letter, 28 January 1937, Marx Memorial Library.
30. Jolly, "Talk by Douglas Jolly," Marx Memorial Library.
31. Coni, *Medicine and Warfare*, 154.
32. D. Jolly, letter, 2 January 1937, Marx Memorial Library.
33. D. Jolly, letter, 6 January 1937, Marx Memorial Library.
34. D. Jolly, letter, 2 January 1937, Marx Memorial Library.
35. D. Jolly, letter, 2 January 1937, Marx Memorial Library.
36. D. Jolly, letter, 28 January 1937, Marx Memorial Library. Emphasis in original.
37. D. Jolly, letter, 12 January 1937, Marx Memorial Library. Emphasis in original.
38. D. Jolly, letter, 28 January 1937, Marx Memorial Library.
39. D. Jolly, letter, 28 January 1937, Marx Memorial Library.
40. D. Jolly, letter, 13 January 1937, Marx Memorial Library.
41. D. Jolly, letter, 28 January 1937, Marx Memorial Library.
42. D. Jolly, letter, 8 March 1937, Marx Memorial Library.
43. D. Jolly, letter, 28 January 1937, Marx Memorial Library.
44. Cochrane and Blythe, *One Man's Medicine*, 37.
45. D. Jolly, letter, l8 February 1937, Marx Memorial Library.
46. D. Jolly, letter, 28 January 1937, Marx Memorial Library.

47. Stridsberg, *My Five Lives*, 233.
48. Coni, *Medicine and Warfare*, 61.
49. D. Jolly, letter, 28 January 1937, Marx Memorial Library.
50. Beevor, *Battle for Spain*, 238.
51. ARMH Cuenca, *Red Tarancón*, 106.
52. Penny (née Phelps) Fyvel interviewed in Arthur, *Real Band of Brothers*, 77–79.
53. Fyvel (née Phelps), *English Penny*, 20.
54. Fyvel interviewed in Arthur, *Real Band of Brothers*, 77–79.
55. Fyvel, *English Penny*, 20.
56. Penny Phelps quoted in Fyrth and Alexander, *Women's Voices*, 78–79.
57. Fyvel interviewed in Arthur, *Real Band of Brothers*, 77–78.
58. Fyvel interviewed in Arthur, *Real Band of Brothers*, 78.
59. Fyvel, *English Penny*, 21.
60. Fyvel interviewed in Arthur, *Real Band of Brothers*, 79.
61. Penny Phelps quoted in Emma Brockes, "It's the Wrong Picasso," *The Guardian* (UK), 18 October 2001, https://www.theguardian.com/culture/2001/oct/18/artsfeatures3.
62. Fyvel, *English Penny*, 22.
63. D. Jolly, letter, 8 March 1937, Marx Memorial Library.
64. D. Jolly, letter, 8 March 1937, Marx Memorial Library.
65. Quoted in Skudder, "'Bringing It Home,'" 110–11.

8. URGENT NEED OF SALVATION

Epigraph: Fraser, "Doctor's Debt to the Soldier," 70.

1. Bethune, in *Daily Clarion* (Toronto), 17 July 1937, 1.
2. Cochrane and Blythe, *One Man's Medicine*, 35.
3. Hannant, *Politics of Passion*, 150.
4. Cochrane and Blythe, *One Man's Medicine*, 35.
5. Coni, *Medicine and Warfare*, 71–74.
6. Bingham de Urquidi, *Mercy in Madrid*, 466.
7. Fyvel, *English Penny*, 25.
8. D. Jolly, 22 March 1937, Marx Memorial Library.
9. Transcript of interview with Irene Grant, BJC.
10. Jolly, "Emergency Abdominal Surgery," 10.
11. "Medical Work for the Republic," *British Medical Journal*, 28 January 1939, 168.
12. Jolly, *Field Surgery in Total War*, 32–33.
13. D. Jolly to Fredericka Martin, 29 January 1972, Fredericka Martin Papers, Tamiment Library.
14. D. Jolly, letter, 22 March 1937, Marx Memorial Library.
15. *News Sheet of the Auxiliary Christian Left* (newsletter), no. 8 (24 April 1937): 7, con. 20, fol. 10, KPDA.

16. D. Jolly, letter, 28 March 1937, Marx Memorial Library. Emphasis in original.
17. D. Jolly, letter, 13 April 1937, Marx Memorial Library.
18. Lustiger, *Shalom Libertad!*, 282. Translation from German by Mark Derby.
19. Basch, "Harc az életért," in Kepes, *Magyar önkéntesek a spanyol*, 94–98.
20. D. Jolly, letter, 13 April 1937, Marx Memorial Library.
21. Lethbridge, *Norman Bethune in Spain*, 111.
22. D. Jolly, letter, 23 April 1937, Marx Memorial Library.
23. Quoted in Fuster Ruiz, *El servicio de sanidad*, 134.
24. Quoted in Fuster Ruiz, *El servicio de sanidad*, 132.
25. Broggi, *Memorias de un cirujano*, 220.
26. Coni, *Medicine and Warfare*, 136.
27. Broggi, *Memorias de un cirujano*, 77.
28. Costello, *John Macmurray*, 271.
29. Beevor, *Battle for Spain*, 254.
30. J. Macmurray, 19 May 1937, quoted in Costello, *John Macmurray*, 272.
31. Lewis, Polanyi, and Kitchin, *Christianity and the Social Revolution*, v.
32. I am grateful to Gabor Basch and other descendants of Anna-Mária Basch for use of this photograph.
33. D. Jolly, letter, 4 May 1937, Marx Memorial Library.
34. Broggi, *Memorias de un cirujano*, 226.
35. D. Jolly, letter, 4 May 1937, Marx Memorial Library.
36. Coni, *Medicine and Warfare*, 114.
37. Kenneth Sinclair-Loutit, "Ambulance in Spain," *Lancet*, 15 May 1937, 1188–89.
38. Fuster Ruiz, *El servicio de sanidad*, 48.
39. Fuster Ruiz, *El servicio de sanidad*, 61.
40. Fuster Ruiz, *El servicio de sanidad*, 63.
41. Coni, *Medicine and Warfare*, 133.
42. Fuster Ruiz, *El servicio de sanidad*, 63.
43. Neugass, *War Is Beautiful*, 7.
44. Broggi, *Memorias de un cirujano*, 212.
45. Jolly, *Field Surgery in Total War*, 32–33.
46. E. Barsky quoted in Johnson, "Healing the Wounds," 48.
47. Quoted in Jirku, *We Fight Death*, 9.
48. Jolly, *Field Surgery in Total War*, 11.
49. Coni, *Medicine and Warfare*, 111.
50. Bingham de Urquidi, *Mercy in Madrid*, 363.
51. Jolly, *Field Surgery in Total War*, 12–13.
52. D. Jolly, letter, 9 August 1937, Marx Memorial Library.
53. Cochrane and Blythe, *One Man's Medicine*, 39.
54. Coni, *Medicine and Warfare*, 124.

55. Broggi, *Memorias de un cirujano*, 202.
56. Broggi, *Memorias de un cirujano*, 203.
57. Stridsberg, *My Five Lives*, 240–42.
58. D. Jolly to E. Jolly, 30 June 1937, Barbara Jolly collection.

9. HE DOES HONOR TO HIS NAME

1. Ryan, *Book of the XV Brigade*, 129.
2. Broggi, *Memorias de un cirujano*, 212.
3. Tony Fox, email to author, 14 November 2021.
4. Broggi, *Memorias de un cirujano*, 213.
5. Noel Carritt, transcript of audio interview, 25 November 1982, International Brigades Memorial Trust, London.
6. Cochrane and Blythe, *One Man's Medicine*, 41–42.
7. Quoted in Preston, *Doves of War*, 146.
8. Aileen Palmer to N. Palmer, 29 July 1937, quoted in Martin, *Ink in Her Veins*, 159–60.
9. *Magyar Nap*, 7 October 1937, 5. This left-wing daily, aimed at emigré Hungarians, was published in Czechoslovakia from 1936 to 1938. Translation from Hungarian by Éva Cserháti.
10. Coni, *Medicine and Warfare*, 124.
11. D. Jolly, quoted in Jirku, *We Fight Death*, 4–5.
12. John Kiszely, audio interview, 21 December 1992, Oral History Collection, Imperial War Museum, London.
13. Fyvel in Arthur, *Real Band of Brothers*, 94.
14. R. Saxton, "Medicine in Republican Spain," *Lancet*, 24 September 1938, 752.
15. Keene, "Spanish Springtime," 82.
16. Palfreeman, *Spain Bleeds*, 77, 82.
17. Broggi, *Memorias de un cirujano*, 214. Translation from Spanish by Reuben Sanderson.
18. Saxton, "Medicine in Republican Spain," 752.
19. Fyvel, *English Penny*, 29.
20. Keene, "Spanish Springtime," 82.
21. Cochrane and Blythe, *One Man's Medicine*, 42.
22. Broggi, *Memorias de un cirujano*, 217.
23. Shafer, "Justice, Justice," 76.
24. Gettelmann, "Robert G. Colodny," 263–71.
25. Broggi, *Memorias de un cirujano*, 217.
26. Broggi *Memorias de un cirujano*, 220–21.
27. Beevor, *Battle for Spain*, 318.
28. Broggi, *Memorias de un cirujano*, 219–20.
29. D. Jolly, letter, 9 August 1937, Marx Memorial Library.

30. Colin Carritt, email communication with Dr. David Lowe, 1 June 2020.
31. Noel Carritt Papers, Spanish Collection SC/VOL/NCA/2. Marx Memorial Library, London.
32. D. Jolly, letter, Fredericka Martin Papers, Tamiment Library.
33. Browne, "Start of Specialisation," 66.
34. Browne, "Start of Specialisation," 75.
35. D. Jolly, letter, 29 August 1937, Marx Memorial Library.
36. Coni, *Medicine and Warfare*, 163.
37. Aurora Fernández, quoted in Fyrth, *Signal Was Spain*, 97.
38. D. Jolly, letter, 30 August 1937, Marx Memorial Library.
39. Wintringham, *English Captain*, 56.
40. D. Jolly, letter, 29 August 1937, Marx Memorial Library.
41. D. Jolly, letter, 29 August 1937, Marx Memorial Library. Emphasis in original.
42. D. Jolly, letter, 30 August 1937, Marx Memorial Library.
43. D. Jolly, unpublished notes for speech, in Fredericka Martin Papers, Tamiment Library, NYU.
44. Coni, *Medicine and Warfare*, 163.
45. Heijnis-Mens and de Leede, "Diamant, Noor." Translation from Dutch by Denise Grobben of Stichting Spanje (Spain Foundation).
46. D. Jolly, letter, 9 August 1937, Marx Memorial Library.
47. Jolly, "Emergency Abdominal Surgery."
48. Preston, *Doves of War*, 152.
49. "Letter from Nurse Dodds," *Cromwell Argus*, 11 April 1938, 5.
50. Green, *Chronicle of Small Beer*, 95.
51. Broggi, *Memorias de un cirujano*, 238–39.
52. Jackson, *Beyond the Battlefield*, 51.
53. Jackson, *"For Us It Was Heaven,"* 63–64.
54. Fyrth and Alexander, *Women's Voices*, 75.
55. Rubin, *Spain's Cause Was Mine*, 117.
56. Coni, *Medicine and Warfare*, 164–66.
57. Quoted in Jackson, *"For Us It Was Heaven,"* 64–65.
58. Lillian Urmston quoted in Jackson, *"For Us It Was Heaven,"* 64.
59. Neugass, *War Is Beautiful*, 109.
60. R. Saxton, "A Hospital near Teruel," *Lancet*, 8 January 1938, 104.
61. Fyrth, *Signal Was Spain*, 80. Aurora Fernández was one of the Spanish *chicas* (girls) who volunteered as nursing assistants. They were trained in rudimentary nursing skills by the British nurses.
62. Aurora (née Fernández) Edenhoffer, Fredericka Martin Papers, Tamiment Library.
63. Fyvel, *English Penny*, 24.
64. Beevor, *Battle for Spain*, 355.

65. D. Jolly to Wendy Grant, 26 December 1937, Núala Grant Collection, Hocken Library Uare Taoka o Hākena, Otago University, Dunedin, NZ (hereafter Núala Grant Collection, Hocken Library); and D. Jolly in *News Sheet of the Auxiliary Christian Left* (newsletter), no. 11 (March 1938): 5–6, con. 20, fol. 10, KPDA.
66. Eby, *Comrades and Commissars*, 273.
67. Fyrth, *Signal Was Spain*, 131.
68. Jolly, *Field Surgery in Total War*, 35.
69. Aileen Palmer, quoted in Martin, *Ink in Her Veins*, 170.
70. Leo Eloesser quoted in Coni, *Medicine and Warfare*, 114.
71. Johnson, "Healing the Wounds," 51.

10. THE SAFEST PLACE IN SPAIN

1. Jolly, *Field Surgery in Total War*, 227.
2. Jolly, *Field Surgery in Total War*, 230.
3. Jolly, *Field Surgery in Total War*, 227–28.
4. Report cited in 545/3/661,80, RGASPI. I am grateful to Peter Verbrugh for this resource.
5. Coni, *Medicine and Warfare*, 114.
6. Jolly, *Field Surgery in Total War*, 232.
7. Coni, *Medicine and Warfare*, 137.
8. Beevor, *Battle for Spain*, 377–79.
9. Jolly, *Field Surgery in Total War*, 228.
10. Beevor, *Battle for Spain*, 386–87.
11. Beevor, *Battle for Spain*, 370.
12. Coni, *Medicine and Warfare*, 75–76.
13. R. Saxton, "Medicine in Republican Spain," *Lancet*, 15 April 1938, 917.
14. Otto F. Apel Jr. and Pat Apel, "MASH in the Spanish Civil War," *Lancet* 352 (17 October 1998): 1317.
15. Fuster Ruiz, *El servicio de sanidad*, 186–89.
16. Roman, *Bajo el cielo de España*, 251–52.
17. Rudolf Neumann quoted in Esteve Torres, "Benicàssim (1937–1938)," 4.
18. Jolly, "Emergency Abdominal Surgery."
19. Powell, reprinted in *The Volunteer*, no. 27 (Autumn 2010).
20. Neugass, *War Is Beautiful*, 242–43.
21. Jolly, "Emergency Abdominal Surgery."
22. Stridsberg, *My Five Lives*, 253.
23. Fuster Ruiz, *El servicio de sanidad*, 18–19.
24. Jackson, *At the Margins*, 42.
25. Hollós and Jalsovszky, "Magyar önkéntesek a spanyol polgárháborúban," 99–148. I am grateful to Éva Cserháti for this material.

26. Green, *Chronicle of Small Beer*, 92; and Jackson, *At the Margins*, 51.
27. Bessie, *Men in Battle*, 183–84.
28. Jackson, *At the Margins*, 52.
29. Jackson, *At the Margins*, 55.
30. Jackson, *Beyond the Battlefield*, 7.
31. Jolly, *Field Surgery in Total War*, 34.
32. Jackson, *"For Us It Was Heaven,"* 103.
33. Palfreeman, *Spain Bleeds*, 114.
34. Jolly, *Field Surgery in Total War*, 34.
35. Quoted in Fyrth and Alexander, *Women's Voices*, 104–5.
36. Jackson, *Beyond the Battlefield*, 56.
37. Jackson, *Beyond the Battlefield*, 49; and Jackson, *At the Margins*, 76–77.
38. Jackson, *Beyond the Battlefield*, 24.
39. Quoted in Fyrth and Alexander, *Women's Voices*, 76–77.
40. Jackson, *At the Margins*, 45.
41. Quoted in Baxell, *Unlikely Warriors*, 325.
42. Beevor, *Battle for Spain*, 393.
43. Coni, *Medicine and Warfare*, 166–68.
44. Petrou, *Renegades*, 96.
45. Jolly, *Field Surgery in Total War*, 234.
46. Palfreeman, *Spain Bleeds*, 114.
47. Jackson, *"For Us It Was Heaven,"* 104.
48. Jackson, *"For Us It Was Heaven,"* 107.
49. Fyrth and Alexander, *Women's Voices*, 69.
50. Jolly, *Field Surgery in Total War*, 34.
51. Rubin, *Spain's Cause Was Mine*, 122–27.
52. Jackson, *"For Us It Was Heaven,"* 109.
53. Jackson, *"For Us It Was Heaven,"* 113.
54. Jackson, *Beyond the Battlefield*, 38.
55. Jackson, *Beyond the Battlefield*, 104–5.
56. Fyrth and Alexander, *Women's Voices*, 76–77.
57. Jackson, *Beyond the Battlefield*, 40.
58. Jackson, *Beyond the Battlefield*, 42.
59. Jackson, *"For Us It Was Heaven,"* 108; and Jackson, *At the Margins*, 114.
60. Fyrth and Alexander, *Women's Voices*, 102–3.
61. Palfreeman, *Spain Bleeds*, 114–15.
62. Palfreeman, *Spain Bleeds*, 114–15.
63. Fyrth and Alexander, *Women's Voices*, 101–3.
64. Jolly, *Field Surgery in Total War*, 234.
65. Fyrth and Alexander, *Women's Voices*, 102–3.

66. Jolly, *Field Surgery in Total War*, 236.
67. Carrió, *Diario personal*, 312–13. Translation from Catalan by Andrea Hepworth.
68. John Edward Longstaff, oral history interview by Conrad Wood, 14 September 1988, catalog number 10382, reel 7, Imperial War Museum, https://www.iwm.org.uk/collections/item/object/80009089; and Duncan Longstaff, email to author, 16 July 2019.
69. Pinkerton, "Reginald Saxton," 3.
70. Jackson, *At the Margins*, 122.
71. Fyrth and Alexander, *Women's Voices*, 76–77.
72. Quoted in Preston, "Two Doctors," 22.
73. Alun Menai Williams quoted in Palfreeman, *¡Salud!*, 149.
74. Jolly, *Field Surgery in Total War*, 236.
75. Beevor, *Battle for Spain*, 399.
76. "Direccion y comisariado de sanidad Ejercito del Ebro a los camarades internacionales," BJC.
77. D. Jolly to Frederika Martin, 29 January 1972, Fredericka Martin Papers, Tamiment Library.
78. Muller, *Hemingway*, 203.
79. Henry Buckley quoted in Preston, *We Saw Spain Die*, 409.
80. D. Jolly to Frederika Martin, 29 January 1972, Fredericka Martin Papers, Tamiment Library.
81. Preston, *Doves of War*, 166.
82. Green, *Chronicle of Small Beer*, 92; and Preston, "Two Doctors," 11–12.
83. Preston, *Doves of War*, 167–68.
84. Preston, *Doves of War*, 167, 173.
85. Testimonial of Lt. Col. Joaquín D'Harcourt, 22 October 1938, BJC.
86. *Diario oficial del Ministerio de Defensa Nacional*, no. 71 (24 March 1938): 850. Translation from Spanish by Alicia García López.
87. Certificate, Medal of Duty, 12 October 1938, BJC.
88. "Caracteristica del Dr Douglas Jolly," C 1092.8.1/103, Archivo General Militar de Ávila, Spain. I am grateful to Alicia García Lopez for supplying this document.
89. "Characterisations of British volunteers of the International Brigades—non-communists," 12 December 1938, 545/6/96/24–25, RGASPI.
90. Masip Gorgori, "La Cova Hospital."

11. CHANGING THE FRONT

Epigraph: Coni, "Medicine and the Spanish Civil War," 147.

1. D. W. Jolly, unpublished autobiographical notes, BJC.
2. Aileen Palmer, 3 April 1938, quoted in Martin, *Ink in Her Veins*, 171.
3. Jackson, *Beyond the Battlefield*, 48–49.

4. Alexander Aitken to D. Jolly, 28 November 1938, BJC.
5. Jolly to F. Martin, 29 January 1972, Imperial War Museum, London.
6. Jackson, *"For Us It Was Heaven,"* 137.
7. Moritz Demant to Jolly, 17 March 1940, BJC.
8. Green, *Chronicle of Small Beer*, 99.
9. Jackson, *Beyond the Battlefield*, 54.
10. *Lancet*, 31 December 1938, 1545.
11. *News Sheet of the Auxiliary Christian Left* (newsletter), November–December 1938, 4A, con. 20, fol. 10, KPDA.
12. Green, *Chronicle of Small Beer*, 99.
13. "The War in Spain," *British Medical Journal*, 28 January 1939, 168–69.
14. Handwritten flyer, Núala Grant Collection, Hocken Library.
15. "Two Years in Spain," *Evening Post*, 17 February 1939, 10.
16. Jolly, unpublished autobiographical notes, BJC.
17. "Engagement Notices," *Press* (Christchurch), 15 March 1939, 2.
18. Ngākawau Miners Union to D. Jolly, 13 March 1939, BJC.
19. Beevor, *Battle for Spain*, 439–40.
20. "For Democracy and Humanity," *Nelson Evening Mail*, 24 April 1939, 10.
21. Derby, *Kiwi Compañeros*, 53–58.
22. Derby, *Kiwi Compañeros*, 79–82.
23. Skudder, "'Bringing It Home,'" 438.
24. *Te Rau Weekly Press* (Gisborne), 19 May 1939, 4.
25. Jolly, "Talk by Douglas Jolly," Marx Memorial Library.
26. *Otago Daily Times*, 15 May 1939, 16.
27. Elsie Freeman, *Woman Today*, June 1939, 15.
28. Dr. Jolly and B. Bryan, "War in Spain: Interesting Addresses," *Hokitika Guardian*, 21 April 1939, 4.
29. *Otago Boys' High School Magazine* 40, no. 1 (April 1939): 11–12.
30. *Otago Daily Times*, 24 March 1939, 4.
31. *Auckland Star*, 15 May 1939, 13.
32. *Evening Post* (Wellington), 8 March 1939, 12.
33. *Workers' Weekly* (NZ), 17 March 1939, 1–2.
34. *Press* (Christchurch), 13 April 1939, 15.
35. *Auckland Star*, 9 February 1940, 3.
36. Jolly, "Unpublished autobiographical notes," n.d., BJC.
37. Jolly, "Unpublished autobiographical notes," n.d., BJC.
38. D. Jolly quoted in *Auckland Star*, 9 February 1940, 3.
39. Allan and Gordon, *Scalpel, the Sword*, 232. I am grateful to Pat Medlicott for drawing this information to my attention.
40. Jolly, *Field Surgery in Total War*, xiv.

41. Alternês and Wainman, *Almas vivas*.
42. Trueta, "Obituary—Maurice Newfield," 111.
43. "Gordon-Taylor, Sir Gordon"; and Sir Gordon Gordon-Taylor to D. Jolly, BJC.
44. Beasley, *Mantle of Surgery*, 60.
45. Costello, *John Macmurray*, 277.
46. McLaughlin, *Royal Army Medical Corps*, 63–64.
47. Ross, "Memoirs," 32.
48. Ross, "Memoirs," 33.
49. McLaughlin, *Royal Army Medical Corps*, 62.

12. THE SYSTEM, NOT THE SURGEON

1. D. Jolly to Irene Grant, 31 December 1940, Núala Grant Collection, Hocken Library.
2. Haldane, *A.R.P.*, 1.
3. Shirlaw and Troke, *Medicine versus Invasion*, 37.
4. Mottram, "Shaping the Inheritance," 80.
5. *Hansard* (UK), 18 June 1940, 58–60.
6. Coni, *Medicine and Warfare*, 138.
7. Bricknell, "Evolution of Casualty Evacuation," 315.
8. Jolly, *Field Surgery in Total War*, 40.
9. Jolly, *Field Surgery in Total War*, 51–54.
10. Broggi, *Memorias de un cirujano*, 228.
11. Bricknell, "Evolution of Casualty Evacuation," 315.
12. Shackleton, *Desert Surgeons*, 39.
13. Quoted in Jolly, *Field Surgery in Total War*, vi.
14. Jolly, *Field Surgery in Total War*, 31–32.
15. Bricknell, "Evolution of Casualty Evacuation," 315.
16. Jolly, *Field Surgery in Total War*, 35–37.
17. Jolly, *Field Surgery in Total War*, xi.
18. Jolly, *Field Surgery in Total War*, xi–xii.
19. *Workers' Weekly* (NZ), 17 March 1939, 1.
20. Jolly, *Field Surgery in Total War*, 45.
21. *British Medical Journal*, 10 December 1938, 1236–38; *British Medical Journal*, 1 July 1939, 35–36; and *British Medical Journal*, 15 July 1939, 130.
22. Jolly, *Field Surgery in Total War*, 107.
23. Trueta, *Trueta*, 63–64, 79.
24. Orwell, *Homage to Catalonia*, 182.
25. Jolly, *Field Surgery in Total War*, 110.
26. Jolly, *Field Surgery in Total War*, 189.
27. Jolly, *Field Surgery in Total War*, 167.
28. Jolly, *Field Surgery in Total War*, 191–92.

29. Dr. G. Gordon-Taylor, quoted in Jolly, *Field Surgery in Total War*, v; and publisher's blurb for Jolly, *Field Surgery in Total War*.
30. Jolly, *Field Surgery in Total War*, 6.
31. Jolly, *Field Surgery in Total War*, 6, 190–91.
32. Lancet, 26 October 1940, 520.
33. Review, *Field Surgery in Total War*, in *Journal of the Royal Army Medical Corps*, 1 January 1941, 59–60.
34. "Surgical Experience in the Spanish Civil War," *British Medical Journal*, 26 October 1940, 560–61.
35. Jolly, *Field Surgery in Total War*, 2nd ed., dust jacket.
36. Komrower, "Obituary, Douglas Waddell Jolly," 798.
37. *Annals of Surgery* 113, no. 6 (June 1941): 1120.
38. Churchill, *Surgeon to Soldiers*, 90–93.
39. Pike, "Contributions to Military Medicine."
40. Bricknell, "Evolution of Casualty Evacuation," 168, 357.
41. Churchill, *Surgeon to Soldiers*, 90–93.
42. Shackleton, *Desert Surgeons*, 48–49.
43. Welch, "War Wounds," 156–68.
44. Bricknell, "Evolution of Casualty Evacuation," 169–70.
45. Apel and Apel, "MASH in the Spanish Civil War," 1317–17.
46. Stealhy and Cannon, *Evolution of Forward Surgery*, 248.
47. Stealhy and Cannon, *Evolution of Forward Surgery*, 281–82.
48. Shackleton, *Operation Vietnam*; and Michael Shackelton, in-person communication with author, 16 April 2011.
49. Bricknell, "Evolution of Casualty Evacuation," 170–71.
50. Bricknell, "Evolution of Casualty Evacuation," 360.
51. Dunn, "East Timor," 810.
52. Shackleton, *Desert Surgeons*, 122–25.

13. THE TOBRUK PLASTER

1. Harrison, *Medicine and Victory*, 34.
2. *British Medical Journal*, 1 July 1939, 35.
3. Gunson and Dodsworth, "Fifty Years of Blood Transfusion," 65–67.
4. *British Medical Journal*, 7 October 1939, 73.
5. Ogilvie, "Surgical Advances," 21–22.
6. McLaughlin, *Royal Army Medical Corps*, 86–87.
7. Irene Grant to Karl Polanyi, 1 September 1940, con. 56, fol. 13, KPDA. Emphasis in original.
8. Tyrer, *Sisters in Arms*, 149–55.
9. Shackleton, *Desert Surgeons*, 40.

10. Shackleton, *Desert Surgeons*, 47–48.
11. Fred Bowerbank quoted in Shackleton, *Desert Surgeons*, 49–50.
12. S. Wilson to I. Wilson, 26 April 1941, Shackleton Family Collection, Wellington, NZ.
13. Edwards, "Contribution of War," 243.
14. Shackleton, *Desert Surgeons*, 58–62.
15. Shackleton, *Desert Surgeons*, 70.
16. Shackleton, *Desert Surgeons*, 89–94.
17. Shackleton, *Desert Surgeons*, 122.
18. *NZEF* [New Zealand Expeditionary Force] *Times* 1, no. 28 (5 January 1942): 1.
19. Shackleton, *Desert Surgeons*, 52–53.
20. Shackleton, *Desert Surgeons*, 125.
21. Stanley Wilson quoted in Shackleton, *Desert Surgeons*, 116–17.
22. Cole, "First Half-Century," 723.
23. Geer, *Mercy in Hell*, location 891.
24. McLaughlin, *Royal Army Medical Corps*, 65–67.
25. McLaughlin, *Royal Army Medical Corps*, 73.
26. Ross, "Traumatic Surgery," 17–18.
27. Geer, *Mercy in Hell*, location 1017.
28. Preston, "Two Doctors," 22.
29. Harrison, *Medicine and Victory*, 35.
30. Ogilvie, "Surgical Advances," 21–22.
31. Fraser, "Penicillin," 1724.
32. Quoted in Harrison, *Medicine and Victory*, 116–17.
33. Fraser, "Doctor's Debt," 68–69.
34. Ross, "Traumatic Surgery," 19–20.
35. Fraser, "Doctor's Debt," 68–69.
36. Bricknell, "Evolution of Casualty Evacuation," 317.
37. Geer, *Mercy in Hell*, location 891.
38. Geer, *Mercy in Hell*, location 998.
39. Beevor, *Second World War*, 224.
40. Harrison, *Medicine and Victory*, 109.
41. Marnham, "Tobruk Plaster," 281–82.
42. D. Jolly to Fredericka Martin, 29 January 1972, Imperial War Museum, London.
43. Harrison, *Medicine and Victory*, 112; and Watts, *Surgeon at War*, 32.
44. Stout, *New Zealand Medical Services*, 264–65.
45. Churchill, *Annals of Surgery*, 271.
46. Churchill, *Annals of Surgery*, 282–83.
47. McLaughlin, *Royal Army Medical Corps*, 69.
48. McLaughlin, *Royal Army Medical Corps*, 73.

49. Churchill, *Surgeon to Soldiers*, 90–93.

14. MERRY HELL

1. McLaughlin, *Royal Army Medical Corps*, 89.
2. Stallard, "War Surgery of the Eye," 111.
3. Jolly to American nurse, Imperial War Museum, London, 35–36.
4. Quoted in Tyrer, *Sisters in Arms*, 159–60.
5. Quoted in Rhodes-Wood, *War History*, 187–88.
6. D. Jolly to Irene Grant, 4 September 1942, Núala Grant Collection, Hocken Library.
7. Bricknell, "Evolution of Casualty Evacuation," 318.
8. Ogilvie, "Surgical Advances," 261.
9. D. Jolly to Irene Grant, 22 November 1942, Núala Grant Collection, Hocken Library.
10. D. Jolly to Irene Grant, 10 January 1943, Núala Grant Collection, Hocken Library.
11. Lesch, *First Miracle Drugs*, 240.
12. Ross, "Memoirs," 34–35.
13. Stammers, "Influence of Environment," 555.
14. Harrison, *Medicine and Victory*, 157.
15. Prof. Florey quoted in Fraser, "Doctor's Debt to the Soldier," ref. RAMC/826.
16. Harrison, *Medicine and Victory*, 156.
17. Florey and Abraham, "Work on Penicillin," 311.
18. Conniff, *Penicillin*.
19. Frøland, *Duel without End*, 512.
20. Record no. WO-373-77-349, War Office, London.
21. D. Jolly to Irene Grant, January 1943, Núala Grant Collection, Hocken Library.
22. Wiltse, *Medical Department*, 553–54.
23. Fraser, "Penicillin," 1725.
24. Fraser, "Penicillin," 1725.
25. Bennett, "Medical Support," 22.
26. Cameron, "Medical Services, Eighth Army," 12–18, emphasis in original; and Ogilvie, "Surgical Advances," 262.
27. Col. L. M. Rowlette, Special Order of the Day, 26 October 1943, BJC.
28. Komrower, "Military Medicine in Italy," 25.
29. Quoted in Bowerbank, *Doctor's Story*, 271–72.
30. McLaughlin, *Royal Army Medical Corps*, 82.
31. Bennett, "Medical Support," 23.
32. Longstaff, oral history interview, Imperial War Museum (see chap. 10, note 68). Note: In this interview, Longstaff misidentifies the Spanish hospital where Jolly treated him as Mataró in Barcelona. His memory here is incorrect, probably because, with his eyes bandaged, in shock from his wound, and later heavily sedated, his

awareness of his surroundings was understandably faulty. I am grateful to Linda Palfreeman for pointing out this factual error in Longstaff's recorded recollections.

33. Longstaff, oral history interview, Imperial War Museum.
34. John Longstaff, "Any Bread, Mister," unpublished memoir, n.d., Duncan Longstaff collection.
35. Ross, "Memoirs," 35–36.
36. Edwards, "Contribution of War," 242–43.
37. Harrison, *Medicine and Victory*, 165.
38. Bricknell, "Evolution of Casualty Evacuation," 315.
39. Poole, "Army Progress with Penicillin," 111.
40. Harrison, *Medicine and Victory*, 170.
41. Edwards, "Contribution of War," 241.
42. Congress of CMF Army Surgeons, Rome, *Proceedings*, held in D. Jolly papers, BJC.
43. Derby, *Petal and Bullets*, 144.
44. Brig. H. Edwards to D. Jolly, 10 November 1945, BJC.

15. PHANTOM PAIN

1. Elizabeth Jolly to Doug Jolly, London, 30 July 1946, BJC.
2. In writing her letter, Anna-Mária referred to her son's name, János, with the French equivalent. A-M. Basch, Brussels, to D. Jolly, London, 9 April 1946, BJC. Translation from French by John Jamieson.
3. A-M. Basch, Brussels, to D. Jolly, London, 9 April 1946, BJC. Translation from French by John Jamieson. Emphasis in original.
4. International Tracing Service Digital Archive, Bad Arolsen: Subcollection: 1.1.35.1, Document ID: 3765989—List material Ravensbrück.
5. International Tracing Service Digital Archive, Bad Arolsen: Subcollection: 1.1.9.11, Document ID: 11187079—List material Gurs; and Subcollection: 1.1.9.1, Document ID: 11182695—List material BdS France.
6. A-M. Basch, Brussels to D. Jolly, London, 9 April 1946, BJC.
7. A-M. Basch, Brussels to D. Jolly, London, 9 April 1946, BJC.
8. *Volunteer* (Journal of the Veterans of the Abraham Lincoln Brigade) 2 (1979): 4.
9. Franz Kriegel, Prague, to D. W. Jolly, London, 30 October 1946, BJC.
10. Stewart, "'Finest Municipal Hospital Service,'" 330; and Desmond Painter, email to author, 20 November 2022.
11. Rivett, "Health Care before the NHS."
12. Royal Cancer Hospital, *Royal Cancer Hospital*, 9.
13. Komrower, "Obituary, Douglas Waddell Jolly," 298.
14. Cope, *Royal College of Surgeons*, 192–93.
15. Cope, *Royal College of Surgeons*, 196–97; and Jones, *Annals*, 238.

16. Brig. W. H. Ogilvie, "Report by Consultant Surgeon MEF for the Period 1 Sep. to 31 March 1943," 12 May 1943, GHQ MEF, p. 5, WO 222/1291, UK National Archives, London. The meaning of the acronym "CDO" is not known to the author.
17. Beasley, *Mantle of Surgery*, 15.
18. Irene Grant to Karl Polanyi, 29 May 1947, KPDA.
19. Cochrane and Blythe, *One Man's Medicine*, 42.
20. D. W. Jolly, unpublished autobiographical notes, BJC.
21. Certificate of title, vol. 4, folio 87, Cromwell Museum Archive, Cromwell, NZ.
22. Barbara Jolly, in-person communication with author, 11 June 2018.
23. *Otago Daily Times*, 10 December 1947, 4.
24. Eunice E. Frost, Penguin Books, to D. W. Jolly, 24 November 1950, BJC.
25. D. W. Jolly to secretary, World Health Organization, Geneva, 16 May 1950; secretary, Nuffield Foundation, to D. W. Jolly, 25 October 1950; A. Landsborough-Thompson, Medical Research Council, to D. W. Jolly, 3 August 1950; and I. Harvey-Flack, *British Medical Journal*, to D. W. Jolly, 1 June 1950—all in BJC.
26. Dale, *Karl Polanyi*, 17.
27. D. Jolly to Karl Polanyi, 27 July 1947, con. 48, fol. 2, KPDA.
28. D. Jolly to Karl Polanyi, 9 September 1947, con. 48, fol. 2, KPDA.
29. D. Jolly to Karl Polanyi, 28 September 1947, con. 48, fol. 2, KPDA. Emphasis in original.
30. Karl Polanyi to Irene Grant, undated but probably 1952, con. 56, fol. 13, KPDA.
31. D. Jolly to Stan and Mollie Jolly, 12 June 1950, BJC. Emphasis in original.
32. D. Jolly to K. Polanyi, 22 August 1950, con. 56, fol. 14, p. 37, KPDA.
33. "Otago Soldiers' Graves near Armentieres," *Otago Daily Times*, 23 October 1950.
34. Weedon et al., *History of Queen Mary's Hospital*, 16–18.
35. Weedon et al., *History of Queen Mary's Hospital*, 29.
36. D. Jolly to Karl Polanyi, 22 August 1950, con. 56, fol. 13, KPDA.
37. "Limb-Fitting History Sheet, 1951," BJC.
38. Quoted in Derby, *Kiwi Compañeros*, 133.
39. H02/QM/A/12/002, Garden party, receptions and other functions, 1960 Dec.–1966 Aug., Queen Mary Hospital records, London Metropolitan Archives.
40. J. G. H. Newfield to D. Jolly, 8 July 1953, BJC.
41. D. Jolly to "To whom it may concern," n.d., BJC.
42. G. Newfield to D. Jolly, 8 August 1953, BJC.
43. D. Jolly to E. Simpson, 1 February 1956, MS 959/418, special collections, Leeds University Library.
44. D. Jolly to Karl Polanyi, 27 July 1947, con. 48, fol. 2, KPDA.
45. David Edmonds, "Esther Simpson—the Unknown Heroine," *Jewish Chronicle* (online ed.), 11 May 2017.

16. LIGHT IN THE DARKNESS

Epigraph: Goodwin and Redfield Jamison, *Manic-Depressive Illness*, 869.

1. Costello, *John Macmurray*, 4.
2. K. Wintringham to D. Jolly, 14 November 1965, BJC.
3. Jay Kain to D. Jolly, 26 October 1959, BJC.
4. Jay Kain to D. Jolly, 9 February 1960 and 12 February 1960, BJC.
5. A-M. Basch to D. Jolly, 17 March 1960, BJC. Translation from French by John Jamieson.
6. Lemesle, "Basch, Anne-Marie."
7. *Mitteilungsblatt der Österreichischen Lagergemeinschaft*, no. 12 (November 1974).
8. Desmond Painter, email to author, 20 November 2022.
9. Weedon et al., *History of Queen Mary's Hospital*, 35.
10. D. W. Jolly, in "A Symposium on the Wheelchair," 20 November 1963, London, 24, BJC.
11. "British Orthopaedic Association," 188.
12. D. Jolly, unpublished lecture notes on "Society and the Amputee," n.d., BJC.
13. D. Jolly to Sir G. Godber, 28 September 1968, BJC.
14. Sir George Godber, Ministry of Health, to D. Jolly, 30 August 1968, BJC.
15. Marriage certificate, Hampstead registry office, 3 April 1968, BJC.
16. Mann and Co., estate agents, E. Horsley, 17 July 1968, BJC.
17. A-M. Basch, Budapest, to D. Jolly, 21 December 1968, BJC.
18. D. Jolly to Sir George Godber, 28 September 1968, BJC.
19. Rudnytsky and Preston, *Her Hour Come Round*, 15.
20. Rudnytsky and Preston, *Her Hour Come Round*, 173.
21. Rudnytsky and Preston, *Her Hour Come Round*, 80.
22. Psychiatrist's report, Dr. Nina Coltart, 7 September 1968, BJC.
23. Psychiatrist's report, Dr. Nina Coltart, 7 September 1968, BJC.
24. Coltart, *How to Survive*, 100.
25. Medication schedule, D. Jolly, BJC.
26. Goodwin and Jamison, *Manic-Depressive Illness*, 869.
27. Goodwin and Jamison, *Manic-Depressive Illness*, 34.
28. Dr. Kay Jamison, telephone communication with author, 6 April 2022.
29. Quoted in Derby, *Kiwi Compañeros*, 133.
30. Irene Grant to D. Jolly, 4 February 1972, BJC.
31. Jacqui O'Donnell, telephone communication with author, 1 June 2021.
32. Barbara Jolly, telephone communication with author, 11 June 2018.
33. Allan Jolly, telephone communication with author, 10 September 2019.
34. Joanna Jones to W. Alexander, 13 April 1983, BJC.
35. Julian Davies, notes for plaque unveiling ceremony, Cromwell, Central Otago, 23 March 2018, BJC.
36. Julian Davies, telephone communication with author, 8 May 2022.

37. Joanna Kain, notes for plaque unveiling ceremony, Cromwell, Central Otago, 23 March 2018, BJC.
38. Joanna Kain per Julian Davies, telephone communication with author, 8 May 2022.
39. D. Jolly to Fredericka Martin, 29 May 1970, BJC.
40. D. Jolly to Fredericka Martin, 24 September 1970, BJC.
41. D. Jolly to Fredericka Martin, 29 January 1972, BJC.
42. Bill Alexander, International Brigade Association, London, to D. W. Jolly, n.d., BJC.
43. Barbara Jolly to Jay Jolly, 8 October 1982, BJC.
44. Social Services Department, West Sussex County Council, to D. W. Jolly, 29 April 1983, BJC.
45. W. Alexander to Joanna Jones, 8 April 1983, BJC.
46. Joanna Jones to W. Alexander, 13 April 1983, BJC.
47. Fredericka Martin to D. Jolly, 13 September 1983, BJC.
48. Joanna Jones to Fredericka Martin, 9 December 1983, BJC.
49. Death certificate, D. W. Jolly, 19 December 1983, BJC.
50. Death notice, D. W. Jolly, *Morning Star*, BJC.
51. Peter de Sarigny to Joanna Jones, 24 December 1983, BJC.

17. SAVING FROM SUBMERSION

Epigraph: D. Jolly, 28 January 1937, personal letter, Marx Memorial Library.

1. Title deed information for certificate of title, vol. 4, fol. 87, Cromwell Museum Archives.
2. Sydney, *Promised Land*, 150.
3. Adams, "Douglas Waddell Jolly," 253–56.
4. Cochrane and Blythe, *One Man's Medicine*, 42; and interview with Alexander Tudor-Hart, accession no. 13771, Sound Archives, Imperial War Museum.
5. Costello, *James Macmurray*, 1.
6. Kuttner, "Man from Red Vienna," 55–57.
7. Joseph Stiglitz, foreword to Polanyi, *Great Transformation*.
8. Jordi Martí-Rueda, email to author, 29 January 2021.
9. Ciuró, "Ciuró."
10. Derby, *Kiwi Compañeros*.
11. Desmond Painter, email to author, 20 November 2022.

BIBLIOGRAPHY

ARCHIVES AND MANUSCRIPT MATERIALS

Archives New Zealand (NZ) Te Rua Mahara o te Kāwanatanga, Wellington.
Archivo General Militar de Ávila, Spain.
Carrit, Noel. Papers. Spanish Collection SC/VOL/NCA/2. Marx Memorial Library, London.
Cromwell Museum Archive, Cromwell, NZ.
Cserháti, Éva. Collection. Budapest.
Grant, Núala. Collection. Hocken Library Uare Taoka o Hākena, Otago University, Dunedin, NZ.
Imperial War Museum. London.
International Brigades Memorial Trust, London.
International Tracing Service Digital Archive, Bad Arolsen, Germany.
Jolly, Barbara. Collection. Auckland, NZ.
Jones, Bidda. Collection. Hocken Library Uare Taoka o Hākena, Otago University, Dunedin, NZ.
Leeds University Library, Special Collections, Leeds, UK.
London Metropolitan Archives.
Martin, Fredericka. Papers. ALBA.001. Tamiment Library and Robert F. Wagner Labor Archive, New York University.
Marx Memorial Library, London.
NZ Student Christian Movement. Papers. Alexander Turnbull Library, Wellington, NZ.
Polanyi, Karl. Digital Archive. Concordia University, Quebec.
Polyani, Michael. Papers. University of Chicago Library.
RGASPI (Russian State Archive of Socio-Political History), Moscow.
Shackleton Family. Collection. Wellington, NZ.
Sinclair-Loutit, Kenneth. Papers. SC/IND/JFY/2/1/7, SC Collection. Marx Memorial Library, London.
Special Collections Research Center, University of Chicago.
Svenska Spanienfrivilligas Vänner (Friends of Swedish Spain Volunteers). Stockholm, Sweden.
UK National Archives, London.

UK War Office, London.
Wellington Medical History Association, NZ. In Archives NZ, Wellington.

PUBLISHED WORKS

Adams, D. B. "Douglas Waddell Jolly as a Pioneer in the Surgical Treatment of Trauma." *Surgery, Gynecology and Obstetrics* 171 (September 1990): 253–56.

Aitken, Alexander. *Gallipoli to the Somme: Recollections of a New Zealand Infantryman.* London: Oxford University Press, 1963.

Allan, Norman. *Ted Allan: A Life.* Online biography. http://www.normanallan.com/Misc/Ted/nT%20ch%202.htm. Last accessed 17 January 2023.

Allan, Ted, and Sydney Gordon. *The Scalpel, the Sword: The Story of Doctor Norman Bethune.* Voyageur Classics. Toronto: Dundurn Press, 2009. First published by Monthly Review Press, 1952.

Alternês, Serge, and Alec Wainman. *Almas vivas: La Guerra Civil Española en imágenes.* Lleida, Spain: Milenio Publicaciones, 2017.

ARMH (Association for the Recovery in Historical Memory) Cuenca. *Red Tarancón: Spaniards and Internationals in a Tarancón at War.* Tarancón: ARMH Cuenca, 2022.

Arnold, T. J., J. O. Lucas, G. H. Fairmaid, M. G. McInnes, and W. J. Patrick. *Centennial Publication: Otago Boys' High School Old Boys' Register.* Dunedin, NZ: Otago High School Old Boys' Society (Inc.), 1963.

Arthur, Max. *The Real Band of Brothers: First-hand Accounts from the last British Survivors of the Spanish Civil War.* London: Collins, 2009.

Austin, Lt. Col. W. S. *Official History of New Zealand Rifle Brigade.* Wellington, NZ: L. T. Watkins, 1924.

Barber, L. H., and R. J. Towers. *Wellington Hospital, 1847–1976.* Wellington, NZ: Wellington Hospital Board, 1976.

Barnes, Kenneth, et al. *Towards a Quaker View of Sex.* Rev. ed. London: Friends Home Service Committee, London, 1964.

Basch, Anna-Mária. "Harc az élert" (1959). In *Magyar önkéntesek a spanyol nép szabadságharcában,* edited by Imre Kepes. Budapest: Zrínyi Katonai Kiadó, 1987. ("A Fight for Life," unpaged, translated from Hungarian by Mary Mowbray.)

Baxell, Richard. "The British Battalion of the International Brigades in the Spanish Civil War 1936–1939." PhD thesis, University of London, 2001.

———. *The Unlikely Warriors: The British in the Spanish Civil War and the Struggle against Fascism.* London: Aurum Press, 2012.

Beasley, A. W. *The Mantle of Surgery: The First Seventy-Five Years of the Royal Australasian College of Surgeons.* Melbourne: Royal Australasian College of Surgeons, 2002.

Beevor, A. *The Battle for Spain: The Spanish Civil War, 1936–1939*. London: Phoenix, 2006.
———. *The Second World War*. London: Weidenfeld & Nicolson, 2012.
Bell, Sir Francis Gordon. *Surgeon's Saga*. Wellington, NZ: A. H. and A. W. Reed, 1968.
Bennett, J. D. C. "Abdominal Surgery in War—the Early Story." *Journal of the Royal Society of Medicine* 84 (September 1991).
———. "Medical Support for the British Eighth Army in Italy during World War II." *Army History* no. 42 (Summer 1977).
Berry, Christine. *The New Zealand Student Christian Movement, 1896–1996: A Centennial History*. Wellington: Student Christian Movement Aotearoa, 1999.
Bessie, Alvah. *Men in Battle*. California: Chandler and Sharp Publishers, 1975. First published by Scribner's, 1939 (New York).
Betts, F. M. *Celebrating a Century, 1865–1965: A History of the Cromwell and Consolidated Schools of Lowburn and Kawarau Gorge: Centennial Celebrations, January 29, 30, 31 1965*. Dunedin, NZ: Printed by the *Otago Daily Times*, 1965.
Bingham de Urquidi, Mary. *Mercy in Madrid: Nursing and Humanitarian Protection during the Spanish Civil War, 1936–37*. Translated by Magdalena Urquidi Bingham. Lanús, Argentina: Ediciones del Sur, 2004. First published as *Misericordia en Madrid* by B. Costa-Amic, 1975 (Mexico).
Bowerbank, Sir Fred. *A Doctor's Story*. Wellington, NZ: Wingfield Press, 1958.
Bricknell, M. C. M. "The Evolution of Casualty Evacuation in the British Army in the 20th Century." Pt. 2. *Journal of the Royal Army Medical Corps* 148 (2002).
"British Orthopaedic Association—Annual Meeting, 1964." *Journal of Bone and Joint Surgery*. 1964.
Brittain, Vera. *The Rebel Passion: A Short History of Some Pioneer Peace-Makers*. London: George Allen & Unwin, 1964.
Broggi, Moisès. *Memorias de un cirujano*. Barcelona: Ediciones Península, 2001.
Browne, J. S. "Anaesthesia and the Spanish Civil War: The Delivery of Anaesthetic Care in a Divided Spain." *History of Anaesthesia Society Proceedings* 46 (2013).
———. "Anaesthetics and the Spanish Civil War: The Start of Specialisation." *European Journal of Anaesthesiology* no. 31 (2014).
Browne, Sebastian. *Medicine and Conflict: The Spanish Civil War and Its Traumatic Legacy*. London: Routledge/Cañada Blanch Studies on Contemporary Spain, 2019.
Brunton, Warwick. *The Medicine of the Future: A History of the Department of Preventative and Social Medicine, University of Otago, 1886–2011*. Dunedin, NZ: Department of Preventative and Social Medicine, University of Otago, 2011.
Burns, Dr. C. R. "Post-Graduate Study." *Digest, Annual Publication of the Medical School, University of Otago* 1, no. 1 (October 1934).
Cameron, Brig. W. M. "Medical Services, Eighth Army: Lessons of the Italian Campaign, 10 July 1943–2 May 1945." RAMC/1321, Royal Army Medical Corps

Muniments, Wellcome Collection, 12–18. Accessed 27 November 2021. https://wellcomecollection.org/works/nd5t439y.

Capa, Robert. *Death in the Making: Reexamining the Iconic Spanish Civil War Photobook*. Bologna: Damiani/International Centre for Photography, facsimile ed., 2020. First published 1938 by Covici Friede (New York).

Carrió, Ricardo Sola. *Diario personal: Julio 1936 Diciembre (Barcelona)—Batalla del Ebro, Barcelona*. Barcelona: E. M., 1978.

Chisholm, Frederick R. "The Otago Medical School 50 Years Ago: Being Dr. Chisholm's Recollections, from His First Year in 1923 to the Finish of His Term as Medical Tutor in 1933." Unpublished manuscript, 1980, Hocken Library, Dunedin.

Churchill, Col. Edward D. *Annals of Surgery* 120, no. 3 (September 1944).

———. *Surgeon to Soldiers: Diary and Records of the Surgical Consultant, Allied Force Headquarters, World War II*. Philadelphia: J. B. Lippincott, 1972.

Ciuró, Lourdes. "Ciuró: 'Volem tancar el dol però no oblidar ni les persones ni els fets que van causar tant dolor'" ("Ciuró: 'We want to close the mourning but not forget either the people or the events that caused so much pain'"). Govern.Cat (Catalan Government website), May 8, 2022. https://govern.cat/salapremsa/notes-premsa/421084/ciuro-volem-tancar-el-dol-pero-no-oblidar-ni-les-persones-ni-els-fets-que-van-causar-tant-dolor. Translation within website.

Clarke, Alison. *A Living Tradition: A Centennial History of Knox College*. Dunedin, NZ: Knox College, 2009.

Cochrane, A. L., and M. Blythe. *One Man's Medicine: An Autobiography of Professor Archie Cochrane*. London: Cardiff University, 1989.

Cole, D. "The First Half-Century of the College [of Surgeons, Australasia] in New Zealand." *Australian and New Zealand Journal of Surgery* 47 no. 6 (December 1977).

Colodny, R. G. *The Struggle for Madrid: The Central Epic of the Spanish Conflict, 1936–1937*. London: Routledge, 2009.

Coltart, Nina. *How to Survive as a Pyschotherapist*. Lanham MD: Jason Aronson, 1993.

Congress of CMF [Congress of Central Mediterranean Forces] Army Surgeons. *Proceedings of the Congress of CMF Army Surgeons*. Rome: British Military Printing Press, February 1945.

Coni, Nicholas. "Medicine and the Spanish Civil War." *Journal of the Royal Society of Medicine* 95 (March 2002).

———. *Medicine and Warfare: Spain, 1936–1939*. London: Routledge/Cañada Blanch Studies in Contemporary Spain, 2008.

Conniff, Richard. "Penicillin: Wonder Drug of World War II." Historynet, March 7, 2017. https://www.historynet.com/penicillin-wonder-drug-world-war-ii.htm.

Cope, Zachary. *The Royal College of Surgeons of England: A History*. London: Anthony Blond, 1959.

Cooper, R. M. *Refugee Scholars: Conversations with Tess Simpson*. Leeds: Moorland Books, 1992.

Costello, John E. *John Macmurray: A Biography*. Edinburgh: Floris Books, 2002.

Cox, Geoffrey. *Defence of Madrid: An Eyewitness Account from the Spanish Civil War*. Dunedin, NZ: Otago University Press, 2007. First published 1937 by Victor Gollancz (London).

Cromwell Schools Jubilee Committee. *Celebrating 125 Years of Education, 1865–1990, in the Cromwell Area: A History of the Bannockburn, Cromwell, Kawarau Gorge, Lowburn, Nevis and St John's Schools*. Cromwell Schools Jubilee Committee, 1990.

Dale, Gareth. *Karl Polanyi: A Life on the Left*. New York: Columbia University Press, 2016.

Derby, Mark, ed. *Kiwi Compañeros: New Zealand and the Spanish Civil War*. Christchurch: Canterbury University Press, 2009. Translated by Cristina Gómez de la Torre Curt as *Compañeros <Kiwis>: Nueva Zelanda y la Españo civil española* (Ediciones de la Universidad de Castilla-La Mancha, 2011).

———. *Petal and Bullets—Dorothy Morris: New Zealand Nurse in the Spanish Civil War*. Eastbourne, UK: Sussex Academic Press, 2015.

Derby, Mark, and David Jorge. "Moisès Broggi i Vallès (1908–2012): Military Surgeon and Catalan Humanitarian." *Journal of Medical Biography* 24, no. 1 (2016): 23–29.

Diario oficial del Ministerio de Defensa Nacional, no. 71 (24 March 1938): 850.

Don, Alexander. *Memories of the Golden Road: A History of the Presbyterian Church in Central Otago*. Wellington, NZ: A. H. and A. W. Reed, 1936.

Dougherty, Ian. *Dunedin: Founding a New World City*. Dunedin, NZ: Saddle Hill Press, 2007.

Dow, Derek A. "Hercus, Charles Ernest." *Dictionary of New Zealand Biography*, 1998. Reprinted in *Te Ara, the Encyclopedia of New Zealand*. Accessed 20 June 2020. https://teara.govt.nz/en/biographies/4h28/hercus-charles-ernest.

Dunn, Andrew C. "East Timor: The Work of the New Zealand Forward Surgical Team from 1999 to 2000." *Military Medicine* 167, no. 10 (October 2002).

Eby, C. D. *Comrades and Commissars: The Lincoln Battalion in the Spanish Civil War*. University Park: Penn State University Press, 2007.

Edwards, Hon. Col. Harold C. "The Contribution of War to the Advancement of Surgery." *Journal of the Royal Army Medical Corps*, no. 102 (1956).

Esteve Torres, Isabel. "Benicàssim (1937–1938)—A través de los recuerdos de brigadistas alemanes." Valencia: Asociación de Amigos de las Brigadas Internacionales, 2014.

Fernández Suárez, Roberto. *Fuencarral durante la 2ª República, la guerra civil y el primer Franquismo*. UNED, 29 September 2018. https://issuu.com/sierracultura/docs/la_guerra_civil_y_el_primer_franqui.

Florey, H. W., and E. P. Abraham. "The Work on Penicillin at Oxford." *Journal of the History of Medicine and Allied Sciences* 6, no. 3 (Summer 1951).

Fraser, Brig. Sir Ian. "The Doctor's Debt to the Soldier." *Journal of the Royal Army Medical Corps* 118, no. 2 (1972). Available in Royal Army Medical Corps Muniments Collection, ref. RAMC/826, https://wellcomecollection.org/works/k5jds4az.

———. "Penicillin: Early Trials in War Casualties." *British Medical Journal* 289 (22–29 December 1984).

Frøland, Stig S. *Duel without End: Mankind's Battle with Microbes*. London: Reaktion Books, 2022.

Fuster Ruiz, F. *El servicio de sanidad de las Brigadas Internacionales*. Albacete: Edicones de la Universidad de Castilla–La Mancha, 2018.

Fyrth, J. *The Signal Was Spain: The Spanish Aid Movement in Britain, 1936–39*. New York: St. Martin's Press, 1986.

Fyrth, Jim, and Sally Alexander. *Women's Voices from the Spanish Civil War*. London: Lawrence Wishart, 1991.

Fyvel, Penelope (Penny Phelps). *English Penny*. Ilfracombe, Devon: Arthur Stockwell, 1992.

Geer, Capt. Andrew. *Mercy in Hell: An American Ambulance Driver with the Eighth Army*. Kindle ed. London: Arcole Publishing, 2017. First published by Whittlesey House, 1943 (New York).

General Medical Council, comp. *UK Medical Registers, 1859–1959*. London: General Medical Council, 1859–1959.

Gettelmann, M. E. "Robert G. Colodny: The Struggle against Fascism at Home and Abroad." *Science and Society* 68, no. 3 (Fall 2004): 263–71.

Goodwin, Frederick K., and Kay Redfield Jamison. *Manic-Depressive Illness: Bipolar Disorders and Recurrent Depression*. 2nd ed. New York: Oxford University Press, 2007.

"Gordon-Taylor, Sir Gordon (1878–1960)." In *Plarr's Lives of the Fellows*. London: Royal College of Surgeons of England, March 7, 2008. https://livesonline.rcseng.ac.uk/client/en_GB/lives/search/results?qu=Gordon-Taylor&te=ASSET.

Gosling, G. C. *Payment and Philanthropy in British Healthcare, 1918–48*. Manchester: Manchester University Press, 2017.

Green, Nan. *A Chronicle of Small Beer: The Memoirs of Nan Green (Radical Recoveries)*. Nottingham: Trent University, 2005.

Gunson, H. H., and H. Dodsworth. "Fifty Years of Blood Transfusion." *Transfusion Medicine* 6, supp. 1 (1996).

Haldane, J. B. S. *A.R.P.* London: Victor Gollancz, 1938.

Hannant, Larry, ed. *The Politics of Passion: Norman Bethune's Writing and Art*. Toronto: University of Toronto Press, 1998.

Harding Rains, A. J. "The Hand Physician: An Historical Perspective of Surgical Training, the FRCS, and Specialism." *Annals of the Royal College of Surgeons of England* 54 (1974).

Harrison, Mark. *Medicine and Victory: British Military Medicine in the Second World War*. Oxford: Oxford University Press, 2004.

Heijnis-Mens, Saskia, and Seran de Leede. "Diamant, Noor." In International Institute for Social Research, *Nedelandse vrijwilloigers in de Spaanse Burgeroorlog* [Dutch volunteers in the Spanish Civil War]. September 8, 2017. https://spanjestrijders.nl/bio/diamant-noor.

Hercus, C. "The Eightieth Anniversary of the Otago Medical School." *NZ Medical Journal* 54, no. 300 (April 1955).

———. "The OUMC." In *The First Fifty Years: A Commentary on the Development of the Royal New Zealand Army Medical Corps from Its Inception in 1908*, edited by Medical Section, NZ Army Headquarters. Wellington, NZ: Medical Section, NZ Army Headquarters, 1958.

Hollós, Alfréd, and Katalin Jalsovszky. "Magyar önkéntesek a spanyol polgárháborúban" [Hungarian volunteers in the Spanish Civil War] (Fényképkatalógus). *Magyar Munkásmozgalmi Múzeum Évkönyve*. Budapest: Múzsák Közm?velési Kiadó, 1983.

Jackson, Angela. *At the Margins of Mayhem: Prologue and Epilogue to the Last Great Battle of the Spanish Civil War*. Torfaen, Wales: Warren and Pell, 2008.

———. *Beyond the Battlefield: Testimony, Memory and Remembrance of a Cave Hospital in the Spanish Civil War*. Torfaen, Wales: Warren and Pell, 2005.

———. *"For Us It Was Heaven": The Passion, Grief and Fortitude of Patience Darton, from the Spanish Civil War to Mao's China*. Eastbourne, UK: Sussex Academic Press, 2012.

Jirku, Gusti. *We Fight Death: The Work of the Medical Service of the International Brigades in Spain*. Madrid: Rivadeneyra, 1937.

Johnson, Ashley. "Healing the Wounds of Fascism: The American Medical Brigade and the Spanish Civil War." BA honors thesis, Mount Holyoke College, 2007.

Jolly, D. "Emergency Abdominal Surgery: Its Significance in an Antifascist Army." *Ayuda Médica Internacional*, no. 7 (April 1938): 10. Marx Memorial Library, London.

———. *Field Surgery in Total War*. London: Hamish Hamilton, 1940.

Jones, Carmalt. *Annals of the University of Otago Medical School, 1875–1939*. Wellington, NZ: Reed, 1945.

Keene, Judith. "A Spanish Springtime." *Labour History* (Liverpool University Press), no. 52 (May 1987).

Kellaway, J., and M. Maryan. *A Century of Care: Palmerston North Hospital, 1893–1993*. Double Bay, Australia: Focus Books, 1993.

Komrower, Lt. Col. G. M. "Military Medicine in Italy: Analysis of One Year's Work in a Medical Division." *Journal of the Royal Army Medical Corps*, no. 87 (1946).

———. "Obituary, Douglas Waddell Jolly." *British Medical Journal* 288 (1984): 298.

Kuttner, Robert. "The Man from Red Vienna." *New York Review of Books*, 21 December 2017, 55–57.
Laytham, P., and E. Laytham. *The Cromwell Gorge: An Historical Guide*. Cromwell: Cromwell and Districts Promotion Group, 1995.
Le Couteur, Claire Elizabeth. "Dentist, Doctor, Dean: Professor Sir Charles Hercus and His Record of Fostering Research at the Otago Medical School, 1921–1958." PhD thesis, University of Canterbury, 2013.
Lemesle, Hervé. "Basch, Anne-Marie." *Le Maitron—dictionnaire biographique mouvement ouvrier, mouvement social* [Biographical dictionary of the social labour movement], 17 December 2019. Revised 3 January 2022. https://maitron.fr/spip.php?article221238.
Lesch, John E. *The First Miracle Drugs: How the Sulfa Drugs Transformed Medicine*. London: Oxford University Press, 2007.
Lethbridge, David. *Norman Bethune in Spain: Commitment, Crisis, and Conspiracy*. Eastbourne, UK: Sussex Academic Press, 2013.
Lewis, John, Karl Polanyi, and Donald Kitchin, eds. *Christianity and the Social Revolution*. London: Victor Gollancz, 1935.
Licence, Amy. *Living in Squares, Loving in Triangles: The Lives and Loves of Virginia Woolf and the Bloomsbury Group*. Stroud: Amberley Publishing, 2016.
Lustiger, Arno. *Schalom Libertad! Juden im spanischen Bürgerkrieg*. Berlin: Aufbau Taschenbuch, 2001. First published by Athenäum, 1989 (Frankfurt).
Macdonald Wilson, D. *A Hundred Years of Healing: Wellington Hospital, 1847–1947*. Wellington, NZ: A. H. and A. W. Reed, 1948.
Mangan, Kate. *Never More Alive: Inside the Spanish Republic*. London: Clapton Press, 2020.
Marnham, R. "The Tobruk Plaster." *Journal of the Royal Army Medical Corps* 85, no. 6 (1945).
Martin, Sylvia. *Ink in Her Veins: The Troubled Life of Aileen Palmer*. Perth: University of Western Australia Publishing, 2016.
Masip Gorgori, Enric. "La Cova Hospital de Santa Llúcia." *Això va Passar* [That happened] (blog), 3 July 2020. www.això-va-passar.eu/news/la-cova-hospital-de-santa-llucia/.
McEldowney, Dennis, ed. *Presbyterians in Aotearoa, 1840–1990*. Wellington, NZ: Presbyterian Church of New Zealand, 1990.
McLaughlin, Raymond. *The Royal Army Medical Corps*. Yorkshire: Leo Cooper, 1972.
Mitteilungsblatt der Österreichischen Lagergemeinschaft, no. 12 (November 1974).
Mottram, David W. "Shaping the Inheritance of the Spanish Civil War on the British Left, 1939–1945." PhD thesis, University of Manchester, 2017.
Muller, Gilbert H. *Hemingway and the Spanish Civil War: The Distant Sound of Battle*. Cham, Switzerland: Palgrave (Springer Nature), 2020.

Neugass, James. *War Is Beautiful: An American Ambulance Driver in the Spanish Civil War*. Edited by Peter N. Carroll and Peter Glazer. New York: New Press, 2008.
Newman, Charles. "The History of Postgraduate Medical Education at the West London Hospital." *Medical History* 4 (October 1966).
Ogilvie, W. H. "Surgical Advances during the War." *Journal of the Royal Army Medical Corps* 85, no. 6 (December 1945).
Orwell, George. *Homage to Catalonia*. New York: Penguin Books, 1984. First published by Secker and Warburg, 1938 (London).
Otago Settlers Association. "Otago's First Catastrophe on the Western Front." *Journey of the Otagos: Retracing the Steps of the Otago Infantry Regiment and Otago Mounted Rifles in WWI* (blog), 18 July 2016. https://journeyoftheotagos.wordpress.com/2016/07/18/otagos-first-catastrophe-on-the-western-front/.
Page, Dorothy. *Anatomy of a Medical School: A History of Medicine at the University of Otago, 1875–2000*. Dunedin, NZ: Otago University Press, 2008.
Palfreeman, Linda. *¡Salud! British Volunteers in the Republican Medical Service during the Spanish Civil War, 1936–1939*. Eastbourne, UK: Sussex Academic Press/Cañada Blanch Series on Contemporary Spain, 2012.
———. *Spain Bleeds: The Development of Battlefield Blood Transfusion during the Civil War.* Eastbourne, UK: Sussex Academic Press, 2016.
Parcell, James C. *Heart of the Desert*. Wellington, NZ: Whitcombe & Tombs, 1951.
Parry, Gordon. *Otago Medical School, 1875–1975—an Historical Sketch*. Dunedin, NZ: Medical School, University of Otago, 1975.
Petrou, Michael. *Renegades: Canadians in the Spanish Civil War*. Torfaen, Wales: Warren and Pell, 2008.
Pike, Dr. W. "Contributions to Military Medicine by Volunteers in the Spanish Civil War." *Volunteer* (organ of Veterans of the Abraham Lincoln Brigade) 4, no. 2 (1982).
Pinkerton, P. "Norman Bethune—and His Contribution to Blood Transfusion in War." *Transfusion Medicine Reviews* 21, no. 3 (July 2007): 255–64.
———. "Reginald Saxton: An Unlikely Pioneer of Battleground Transfusion." *Transfusion Medicine*, 2021, 3.
Polanyi, Karl. *The Great Transformation: The Political and Economic Origins of Our Time*. Boston: Beacon Press, 2001. First published by Farrar and Rinehart, 1944 (New York).
Poole, Maj.-Gen. L. T. "Army Progress with Penicillin." *British Journal of Surgery* 32, no. 125 (1944).
Powell, Margaret. "Notes from the Aragón Front." *The Volunteer* (newsletter of the International Brigades Memorial Trust), no. 27 (Autumn 2010): 9. First published in *British Nursing Journal*, April 1938.
Preston, Paul. *Doves of War: Four Women of Spain*. New York: HarperCollins, 2002.

———. "Two Doctors and One Cause: Len Crome and Reginald Saxton in the International Brigades." *International Journal of Iberian Studies* 19, no. 1 (2006).
———. *We Saw Spain Die: Foreign Correspondents in the Spanish Civil War*. London: Constable, 2008.
Pyke, V. *History of the Early Gold Discoveries in Otago*. Dunedin, NZ: *Otago Daily Times* and Witness Newspapers, 1887.
Raeburn, James Fraser George. "Hammering the World into Shape: Scottish Volunteers in the International Brigades, 1936–9." PhD thesis, University of Edinburgh, 2018.
Rhodes-Wood, Maj. E. H. *A War History of the Royal Pioneer Corps, 1939–1945*. Aldershot, UK: Gale and Polden, 1960.
Ricolas UK (Irene Grant's great-granddaughter). "Irene Grant and Brecht's Daughter." Soundcloud, sound recording, 2013. (Originally broadcast on BBC radio in the 1970s.) https://soundcloud.com/richard-rowe-4/irene-brechts-daughter.
Rivett, Geoffrey. *The Development of the London Hospital System, 1823–1982*. Historical Series No. 4. London: King Edward's Hospital Fund, 1986. https://www.nuffieldtrust.org.uk/sites/default/files/development-of-the-london-hospital-system-navigable-version.pdf.
———. "Health Care before the NHS." *From Cradle to Grave: The History of the NHS, 1948–1987*. London: Nuffield Trust, 2014. https://www.nuffieldtrust.org.uk/chapter/inheritance#hospital-services.
Robinson, R. G. "The Otago Medical School, 1875–1975." *British Medical Journal* 1 (1975).
Rogoyska, Jane. *Gerda Taro: Inventing Robert Capa*. London: Jonathon Cape, 2013.
Roman, Valter. *Bajo el cielo de España: Memorias de un brigadista internacional rumano*. Translated by J. L. Forneo. Zaragoza: Cierzo Rojo, 2018. First published in Romanian as *Sub cerul Spaniei: Cavalerii sperantei*. Bucharest: Editura Militaria, 1972.
Ross, James A. "Memoirs of an Army Surgeon." McCombe lecture. *Journal of the Royal Army Medical Corps* 125 (1979).
———. "Traumatic Surgery on the Line of Communication: A Clinical Record." *Journal of the Royal Army Medical Corps*, no. 83 (1944).
Rothman, K. "Christmas and New Year with the Internationals." *Solidarity*, no. 5 (1938): 4. Collection of Svenska Spanienfrivilligas Vänner.
Royal Cancer Hospital. *The Royal Cancer Hospital, Fulham Road, London, 1851–1951: A Short History of the Royal Cancer Hospital Prepared for the Centenary, 1951*. London: Royal Cancer Hospital, 1951.
Rubin, Hank. *Spain's Cause Was Mine: A Memoir of an American Medic in the Spanish Civil War*. Carbondale: Southern Illinois University Press, 1997.
Rudnytsky, Peter L., and Gillian Preston, eds. *Her Hour Come round at Last: A Garland for Nina Coltart*. London: Karnac Books, 2011.
Ryan, Frank, ed. *The Book of the XV Brigade*. Torfaen, Wales: Warren and Pell, 2003.

Shackleton, Michael. *Desert Surgeons: New Zealand's Mobile Surgical Unit in World War II.* Wellington, NZ: Ngaio Press, 2011.

———. *Operation Vietnam*. Dunedin, NZ: University of Otago Press, 2004.

Shafer, Leslie. "Justice, Justice, Shall Ye Seek: Jewish Warriors in Spain, 1936–1938." MA thesis, Florida Atlantic University, 1998.

Shirlaw, G. B., and Clifford Troke. *Medicine versus Invasion: The Home Guard Medical Service in Action*. London: Secker and Warburg, 1941.

Skudder, Susan. "'Bringing It Home': New Zealand Responses to the Spanish Civil War, 1936–1939." PhD thesis, University of Waikato, 1986.

Spiegel, Irene Goldin. *Gegen den Faschismus kämpfen: Spanien und Frankreich, 1937–1947* [Fighting fascism: Spain and France 1937–1947]. Vienna: Theodor Kramer Gesellschaft, 2022.

Stallard, H. B. "War Surgery of the Eye: An Analysis of 102 Cases of Intra-Ocular Foreign Bodies." *British Journal of Ophthalmology*, March 1944.

Stammers, F. A. R. "Influence of Environment on Surgery." *British Medical Journal*, 7 September 1957.

Steahly, Lance P., and D. W. Cannon, eds. *The Evolution of Forward Surgery in the US Army: From the Revolutionary War to the Combat Operations of the 21st Century*. Sam Houston: Borden Institute, 2018.

Stewart, John. *"The Battle for Health": A Political History of the Socialist Medical Association 1930–51.* Farnham, UK: Ashgate, 1999.

———. "'The Finest Municipal Hospital Service in the World'? Contemporary Perceptions of the London County Council's Hospital Provision, 1929–39." *Urban History* (Cambridge University Press) 32, no. 2 (2005).

———. "'For a Healthy London': The Socialist Medical Association and the London County Council in the 1930s." *Medical History* 42 (1997).

Stout, Duncan M. *New Zealand Medical Services in Middle East and Italy*. Wellington, NZ: Historical Publications Branch, NZ Department of Internal Affairs, 1956.

Stridsberg, G. F. *My Five Lives*. Translated by A. J. Pomerans. London: Heinemann, 1963.

"Surgical Experience in the Spanish Civil War." *British Medical Journal*, 26 October 1940, 560–61.

Sutton, P. E. "The NZ Student Christian Movement, 1896–1936." MA thesis, University of Canterbury, 1946.

Sweetman, R. *Above the City: Otago Boys' High School History, 1863–2013*. Dunedin, NZ: OBHS Foundation, 2013.

Sydney, Grahame. *Promised Land: From Dunedin to the Dunstan Goldfields*. North Shore, NZ: Penguin Books, 2009.

Thomas, Hugh. *The Spanish Civil War*. London: Eyre and Spottiswoode, 1961.

Townshend-Stephens, Capt. R. "John Melly of the British Ambulance Service in Ethiopia." *St. Bartholomew's Hospital Journal* 43 (September 1936).
Tremlett, Giles. *The International Brigades: Fascism, Freedom and the Spanish Civil War*. London: Bloomsbury, 2020.
Trueta, J. "Obituary: Maurice Newfield." *Eugenics Review* 41, no. 3 (October 1949): 111.
———. *Trueta: Surgeon in War and Peace*. Translated by Amelia Stubell and Michael Stubell, London: V. Gollancz, 1980.
Tyrer, Nicola. *Sisters in Arms: British Army Nurses Tell Their Story*. London: Phoenix, 2009.
Vaill, Amanda. *Hotel Florida: Truth, Love and Death in the Spanish Civil War*. London: Bloomsbury, 2014.
Watts, Lt. Col. J. C. *Surgeon at War*. London: Allen & Unwin, 1955.
Webster, Charles. *The National Health Service: A Political History*. London: Oxford University Press, 2002.
Weedon, Brenda, et al. *A History of Queen Mary's Hospital, Roehampton*. London: Richmond, Twickenham, and Roehampton Healthcare NHS Trust, 1996.
Welch, C. E. "War Wounds of the Abdomen." *New England Journal of Medicine* 237:156–68.
Wiltse, Charles M. *Medical Department: Medical Service in the Mediterranean and Minor Theaters*. Washington DC: Office of the Chief of Military History, Department of the Army, 1965. https://collections.nlm.nih.gov/catalog/nlm:nlmuid-9203417-bk.
Wintringham, T. *The Coming World War*. London: Wishart Books, 1935.
———. *English Captain*. London: Faber and Faber, 1939.
Ziff, Trisha (director). *The Mexican Suitcase* (documentary film), prod. 212. Berlin: Mallerich Films, Alicorn Films, 2011.
Zuehlke, Mark. *The Gallant Cause: Canadians in the Spanish Civil War, 1936–1939*. Vancouver: Whitecap Books, 1996.

INDEX

Page numbers with F indicate illustrations

www.ingramcontent.com/pod-product-compliance
Ingram Content Group UK Ltd.
Pitfield, Milton Keynes, MK11 3LW, UK
UKHW012143120726
472909UK00002B/16

9 781496 213389